COMPREHENSIVE GYNECOLOGY REVIEW

FOURTH EDITION

FRANK W. LING, MD
UT Medical Group Professor and Chair
Department of Obstetrics and Gynecology
University of Tennessee College of Medicine
Memphis, Tennessee

LOUIS A. VONTVER, MD, MEd
Professor Emeritus
Department of Obstetrics and Gynecology
University of Washington School of Medicine
Seattle, Washington

ROGER P. SMITH, MD
Professor, Vice Chair, and Program Director
University of Missouri–Kansas City, Truman Medical Center
Kansas City, Missouri

SHARON T. PHELAN, MD
Professor
Department of Obstetrics and Gynecology
University of New Mexico School of Medicine
Albuquerque, New Mexico

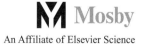
Mosby
An Affiliate of Elsevier Science

St. Louis, Missouri 63146

COMPREHENSIVE GYNECOLOGY REVIEW   ISBN 0–323–01798–3
Copyright © 2003, 1997, 1992, 1988, Mosby, Inc. All rights reserved.

Notice

Obstetrics and Gynecology is an ever-changing field. Standard safety precautions must be followed, but as new research and clinical experience broaden our knowledge, changes in treatment and drug therapy may become necessary or appropriate. Readers are advised to check the most current product information provided by the manufacturer of each drug to be administered to verify the recommended dose, the method and duration of administration, and contraindications. It is the responsibility of the treating physician, relying on experience and knowledge of the patient, to determine dosages and the best treatment for each individual patient. Neither the Publisher nor the author assumes any liability for any injury and/or damage to persons or property arising from this publication.

The Publisher

Library of Congress Cataloging-in-Publication Data

Comprehensive gynecology review/Frank W. Ling ... [et al.].—4th ed.
    p.   cm.
  ISBN 0–323–01798–3
    1. Gynecology—Examinations, questions, etc. I. Ling, Frank W.
RG101 .C726 2003
618.1'0076—dc21   2002029540

Acquisitions Editor: Judith Fletcher
Project Manager: Peter Faber
Book Designer: Karen O'Keefe Owens

CE/MVY

Printed in the United States of America.

Last digit is the print number: 9 8 7 6 5 4 3 2 1

Preface

The authors are honored to be offering the readers this fourth edition of *Comprehensive Gynecology Review*. Its "parent" book, *Comprehensive Gynecology*, has proved to be the leader in its field of reference textbooks in gynecology. The opportunity to work with this material, helping the reader identify clinically significant questions and answers, is one that is a privilege. It is recognized that adult learners have many ways of approaching the educational process. Using a test format is one that has survived the test of time. It is with this in mind, and the desire to help reinforce the outstanding presentation in the "parent" text, that this fourth edition is offered. Its intended audience is practicing physicians, residents, and students interested in gynecology. It can be used to identify areas of weakness, to reinforce new information obtained by reading the textbook, or to reassure oneself that the subject matter is understood. The format should be familiar; it is standard testing format utilizing only single-answer multiple choice questions and matching sets. *Comprehensive Gynecology Review* chapters follow the textbook chapters exactly. The questions within the chapters have been scrambled, and the answers appear in a separate section. Each answer includes a page reference in *Comprehensive Gynecology*, ed. 4, occasionally an additional reference, and a comment.

Questions were chosen for a variety of reasons. Because the book is to help the learner, the questions are not always of the same difficulty that a final summative or certifying examination would accept. The purpose of these examinations is to assure an agency or school that the examinee has attained a requisite amount of knowledge. The examination must discriminate between those who know and those who do not know. Questions that everyone should be able to answer are not included on those examinations. Because *Comprehensive Gynecology Review* is not written with a specific "level" of physician in mind, it was impossible to eliminate questions to which everyone might know the answer. Besides, one purpose of this book is to reinforce knowledge. Thus, easy questions are included. Likewise, in a final or certifying examination, one must avoid the controversial; such questions are not avoided in this book. In practice, one has to treat the controversial. For this reason some readers will disagree with some of the answers, but this is a self-assessment instrument.

An attempt has been made to put the subject in a clinical perspective and to clarify the material. Many illustrations are included that require interpretation. There is a certain amount of cueing in each chapter that would not exist in a final or certifying examination. In organizing the book by chapters, this could not be avoided because the most conceivable answer for a question in the chapter on endometriosis is likely to be endometriosis.

To simulate test conditions, an examinee should take 45 to 60 seconds to answer each question. All the questions in a chapter should be answered before verifying the answers. Reading all the comments will help to reinforce the material.

In this fourth edition, all of the questions have been reviewed and formatted to fit only two question types. Questions have been written on new material added to the fourth edition of *Comprehensive Gynecology*.

We wish to thank the authors of *Comprehensive Gynecology*, ed. 4, Morton A. Stenchever, William Droegemueller, Arthur L. Herbst, and Daniel R. Mishell, Jr., for cooperating with the writing of this fourth edition of *Comprehensive Gynecology Review*. Our thanks to our families for their patience and support, and our gratitude to the people at Mosby, Judith Fletcher, Heather Krehling, and Donna Ciccotelli, for their encouragement.

Frank W. Ling

Louis A. Vontver

Roger P. Smith

Sharon T. Phelan

Contents

Part Four   Gynecologic Oncology

PART ONE

Basic Sciences

Fertilization and Embryogenesis

for Questions 1–19: Select the one best answer or completion.

1. Human chorionic gonadotrophin (hCG) reaches its peak at which week of pregnancy?

   A. 3–4
   B. 7–9
   C. 20–21
   D. 28–30
   E. 38–40

2. Germ cells are derived from the

   A. primitive coelomic epithelium
   B. yolk sac
   C. bone marrow
   D. germinal epithelium
   E. ovarian stroma

3. The first functioning organ system in the embryo is the

   A. nervous system
   B. digestive system
   C. cardiovascular system
   D. genitourinary system
   E. skeletal system

4. Blood formation in the embryo first occurs in the

   A. liver
   B. spleen
   C. bone marrow
   D. lymph nodes
   E. heart

5. An oocyte undergoing meiosis has an arrest phase

   A. at no time during the two meiotic divisions
   B. only once during the two meiotic divisions
   C. once during each of the two meiotic divisions
   D. two times during the first meiotic division
   E. two times during the second meiotic division

6. Which of the following events *does not* occur during meiosis?

   A. pairing of homologous chromosomes
   B. ovulation
   C. fertilization
   D. tubal migration
   E. implantation

7. Fertilization usually occurs in the

   A. vas deferens
   B. ampulla of the fallopian tube
   C. ovary
   D. cervix
   E. fundus of the uterus

8. Which of the following is the most important factor contributing to the development of a specific anomaly by a known teratogen?

   A. dose of the teratogen
   B. timing of the exposure to the teratogen
   C. genetic makeup of the embryo
   D. presence of other environmental factors
   E. duration of action of the teratogen

9. During the development of the excretory system, the sequence of the three sets of excretory ducts and tubules is

   A. pronephric, mesonephric, and metanephric
   B. mesonephric, metanephric, and pronephric
   C. pronephric, metanephric, and mesonephric
   D. metanephric, pronephric, and mesonephric
   E. mesonephric, pronephric, and metanephric

10. In the female, part of the mesonephric duct may form a

    A. Bartholin gland
    B. pelvic kidney
    C. Gartner duct cyst
    D. nabothian cyst
    E. round ligament

11. In the human embryo, absence of the müllerian-inhibiting factor (MIF) results in the formation of

    A. testes
    B. ovaries
    C. a uterus
    D. a prostate
    E. seminal vesicles

12. It is currently thought that suppression of meiosis in the dictyate stage is caused by a substance produced in the

    A. granulosa
    B. theca
    C. rete cords
    D. pituitary gland
    E. hypothalamus

13. During the embryologic formation of a male fetus, the müllerian system is suppressed by antimüllerian hormone produced by the

    A. pituitary
    B. ovarian graafian follicle
    C. ovarian theca cells
    D. testicular Leydig cells
    E. testicular Sertoli cells

14. The urethral sphincter is important in the control of urinary continence and is composed of

    A. longitudinal striated muscle
    B. horseshoe-shaped striated and smooth muscle
    C. circular smooth muscle
    D. longitudinal smooth muscle
    E. circular striated and smooth muscle

15. During the first 7 to 9 weeks of pregnancy, human chorionic gonadotrophin (hCG) doubles every

    A. day
    B. 1.2–2 days
    C. 2–3 days
    D. 3.4–4 days
    E. 5–6 days

16. One theory of sexual differentiation is that genes on the Y chromosome activate the production of H-Y antigen. An alternative theory describes the presence of two genes: one on the Y chromosome, producing a testes-defining factor (TDF), and one an ovarian-determining (Od) gene on the X chromosome or an autosome. According to this theory,

    A. Od gene activation suppresses TDF
    B. TDF activation suppresses the Od gene
    C. both TDF and Od are activated in the male
    D. both TDF and Od are activated in the female
    E. TDF is activated only if H-Y antigen is present

17. In the human, teratogen exposures are most likely to cause specific organ malformations if that exposure occurs

    A. just before conception
    B. within 7 days after conception
    C. 8–49 days after conception
    D. 50–90 days after conception
    E. greater than 3 months after conception

18. Sperm may be attracted to an egg because of binding of a surface receptor on the sperm by

    A. testosterone
    B. progesterone
    C. estrogen
    D. aldosterone
    E. corticosterone

19. The urethral sphincter has which of the following cell types?

    A. smooth muscle only
    B. striated muscle only
    C. stromal cells only
    D. both smooth and striated muscle

DIRECTIONS:

for Questions 20–29: For each numbered item, select the one heading most closely associated with it. Each lettered heading may be used once, more than once, or not at all.

20–21: Match the postovulatory day with the appropriate event.

    A. 3–4
    B. 6–7
    C. 9–12
    D. 12–13
    E. 15–16

20. implantation

21. trophoblastic venous sinuses formed

22–26: Match the male and female homologous structures.

    A. vagina
    B. labia majora
    C. ovarian follicles
    D. clitoris
    E. round ligament

22. scrotum

23. penis

24. prostatic utricle

25. seminiferous tubules

26. gubernaculum testis

27–29: Match the congenital abnormality with the embryonic developmental failure.

    A. Sinovaginal bulb fails to canalize.
    B. Paramesonephric duct does not develop.
    C. Paramesonephric duct does not fuse.
    D. Anal membrane fails to rupture.

27. absence of uterus

28. uterus didelphys

29. transverse vaginal septum

ANSWERS

1. **B,** Page 8. hCG doubles every 1.2 to 2 days in pregnancy, with its peak reached at 7 to 9 weeks of pregnancy.
2. **B,** Page 4. Germ cells are derived from the endoderm in the wall of the yolk sac; they migrate to the germinal ridge, which later forms the gonads. The "germinal" epithelium is derived from the primitive coelomic epithelium and invests the ovary but does not produce germ cells.
3. **C,** Page 9. Blood vessel formation (angiogenesis) occurs in the extraembryonic mesoderm by day 15 or 16. By day 21, the primitive heart is connected with blood vessels of the embryo to become the first functioning organ system.
4. **A,** Page 9. In the embryo, blood formation does not begin until the second month of gestation, occurring first in the developing liver. Blood vessel formation begins in the extraembryonic mesoderm of the yolk sac by day 15 or 16. Embryonic vessels appear approximately 2 days later.
5. **C,** Page 4. At approximately 5 months' gestation, oocytes of the female fetus enter the process of meiosis and progress to the prophase of the first meiotic division before entering the first arrest, which lasts for several years. After puberty,

maturation of selected follicles continues to the second meiotic metaphase, when the second arrest occurs. This arrest lasts until the oocyte is activated by fertilization.

6. **E,** Pages 4–6. One of the first events in meiosis is the tight pairing of homologous chromosomes. This is followed by the formation of a tetrad as each chromosome of the pair splits longitudinally, forming two chromatids. Meiosis is arrested at this point until after puberty. During each menstrual cycle, a few follicles ripen, and in those follicles the oocyte resumes meiosis. Ovulation occurs while the egg is in the second meiotic division, and the final steps of the second meiotic division are completed after fertilization, while the egg is being transported through the fallopian tube. Meiosis is completed in the fallopian tube, and cellular division begins. Implantation in the endometrium usually occurs 5 to 7 days after fertilization, at which time a blastocyst has formed.

7. **B,** Pages 6–7. Fertilization usually occurs in the fallopian tube. The spermatozoa undergo capacitation and acrosome reaction during their transportation through the female genital tract. This activates enzyme systems to make it possible

for a sperm to penetrate the zona pellucida, after the sperm is attracted to the egg. The sperm then enters the cytoplasm of the egg, and the head swells, giving rise to the male pronucleus. The egg casts off the second polar body, and the female pronucleus is formed. These pronuclei contain the haploid sets of chromosomes of maternal and paternal origin. The nuclear membrane surrounding them disappears and establishes the diploid complement of chromosomes in preparation for mitosis and cleavage. Because of failure of chromosome arrangement on the spindle, gene defects, and environmental factors, a significant number of fertilized ova do not complete cleavage. Teratogens present during fertilization usually either cause no effect or result in complete destruction of the fertilized ovum. Monozygotic twinning may occur at any stage until the formation of the blastula because, before this time, each cell is totipotential.

8. **B,** Page 9. Although all of these factors may contribute to the formation of a given anomaly, the timing of the exposure to the teratogen during the embryonic period of development of a particular organ system is the most likely to cause a specific anomaly of that organ system. All the organ systems are formed between the third and the seventh weeks of gestation. A teratogenic event occurring during this time results in a malformation related to the organ systems developing at the time of the insult. Therefore, cardiovascular abnormalities are expected if a teratogen is given during the early embryonic period, when the heart and blood vessels are forming. In addition, the effects of a teratogen depend on the dose and duration of exposure as well as on the genetic makeup; they may be influenced by other environmental factors in operation at that time, including physical conditions such as temperature and irradiation. Sometimes the teratogen's byproducts are also damaging. Before day 7 or after day 49, teratogens usually do not cause specific malformations. They may kill the embryo or injure cells, leading to cellular malfunction or growth retardation.

9. **A,** Page 10. Pronephric ducts form first at about the fourth week after conception. They are not known to have any excretory function. Late in the fourth week, the mesonephric tubules and their accompanying ducts develop. These mesonephric ducts produce urine for 2 or 3 weeks. The metanephric duct begins its development early in the fifth week of gestation. It starts to function 2 to 3 weeks thereafter. The duct begins as a pelvic organ, and through differential growth it ultimately relocates in the lumbar region. Although the fetus produces urine, which contributes to the amniotic fluid, the placenta handles the excretory functions of the fetus.

10. **C,** Pages 10–12; Table 1–2 (in Stenchever). Gartner's duct cyst may occur in the broad ligament next to the uterus or cervix and is most common on the lateral wall of the vagina. The differential diagnosis for such a cyst includes congenital anomalies, such as a blind vaginal pouch, and acquired cysts, such as inclusion cysts after surgery.

11. **C,** Page 16. MIF, or antimüllerian hormone, is produced by the Sertoli cells of the testes. If production does not occur because of the absence of a Y chromosome—and therefore no testes (as in the female)—or because of a failure of the Sertoli cell production, the müllerian anlage is not suppressed and the müllerian duct (paramesonephric ducts) develop into the structures of the female internal genital tract. These include the fallopian tubes and the uterus, including the cervix. The gonad, either testes or ovary, is already formed. The prostate and the seminal vesicles form from the mesonephric, or wolffian, ducts.

12. **A,** Page 5. Meiosis is stimulated by a meiotic-inducing substance produced by the rete cords. As the ovary develops, the granulosa cells surround the ova and separate them from the rete. The granulosa produces an inhibiting substance. Loss of contact with the rete cords allows the granulosa-produced inhibiting substance to suppress meiosis in the dictyate stage. Meiosis resumes after puberty, when each set of follicles begins to grow. The theca, the pituitary, and the hypothalamus are not known to participate in this process.

13. **E,** Pages 11–12. Antimüllerian hormone is produced by the Sertoli cells of the testes. The Leydig cells produce testosterone. Neither the pituitary nor the ovary produces müllerian-suppressive substances, and ovaries are not present in the male fetus. It was originally thought that female müllerian ducts would develop passively in the absence of testes. However, the presence of far more estrogen receptor in the anlage of the female than in the male external genitalia suggests that maternal estrogen may play a role in the development of the female external genitalia and that the process is not totally passive.

14. **B,** Page 10. The urethral sphincter develops at about 15 weeks' gestation from both smooth and striated muscle, primarily from the anterior wall of the urethra. The sphincter develops in a horseshoe shape. Later, the sphincter is under both voluntary and sympathetic α-adrenergic control.

15. **B,** Page 8. hCG has been detected as early as 6 days after ovulation. It doubles every 1.2 to 2 days during the first 7 to 9 weeks of pregnancy. This important fact helps differentiate an abnormally

progressing pregnancy from a normally progressing one through observation of serial quantitative hCG levels in the maternal serum.

16. **B,** Page 16. This alternative theory of sexual differentiation holds that because it is located on the Y chromosome, TDF is present only in the male and that, if present, it suppresses the Od gene. If TDF is not present, the Od gene is expressed and an ovary develops.

17. **C,** Page 9. Exposure to teratogens during the first 7 postconceptual days usually causes complete destruction or has little effect. The same is true until after implantation. The time of specific organ formation is approximately 8 to 49 days after conception. During this time, exposure to teratogens may affect developing organ systems.

18. **B**, Page 6. Recent studies have shown that attraction of sperm to ova (chemotaxis) may be aided by the binding of progesterone, which is found in follicular fluid, to a surface receptor on the sperm. Sperm motility is increased by this process.

19. **D**, Page 10. The urethra is formed by smooth muscle and peripheral striated muscle. The urethral sphincter is located mainly in the anterior urethra and takes a horseshoe shape. This muscle—plus the epithelial lining of the urethra, the voluntary muscles of the genitourinary diaphragm and levators, and the transmitted interperitoneal pressure—increases the urethral pressure above that of the bladder and therefore maintains continence unless these muscles are relaxed or the intervesicular pressure exceeds the combined pressures created within the urethra.

20–21. 20, **B;** 21, **C;** Pages 6–7. Subsequent to the first mitotic division, the cells continue to divide as the embryo passes along the fallopian tube and into the uterus. This takes 3 to 4 days after fertilization. The embryo enters the uterus in any form from 32 cells to the early blastula stage. Implantation typically occurs 3 days after the embryo enters the uterus (Table 1–1). The invading syncytiotrophoblast

TABLE 1–1
Events of Implantation

Event	Days After Ovulation
Zona pellucida disappears	4–5
Blastocyst attaches to epithelial surface of endometrium	6
Trophoblast erodes into endometrial stroma	7
Trophoblast differentiates into cytotrophoblastic and syncytial trophoblastic layers	7–8
Lacunae appear around trophoblast	8–9
Blastocyst burrows beneath endometrial surface	9–10
Lacunar network forms	10–11
Trophoblast invades endometrial sinusoids, establishing uteroplacental circulation	11–12
Endometrial epithelium completely covers blastocyst	12–13
Strong decidual reaction occurs in stroma	13–14

comes into intimate contact with endometrial capillaries to form venous sinuses 9 to 12 days after ovulation.

22–26. 22, **B;** 23, **D;** 24, **A;** 25, **C;** 26, **E;** Table 1–2 (in Stenchever); Page 13. There are homologous male and female derivatives for each embryonic structure. Paired structures include scrotum/labia majora, penis/clitoris, prostatic utricle/vagina, seminiferous tubules/ovarian follicles, and gubernaculum testis/round ligaments.

27–29. 27, **B;** 28, **C;** 29, **A;** Page 15. Abnormalities in specific developmental processes can result in discrete congenital abnormalities. If the paramesonephric duct does not develop, absence of the uterus occurs. Uterus didelphys is a result of lack of fusion of the paramesonephric duct. A transverse vaginal septum results from failure of the sinovaginal bulb to canalize.

CHAPTER

2

Reproductive Genetics

DIRECTIONS:

for Questions 1–13: Select the one best answer or completion.

1. The pedigree in Figure 2–1 suggests the inheritance of a trait that is

    A. autosomal dominant
    B. autosomal recessive
    C. X-linked recessive
    D. X-linked dominant
    E. male-limited autosomal dominant

2. Assume the trait is fully penetrant. The pedigree in Figure 2–2 is most consistent with a gene that is

    A. autosomal dominant
    B. autosomal recessive
    C. X-linked recessive
    D. X-linked dominant
    E. male-limited autosomal dominant

3. A couple who had a barren marriage for 10 years now have experienced two spontaneous abortions at 6 and 8 weeks. Karyotyping was performed on both the husband and the wife. He is 46,XY, and her karyotype is reproduced in Figure 2–3. She is age 30 and he is 32. Based on this information, the woman is at significantly increased risk for

    A. preterm labor
    B. infertility
    C. a child with aneuploidy
    D. a child with a trisomy
    E. multiple pregnancy

FIGURE 2–1

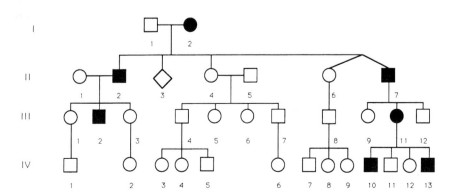

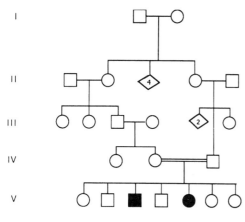

FIGURE 2–2

5. Figure 2–4 represents a(n)

A. robertsonian fusion (translocation)
B. isochromosome
C. reciprocal translocation
D. pericentric inversion
E. paracentric inversion

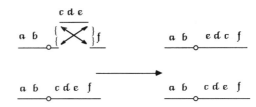

FIGURE 2–4

4. A couple who have experienced recurrent abortions had a karyotype performed on the last abortus. The karyotype was 47,XX,+16. Given this information, you would tell the couple that the chance of delivering a live-born infant with a trisomy is approximately

A. 0.1%
B. 1%
C. 5%
D. 10%
E. 25%

6. The karyotype of a prenatal patient contains a robertsonian fusion involving chromosome 21. Theoretically, the likelihood of her having a live-born infant with a trisomy is

A. zero
B. 25%
C. 33%
D. 50%
E. 100%

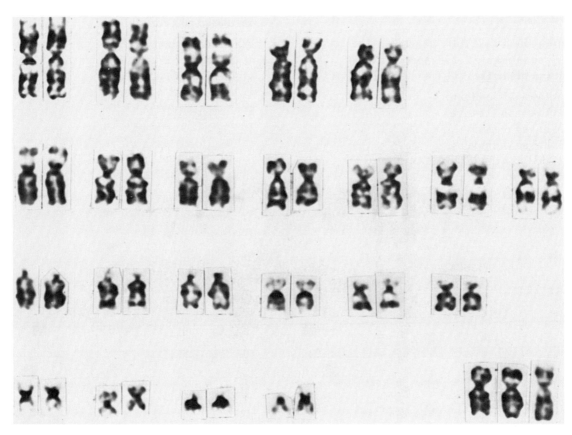

FIGURE 2–3

7. The actual risk of giving birth to a trisomic infant in the situation mentioned in question 6 is

   A. 1%
   B. 5%
   C. 10%
   D. 25%
   E. 33%

8. The spontaneous abortion rate (all embryos that do not result in live-born infants) is

   A. 10%–20%
   B. 21%–30%
   C. 31%–40%
   D. 41%–50%
   E. >50%

9. A sonogram is obtained because the uterine fundus of a patient thought to be 24 weeks pregnant measures 21 cm. In addition to what appears to be cerebral ventriculomegaly, there are oligohydramnios and a hydropic-appearing placenta. This sonogram should suggest that the karyotype of the fetus is

   A. 45,X
   B. 47,XX,21
   C. 47,XYY
   D. 45,X/46,XY
   E. 69,XXX

10. A couple, both of whom have neurofibromatosis, seek genetic counseling. You should tell this couple that

    A. 100% of the offspring will either have the disease or be carriers
    B. 75% of the offspring will have the disease
    C. 50% of the offspring will be homozygous for the gene
    D. 25% of the males will have the more severe form of the disease

11. The most likely outcome of a pregnancy with the karyotype depicted in Figure 2–5 is

    A. severe mental retardation
    B. uniform pregnancy loss
    C. intrauterine fetal demise near term
    D. a fetal intersex condition
    E. a congenital heart defect

12. A 23-year-old gravida 3 para 0-0-3-0 is married to a 27-year-old man who has never fathered a pregnancy that went to term. The couple seeks your advice. Before you recommend that each spouse obtain a karyotype, you would explain that the most likely abnormal finding is

    A. a robertsonian fusion
    B. 47,XXY
    C. 47,XXX
    D. mosaicism
    E. deletion of a somatic chromosome

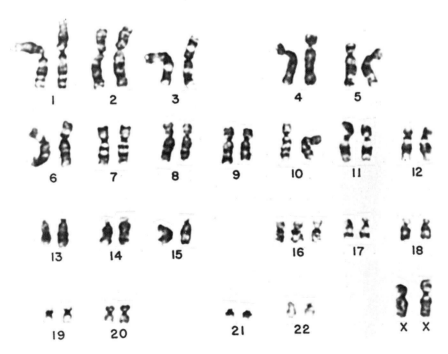

FIGURE 2–5

13. **A fetus who carries the genes for cystic fibrosis can be identified by**

    A. determining the fetal karyotype
    B. using restriction endonucleases to isolate the gene sequence
    C. determining the sodium chloride content of the amniotic fluid between 16 and 20 weeks' gestation
    D. performing a Southern blot test directly on material obtained from a chorionic villus biopsy

DIRECTIONS:

for Questions 14–20: For each numbered item, select the one heading most closely associated with it. Each lettered heading may be used once, more than once, or not at all.

14–15.

    A. nondisjunctional event identified in abortus material
    B. nondisjunctional event not identified in living or abortus material
    C. Patau syndrome
    D. Edwards syndrome
    E. Down syndrome

14. **Trisomy 13**

15. **Trisomy 17**

16–17. **Partial deletions of chromosome**

    A. 4
    B. 5
    C. 18
    D. Short arm of X
    E. Short arm of Y

16. **Wolf-Hirschhorn syndrome**

17. **Cri du chat syndrome**

18–20. **Match the specific chromosomal abnormality with its frequency of occurrence in chromosomally abnormal abortus material.**

    A. 50%
    B. 20%
    C. 15%
    D. 5%
    E. 1%

18. **Turner syndrome**

19. **Triploidy**

20. **Trisomy**

DIRECTIONS:

for each numbered item 21–23, indicate whether it is associated with:

    A. only meiosis
    B. only mitosis
    C. both meiosis and mitosis
    D. neither meiosis nor mitosis

21. nondisjunction

22. 47,XYY

23. 46,XY/45,X

DIRECTIONS:

for Questions 24–30: Select the one best answer or completion.

24. A 35-year-old primigravida underwent amniocentesis 3 weeks ago. The karyotype is reproduced in Figure 2–6. A description of the phenotype should state that

    A. the sex is male
    B. the adult is usually short
    C. adult intellect is usually above normal
    D. gamete function is generally normal
    E. abnormal breast enlargement is present in two thirds of patients

25. A family is suspected of carrying an X-linked recessive abnormality. One female member exhibits the trait. If this *is* an X-linked recessive abnormality, the possible explanation is that this condition

    A. represents inactivation of the abnormal gene in the affected member of the family
    B. represents a female who is homozygous
    C. is an example of complete penetrance
    D. is a polygenic process

26. An 18-year-old paraplegic seeks genetic counseling during the 21st week of her pregnancy. She had a meningomyelocele repaired at birth. There is no history of a neural tube defect (NTD) on the husband's side of the family or for any other member of the woman's family. You should advise this patient

    A. that she should begin taking folate to decrease the risk of recurrence
    B. that her risk of an NTD in this pregnancy is approximately 2%
    C. to undergo a serum determination of α-fetoprotein
    D. to undergo transabdominal umbilical cord blood sampling for karyotyping
    E. to forgo ultrasound studies until term

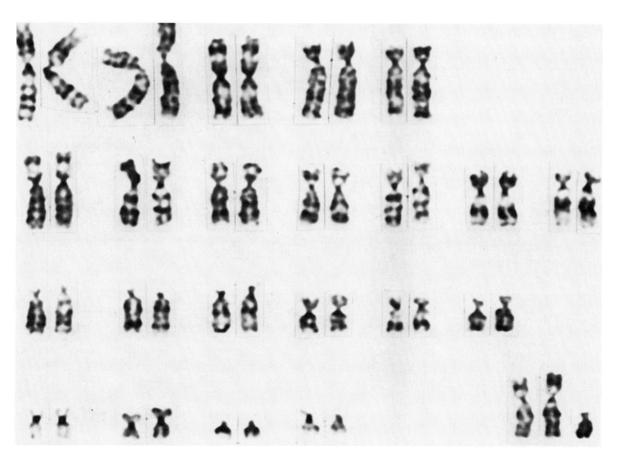

FIGURE 2–6

FIGURE 2–7

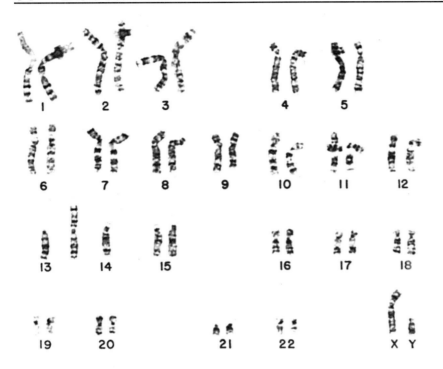

27. A woman who has had three spontaneous abortions is found to have the karyotype shown in Figure 2–7. Rational options available to this couple include

    A. amniocentesis and selective abortion
    B. ovum harvesting and embryo transplantation after the 32-cell stage
    C. donor insemination
    D. reassurance with no further intervention indicated

28. When triploidy is associated with a partial mole,

    A. the likelihood of subsequent development of a choriocarcinoma is increased compared with when the association is with a complete mole
    B. the fetal chromosomes are of paternal origin
    C. follow-up need not include monitoring of β-human chorionic gonadotrophin (β-hCG)
    D. hydropic degeneration of the placenta is unlikely

29. Human cancer is

    A. always the result of multiple point mutations in an oncogene
    B. due to altered cell-cell interactions controlling growth
    C. the result of a stabilized cell skeleton
    D. responsible for the inactivation of tumor suppressor genes in adjacent cells
    E. the result of simultaneous changes in the genetic function of a group of adjacent cells

30. Mutation of the BRCA-1 gene is associated with a lifetime risk of cancer that is approximately

    A. 85%
    B. 75%
    C. 55%
    D. 45%
    E. 35%

ANSWERS

1. **A,** Page 25. Usually, if 50% of the protein produced by the gene pair is enough to give the usual phenotype, the condition is dominant. In this case, no generation is spared, the condition is equally represented between males and females, and all affected individuals have at least one affected parent. Male-to-male transmission rules out X-linked dominant inheritance.

2. **B,** Pages 25–26. Since there is full penetrance, an autosomal dominant trait is unlikely. Both sexes are affected, making X-linked inheritance extremely unlikely. The parents are consanguineous and must be presumed carriers. Two of seven children are affected. With an autosomal recessive trait, one would expect 25% of the children to be affected on the basis of segregation.

3. **B,** Page 28. The karyotype is 47,XXX. Fifty percent of such women are fertile. While most of the offspring produced are normal, there is a slightly increased probability of an offspring being produced with nondisjunctional events involving both the sex chromosomes and the autosomes.

4. **B,** Pages 31–32. Roughly 50% of abortuses with chromosome abnormalities have autosomal trisomy. A trisomy of chromosome 16 has been noted in about one third of cases, but since this condition has never been seen in living persons, it must be considered universally lethal. In women who have produced a conception that is trisomic, the risk of a subsequent trisomic event is 1% to 2%, being somewhat less for women younger than 35 and higher for women older than 35.

5. **E,** Page 30. In robertsonian translocation (central fusion), two acrocentric chromosomes, such as 14 and 21, are involved. An isochromosome is the result of a transverse split (rather than a longitudinal split) of a metacentric chromosome during meiosis. The daughter chromosome has either two long or two short arms. With a reciprocal translocation, chromatin material is exchanged but the chromosomal number does not change. When a chromosome breaks and turns on its axis, as in this question, there is an inversion. In this example, the centromere was not involved, so the inversion is called *paracentric*. When the centromere is included, it is a *pericentric* inversion.

6. **C,** Pages 28–30. One would expect that 25% would be normal; 25%, carriers; 25%, unbalanced and affected; and 25%, monosomic. If this condition involved the 21 chromosome, one would be dealing with Down syndrome. Since monosomy is lethal, the theoretical live-born risk is 33% normal, 33% carriers, and 33% with Down syndrome.

7. **C,** Pages 28–30. The numbers in question 6 do not turn out to be the case. The observed live-born risk of Down syndrome is 10% to 15% if the mother has the translocation and 1% to 2% if the father is the carrier.

8. **E,** Page 31. It has been estimated that about 15% of ova penetrated by sperm fail to divide. Another 15% fail to implant, and 25% to 30% are aborted spontaneously at previous stages. Of the roughly 40% of fertilized ova that survive the first missed menstrual period, as many as 25% are aborted spontaneously, so that only about 30% to 35% of all ova penetrated by sperm actually result in live-born infants. This information is being refined as more information is gained about in vitro fertilization.

9. E, Page 32. Given these findings, one should predict that the karyotype is a polyploidy such as triploidy. The latter is associated with a partial hydatidiform mole. This patient should be followed up as if she had a complete hydatidiform mole.

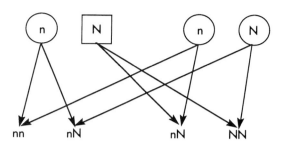

FIGURE 2–8

10. **B,** Pages 24–26. Each parent carries this autosomal dominant gene. It is highly unlikely that either is homozygous for the gene. The gene is not on the X or the Y chromosome; it is on chromosome 17. The sex ratio for heterozygotes, therefore, is one male to one female. The gametes will be as pictured in Figure 2–8. Twenty-five percent will be normal (nn), 75% will be abnormal (NN or nN), 50% will have neurofibromatosis (nN), and 25% will be homozygous for this dominant gene and will have the lethal form (NN).

11. **B,** Pages 31–32. Figure 2–5 depicts a 47,XX+16 karyotype. A trisomy of chromosome 16 has been noted in about one third of trisomic abortus material. Since this condition has never been seen in living persons, it must be considered universally lethal.

12. **A,** Pages 33–34. The diagnosis of a chromosome abnormality in couples with chronic pregnancy wastage is important to rule out an abnormality incompatible with normal gestation, such as homologous translocations between identical members of the same group of chromosomes—for example, 21–21. Roughly 1 in 200 couples suffers from multiple abortions. Simpson discovered that the prevalence of chromosome abnormalities in women with chronic spontaneous abortion problems is about twice that of males (4.8% vs. 2.4%). In counseling a couple, it is important to try to prevent either partner from placing the blame on self or partner. Although occasional sex chromosome abnormalities, such as 47,XXX and 47,XYY, as well as a variety of mosaic representations, are present among such couples, the majority demonstrate either balanced reciprocal translocations or robertsonian fusion.

13. **B,** Page 24. Cystic fibrosis results from an abnormal gene, not a chromosomal abnormality. Identification of an affected individual or carrier may be accomplished by specifically identifying the mutant gene. The key to the localization of genetic information on the DNA molecule has been the discovery of a group of more than 200 bacterial enzymes, called *restriction endonucleases,* that recognize and cut specific nucleotide sequences in the double-stranded DNA molecule. In cases of cystic fibrosis, it is possible to identify

more than 230 different alleles of the single gene responsible for cystic fibrosis. Although the "sweat test" was one of the first tests used for diagnosis in children, it could not be applied to amniotic fluid. There is usually not enough DNA from a chorionic villus biopsy to determine a nucleotide sequence by Southern blot test. Therefore, a cell culture or amplification of the DNA molecule (polymerase chain reaction) is needed.

14–15. 14, **C;** 15, **B;** Page 28. Trisomy 13 and trisomy 15 are usually considered together. Trisomy 13 is known as *Patau syndrome* and is incompatible with extended life. Trisomy 18 is *Edwards syndrome* and is also incompatible with extended life. Trisomy 21 is the more common and familiar Down syndrome. Nondisjunctional events resulting in a trisomy have been described in every autosome except 1 and 17.

16–17. 16, **A;** 17, **B;** Page 30. Wolf-Hirschhorn syndrome is due to the loss of a portion of the short arm of chromosome 4. Cri du chat syndrome is a result of the loss of the short arm of chromosome 5.

18–20. 18, **B;** 19, **C;** 20, **A;** Pages 31–32. Half of abortuses with chromosomal abnormalities have an autosomal trisomy; 20% have the karyotype 45,X; 14% to 19% have triploidy; 3% to 6% have tetraploidy; and 3% to 4% have chromosome rearrangements.

21–23. 21, **C;** 22, **A;** 23, **B;** Pages 22, 27–28. Nondisjunction is the faulty separation of chromosome pairs at anaphase in either meiosis or mitosis. Nondisjunction during spermatogenesis (meiosis) involving the Y chromosome can lead to the karyotype 47,XYY. Nondisjunctional events during mitosis in the early embryo frequently produce individuals with cell populations containing different chromosome numbers (mosaicism).

24. **A,** Page 28. The karyotype is that of 47,XXY, Klinefelter syndrome. Affected men are characterized by tall stature and azoospermia. Although they may be mentally retarded, the condition is usually not severe. Gynecomastia is present in about one third of cases.

25. **B,** Pages 22, 26. *Penetrance* is the percentage of persons in a population with the mutation who actually demonstrate the phenotypic change. In this case, either the female has the recessive gene on both chromosomes or the normal X is the one deactivated during lyonization. Usually, the abnormal X is inactivated.

26. **B,** Page 27. Although it has been suggested that NTDs might be prevented by folate supplements, these must be given preconceptually and during early gestation. The neural tube is formed by 4 weeks post conception. NTD is a multifactorial disorder. In the United States, the risk of recurrence is 11 times the population risk, which is approximately 2%. The sensitivity of amniotic fluid α-fetoprotein is better than that of maternal serum. Maternal serum α-fetoprotein is meant to be a screening test for a low-risk population between 16 and 20 weeks' gestation. Amniocentesis is preferred for patients at risk, especially this late in pregnancy. Another possibility at 20 weeks is ultrasound evaluation, which can reliably detect NTDs at this stage of pregnancy.

27. **A,** Pages 30–33. The karyotype is of a robertsonian fusion (translocation), 45,XY,t(13q14q). There is a 33% theoretical chance that this woman would give birth to an infant with trisomy 13. The actual risk is listed as 10%. This is an abnormal maternal karyotype, so donor insemination will not help. Identifying an abnormal fetus and selective abortion or bypassing the abnormal mother using ovum donation are the only logical options listed.

28. **B,** Pages 33–34. Choriocarcinoma has occurred after a partial mole, but it is much less likely than after a complete mole. Nevertheless, the patient should be followed up as if she had a complete hydatidiform mole. This includes obtaining serial determinations of β-hCG. (See Chapter 35, Comprehensive Gynecology.) In cases of triploidy in which the nuclear material is of paternal origin, the placenta undergoes molar change.

29. **B,** Pages 22, 34–35. Current theories suggest that the majority of human cancers may arise from a genetic change in a single cell. Such genetic alterations may be of various types, but essentially they involve either (1) somatic activation of cell oncogenes through point mutations, rearrangements, or amplifications or (2) inactivation of tumor suppressor genes by point mutation or deletion in either germ or somatic cells. The tumor suppressor gene may play a role in the pathogenesis of the cancer, perhaps through the alteration of normal cell-cell interactions controlling growth. Oncogenes may also exert their effect through alteration of the cell's skeleton.

30. **C,** Page 843. Mutations in the BRCA-1 or BRCA-2 genes are associated with a lifetime risk of breast cancer that approaches 90%. Despite this high rate of occurrence, abnormalities of this gene are detected in only about 45% of families with a significant history of breast cancer. Any alteration in the structure of the gene, including base deletions, insertions, or a missense substitution, may result in altered gene function and an increase in the risk of breast cancer. An increased risk of ovarian cancer in these patients has also been documented.

CHAPTER
3

Reproductive Anatomy

DIRECTIONS:

for Questions 1–15: Select the one best answer or completion.

1. On examination you find that a 40-year-old patient's uterus is anteflexed, firm, and approximately 9 cm long, 6 cm wide, and 4 cm thick, with an estimated weight of approximately 110 g. From this information *alone* you would be able to say that the patient was

   A. nulligravid
   B. multigravid
   C. 8 weeks' pregnant
   D. afflicted with adenomyosis
   E. none of the above

2. The femoral triangle is bounded by the

   A. sartorius, adductor longus, and inguinal ligament
   B. femoral nerve, artery, and vein
   C. rectus abdominis muscle, inguinal ligament, and inferior epigastric vessels
   D. inguinal ligament, inferior epigastric vessels, and transversus abdominis
   E. layers of the abdominal wall

3. At term, the pregnant uterus will have increased in weight over the normal nonpregnant uterine weight approximately

   A. 2–3 times
   B. 4–5 times
   C. 10–20 times
   D. 30–50 times
   E. 100 times

4. A 24-year-old patient is seen for a routine examination, and a 2-cm asymptomatic cystic structure is found submucosally at the junction of the lower and middle thirds of the vagina at approximately the 10 o'clock position. The most likely cause is

   A. vaginal inclusion cyst
   B. clear cell adenocarcinoma
   C. Gartner duct cyst
   D. Skene duct cyst
   E. Bartholin duct cyst

5. After a radical hysterectomy, a patient complains of numbness over the medial aspect of her thigh. No muscle weakness is noted. This condition is most likely due to

   A. transection of the obturator nerve
   B. nonpermanent injury to the obturator nerve
   C. transection of the femoral nerve
   D. nonpermanent injury to the femoral nerve
   E. nonpermanent injury to the pudendal nerve

6. The correct sequence of the arterial blood supply to the uterus begins with the aorta and continues through the

   A. internal iliac, common iliac, uterine
   B. common iliac, hypogastric, uterine
   C. external iliac, internal iliac, uterine
   D. obturator, hypogastric, uterine
   E. common iliac, pudendal, uterine

7. **A patient is most apt to undergo trachelectomy if she**

   A. is of Greek heritage
   B. has undergone a prior subtotal hysterectomy
   C. has a benign ovarian tumor
   D. has an unusual retroperitoneal pelvic mass
   E. has repeated episodes of dysfunctional uterine bleeding, unresponsive to dilatation and curettage

8. **A woman who has endometrial cancer can experience metastases to the inguinal nodes, transported via which lymphatic chain?**

   A. paraaortic
   B. obturator
   C. round ligament
   D. lumbar
   E. iliac

9. **A woman who has a vasovagal response during dilation of the cervix for a suction paraaortic performed in the office is responding to stimulation of which of the following nerves?**

   A. pudendal
   B. obturator
   C. sciatic
   D. femoral
   E. Frankenhäuser's (paracervical) ganglion

10. **The fallopian tube is anatomically divided into four segments. The longest segment is the**

    A. interstitial
    B. isthmic
    C. ampullary
    D. infundibular

11. **The major blood supply to each ovary arises from the**

    A. common iliac artery
    B. internal iliac artery (hypogastric)
    C. obturator artery
    D. external iliac artery
    E. aorta

12. **A woman complains of sudden onset of pain beneath the umbilicus, which then moves to the right lower quadrant. She denies nausea, vomiting, or fever. Her last menstrual period was 7 weeks ago, and she has been sexually active without contraception. Assuming she has a right tubal pregnancy, how do you account for the initial subumbilical pain?**

    A. The tube was located anatomically in the midline.
    B. Tubal pain is transmitted via L2, 3, 4.
    C. Tubal pain is transmitted via S2, 3, 4.
    D. Tubal pain is transmitted via T11–12.
    E. Tubal pain is transmitted via T8–10.

13. **Cystocele and rectocele occur because of weakness of the**

    A. uterosacral ligaments
    B. anal sphincter
    C. endopelvic fascia
    D. cardinal ligaments
    E. ischiocavernosus muscle

14. **Urethral diverticula arise from**

    A. mesonephric duct remnants
    B. an infection of the periurethral glands
    C. urethroceles
    D. straddle injury to the urethra
    E. repetitive increase of intraabdominal pressure

15. **The inferior epigastric artery is a direct branch of the**

    A. pudendal
    B. internal iliac
    C. external iliac
    D. inferior mesenteric
    E. internal mammary

DIRECTIONS:

for Questions 16–30: For each numbered item, select the one heading most closely associated with it. Each lettered heading may be used once, more than once, or not at all.

16–18. Match the female genital structure with the homologous male structure.

(A) prostate
(B) penis
(C) scrotum
(D) penile urethra
(E) Cowper's gland

16. Labia majora

17. Skene glands

18. Labia minora

19–21. Match the following with the labeled portions in Figure 3–1.

19. zona basalis

20. myometrium

21. endometrium

22–24. Match the following structures with the labeled portions of Figure 3–2.

22. ovarian ligament

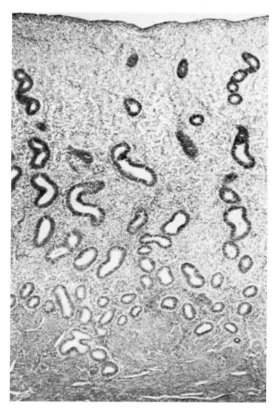

FIGURE 3–1 Histologic view of endometrium during proliferative phase, demonstrating strata in endometrium. (From Demopoulos RI: Normal endometrium. In Blaustein A, ed: *Pathology of the Female Genital Tract*, 2nd ed. New York, Springer-Verlag, 1982, p 216.)

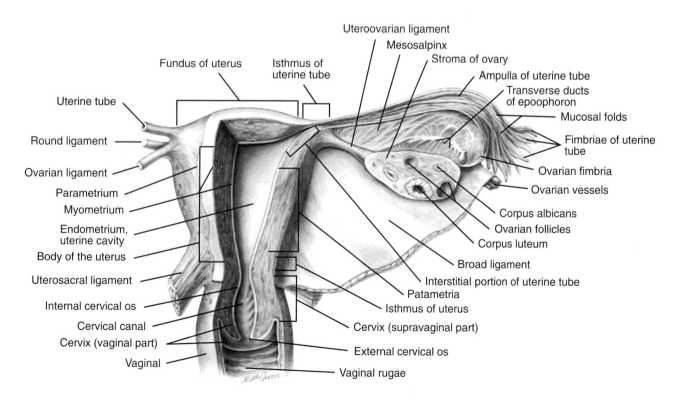

FIGURE 3–2 Schematic drawing of posterior view of cervix, uterus, fallopian tube, and ovary. (Redrawn from Clemente CD: *Anatomy: a Regional Atlas of the Human Body*, 3rd ed. Baltimore, Urban & Schwarzenberg, 1987.)

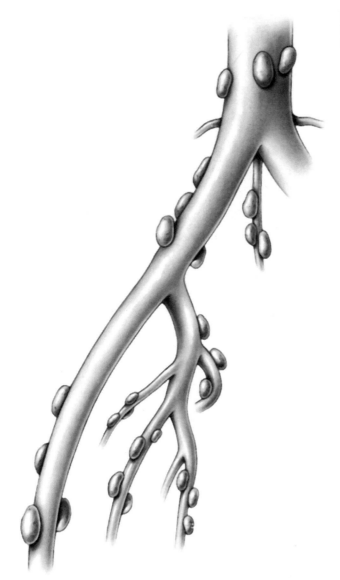

FIGURE 3–3 Schematic view of pelvic lymph nodes. (From Plentl AA, Friedman EA: Lymphatic System of the Female Genitalia. Philadelphia, WB Saunders, 1971, p 13.)

23. cervical portio

24. fimbria ovarica

25–27. **Match the anastomotic connection with the following pelvic vessels**

    A. superior gluteal artery
    B. uterine artery
    C. middle hemorrhoidal artery
    D. inferior vesical artery
    E. obturator artery

25. inferior mesenteric artery

26. deep iliac circumflex artery

27. medial femoral circumflex artery

28–30. **Match the nodes with the labeled areas in Figure 3–3.**

28. internal iliac

29. common iliac

30. aortic

DIRECTIONS:

for Questions 31–38: Select the one best answer or completion.

31. Which of the following muscles is *not* part of the pelvic diaphragm?

A. coccygeus
B. pubococcygeus
C. puborectalis
D. iliococcygeus
E. deep transverse perineal

32. The normal cervix

A. will store living sperm for more than 2 weeks
B. is made up of 40% smooth muscle and 60% connective tissue
C. has its blood supply from both the uterine artery and vaginal arteries
D. is approximately 5 cm long
E. has more nerves in the exocervix than in the endocervix

33. A woman who has noted a sudden increase in body hair has a measured clitoral diameter of 1.5 cm. This is a sign of

A. defeminization
B. masculinization
C. menopause
D. previous childbearing
E. oral contraceptive use

34. A midline plexus that contains pelvic autonomic nerves is the

A. celiac
B. cervical
C. presacral
D. pudendal
E. obturator

35. A female has a uterus measuring 6 cm in length, 3 cm in width, and 1.5 cm in thickness, with a weight of approximately 30 g. This is most consistent with

A. menopause
B. hypermenorrhea
C. adenomyosis
D. uterine fibroids
E. pregnancy

36. Sympathetic nerve fibers to the pelvis

A. are part of the somatic nervous system
B. generally cause vasoconstriction
C. originate from the cranial and sacral nerve roots
D. use acetylcholine as their principal neuro-transmitter
E. may cause vasovagal reaction in a patient when stimulated

37. The main chain of lymph nodes through which the ovaries drain are the

A. sacral nodes
B. common iliac nodes
C. external iliac nodes
D. periaortic nodes
E. superior gluteal nodes

38. Arteriovenous malformations in the female pelvis are usually treated by

A. electrical coagulation
B. embolization followed by ligation
C. ligation only
D. radiation
E. surgical excision

ANSWERS

1. **E,** Page 46. Although the size, shape, and consistency suggest a multigravid uterus, any of the listed possibilities could be true because of the great individual variation in anatomic size and configuration. It would not be possible to state that any one of the given reasons, or some other entity such as leiomyoma or a tumor, was the reason for the upper limits of normal size and weight of this uterus.

2. **A,** Page 56. The femoral triangle's boundaries are the sartorius muscle, the adductor longus muscle, and the inguinal ligament. From medial to lateral, the triangle contains the femoral nerve, artery, and vein. The rectus abdominis muscle, the inguinal ligament, and the inferior epigastric vessels define Hesselbach's triangle, through which a direct inguinal hernia develops. The inguinal ligament, inferior epigastric vessels, and transversus abdominis muscle define the inguinal ring, through which the processus vaginalis runs. The inguinal canal is a space between layers of the abdominal wall that begins at the external inguinal ring and through which an indirect inguinal hernia develops, starting lateral to the inferior epigastric vessels.

3. **C,** Page 46. The normal nonpregnant uterus weighs 40 to 100 g. At term pregnancy, the uterus weighs 800 to 1000 g, which is a 10- to 20-fold increase. This increase is due to both hypertrophy and hyperplasia of muscle fibers, as well as an increase in decidua and the blood volume contained within the uterus. Post partum, the uterus decreases in both size and weight, so that by 6 to 10 weeks post partum it is back to a normal prepregnancy weight, though usually slightly larger than a nulligravid uterus.

4. **C,** Page 44. The anterior lateral position, size, lack of symptoms, and age of the patient make the most likely diagnosis a Gartner duct cyst. Skene's ducts and glands are more anterior and distal in the vagina. Bartholin's gland is distal and posterior. Inclusion cysts generally are found in areas of prior trauma, such as childbirth tears or episiotomy. The patient's age and the description of the cyst make clear cell adenocarcinoma unlikely. A Gartner duct cyst is a dilation of a remnant of the embryonic mesonephros.

5. **B,** Page 59. The obturator nerve is motor to the adductor muscles of the thigh and sensory to the medial thigh. If this nerve had been transected, motor weakness of the adductors would be present. Pressure injury, which involves the sensory fibers only or causes mild muscle weakness, usually disappears in a few days or weeks. The femoral nerve is motor to the extensors of the leg and to the skin of the anterior thigh. The pudendal nerve is sensory to the perineum.

6. **B,** Page 52. The blood flows from the aorta to the common iliac to the hypogastric. The hypogastric (or internal iliac) has several branches that should be known by pelvic surgeons. They are superior gluteal, inferior gluteal, lateral sacral, uterine, internal pudendal, middle vesical, inferior vesical, iliolumbar, middle hemorrhoidal, and vaginal. The obturator and superior vesical arteries may also arise from the hypogastric artery. The hypogastric artery ends as the obliterated umbilical artery. Arterial blood that supplies the uterus does not flow directly through the external iliac, obturator, or pudendal artery.

7. **B,** Page 44. The Greek word for neck is *trachelos.* The word *cervix* originates from the Latin word for neck. Therefore, the surgical removal of the cervix is called *trachelectomy,* which is most apt to be performed in a woman whose cervix was left behind during a prior subtotal hysterectomy. Subtotal hysterectomies are done infrequently now and only if severe problems mandate rapid completion of surgery or if massive adhesions or other conditions prevent total removal of the uterus. These situations are rare. Removal of a normal residual cervix is unnecessary.

8. **C,** Page 55. The inguinal nodes are not commonly involved with endometrial cancer, but the potential is present via the round ligament lymphatics. More commonly, the mode of spread is laterally through the lymphatics surrounding the iliac vessels and extending into the paraaortic chain. Direct extension can also occur if the tumor penetrates the myometrium.

9. **E,** Page 57. The nerve supply to the cervix is via a plexus of nerves in the uterosacral ligaments, known as the *paracervical* (or *Frankenhäuser*)

ganglion. These then innervate the endocervix. The efferent pathway from Frankenhäuser's ganglion is to the hypogastric plexus and enters the spinal cord at T11–12. The vasovagal response of bradycardia—with nausea, sweating, and sometimes syncope—occasionally occurs with cervical or intrauterine manipulation because parasympathetic fibers run together with the sympathetics.

10. **C,** Page 48. The whole fallopian tube is approximately 10 to 14 cm long. The ampullary portion is 4 to 6 cm long and is the segment where fertilization usually occurs. This portion has prominent folds, or *plicae,* which if disrupted by infection, inflammation, or trauma can result in blind pouches that can trap a fertilized ovum, leading to a tubal pregnancy. The other segments are shorter and have the following lengths: interstitial, 1 to 2 cm; isthmic, 2 to 4 cm; infundibular, 1 to 2 cm.

11. **E,** Page 51. The major blood supply of each ovary arises from the aorta. In embryonic development, the gonads migrate caudally from their origin, bringing their blood supply, lymphatics, and nerves along with them. The right ovarian vein enters the inferior vena cava, and the left ovarian vein enters the left renal vein. The lymphatics course cephalad in the infundibulopelvic chain and join the paraaortic nodes at the level of the renal pedicle. Approximately 20% of early ovarian cancer spreads microscopically to the paraaortic nodes.

12. **D,** Pages 49. Pain fibers in the tube are stimulated by tubal distention, with referred pain in the dermatomes supplied by the T11–12 cord segment because the tube developed as a midabdominal structure. Therefore, initial midabdominal pain can be appreciated during tubal distention. When inflammation or rupture occurs, the overlying peritoneum is irritated and pain is localized to the right lower quadrant. The same sequence may occur with appendicitis.

13. **C,** Page 44. Vaginal support is mainly derived from the endopelvic fascia surrounding it. The ischiocavernosus muscle is lateral and is not involved in vaginal wall support. The ligaments support the uterus and the apex of the vagina but not the anterior and posterior walls.

14. **B,** Page 42. Chronic infection of the periurethral glands is thought to be the cause of urethral diverticula. The symptoms may be similar to those of a lower urinary tract infection (eg, frequency, urgency, and dyspareunia). A small amount of urine may leak after voiding as the diverticulum empties when the subject stands.

15. **C,** Page 53; Table 3–1 in Stenchever. The inferior epigastric is a branch of the exterior iliac. It runs in the rectus muscle and may be lacerated at the time of amniocentesis or insertion of a trocar during

laparoscopy. Such a laceration can cause a rectus muscle hematoma.

16–18. 16, **C**; 17, **A**; 18, **D**; Pages 40–42. The homologous anatomic structures in the male are the scrotum, prostate, and penile urethra for the labia majora, Skene's glands, and labia minora, respectively. Embryologic development of genital structures is influenced by the presence of testosterone. The earlier that excess androgen is present in embryonic development, the more likely it is that the configuration of the female genitalia will resemble the genitalia of a male. Knowledge of the homologous structures serves to remind us of this truism.

19–21. 19, **C**; 20, **A**; 21, **B**; Page 47. The zona basalis, myometrium, and endometrium are as shown in Figure 3–1. The endometrium does not have a basement membrane separating it from the myometrium. Rather, the basal endometrium inserts itself in the interstices between the muscle fibers of the myometrium. This results in the gritty sensation and sound when curettage is performed. The visceral peritoneum envelops the uterus, so the uterus is, in fact, a retroperitoneal structure. During the menstrual cycle, the endometrium varies from 1 to 6 mm in thickness, with most of the change occurring in the zona functionalis.

22–24. 22, **B**; 23, **C**; 24, **E**; Figure 3–5 (in Stenchever); Page 47. The ovary is suspended by three ligaments: the *infundibulopelvic ligament*, which attaches the ovary to the pelvic side wall and contains the ovarian arteries, nerves, and lymphatics; the *ovarian ligament*, which attaches the ovary to the uterus; and the *mesovarium*, which is part of the broad ligament and contains anastomotic branches from the uterine artery. The cervical portio is that part of the cervix that extends freely into the vaginal canal and is covered by squamous epithelium. Varying amounts of columnar epithelium may extend onto the surface of the cervical portio. The fimbria ovarica is the long tubal fimbria that attaches the infundibulum of the fallopian tube to the ovary.

25–27. 25, **C**; 26, **A**; 27, **E**; Table 3–1 (in Stenchever); Pages 51–53. The high number of anastomoses in the pelvis allows many blood vessels to be sacrificed without ischemic compromise of the pelvic organs, particularly in younger women. For example, the inferior mesenteric artery can be ligated near the aorta without causing anoxic damage to the bowel because anastomoses through the middle and inferior hemorrhoidal arteries maintain the blood supply. The deep iliac circumflex artery anastomoses with the superior gluteal and iliolumbar artery of the hypogastric, and the medial femoral circumflex artery anastomoses with the inferior hemorrhoidal artery and the inferior gluteal

artery of the hypogastric. Venous return has an even greater number of anastomotic channels.

28–30. 28, **C**; 29, **A**; 30, **D**; Figure 3–14 (in Stenchever); Page 55. The lymphatics of the pelvis are important because pelvic malignancies metastasize along their path. Therefore, the lymphatics must be sampled in cases of pelvic malignancy to determine optimum treatment. The internal iliac nodes are found in the anatomic triangle made up of the external iliac artery, hypogastric artery, and pelvic sidewall. Deep femoral nodes are located in the femoral sheath and feed into the iliac and internal iliac chains. Common iliac nodes are located adjacent to the common iliac artery. Aortic nodes are adjacent to the aorta and require meticulous technique for safe sampling. Para-uterine nodes are found immediately lateral to the uterus and are removed during radical hysterectomy.

31. **E**, Page 59. The pelvic diaphragm consists of the coccygeus and the levator ani. The levator ani is made up of the pubococcygeus, the puborectalis, and the iliococcygeus muscles. The deep transverse perineal muscle is not part of the pelvic diaphragm.

32. **C**, Pages 44–45. The cervix has a complex blood supply from the descending branch of the uterine artery and anastomoses from the vaginal arteries and the middle hemorrhoidal arteries. The cervix contains approximately 85% connective tissue and is approximately 2 to 3.5 cm long. More nerves are contained in the endocervix than in the exocervix. Sperm can live in the cervical crypts for several days at midcycle, but not for longer than 2 weeks.

33. **B**, Page 42. The usual clitoral diameter is less than 1 cm. Any sudden increase in clitoral size, particularly when combined with increased hair growth, should prompt a search for increased androgens from either a tumor of the ovaries (or, much less likely, the adrenals) or some exogenous source. Childbirth may change the clitoral size, but not to this extent. Use of birth control pills and menopause does not enlarge the clitoris. Defeminization is the loss of female characteristics, such as body fat distribution and breast fullness; masculinizing changes include deepening of the voice and clitoromegaly.

34. **C**, Page 57. The presacral plexus contains important components of the autonomic nerves to the pelvis. The plexus is located in the retroperitoneal connective tissue from L4 to the sacral hollow. It is also called the *hypogastric plexus*. Celiac and cervical plexuses of the autonomic nervous system do not supply the pelvis. The pudendal and obturator nerves are sensory and motor nerves of the somatic nervous system.

35. **A**, Page 46. A small uterus such as this is consistent with a state of menopause or other causes of

ovarian failure. Uteri from women with hypermenorrhea, adenomyosis, uterine fibroids, or pregnancy all should be larger. A uterus of a normal menstruating woman would also be larger in all dimensions and would weigh approximately 50 to 80 g. The upper limit of normal nonpregnant uterine size is approximately 110 g.

36. **B,** Page 57. The sympathetic and parasympathetic nerves make up the autonomic nervous system. Parasympathetic nerves originate in the cranial and sacral segments of the central nervous system and have ganglia near the visceral organs they serve; they generally cause vasodilation and muscle relaxation. The sympathetic fibers originate from the thoracic and lumbar regions of the spinal cord; they cause constriction of the vessels and muscle contraction. Both elements of the autonomic nervous system enter the pelvis through rather ill-defined plexuses.

37. **D,** Page 56. The ovary arises in the abdomen and descends into the pelvis, bringing its nerve, blood, and lymphatic supply. Therefore, if ovarian cancer metastasizes through lymphatics from the ovary, it tends to go to the periaortic nodes. The other nodes receive lymphatic drainage from both the vagina and the cervix.

38. **B,** Page 54. Arteriovenous malformations in the pelvis are rare. They may be found incidentally with ultrasound imaging in an asymptomatic woman or because of symptoms of bleeding or cardiac compromise, or both. Usually, treatment consists of imaging-guided embolization followed by ligation. Radiation would destroy other tissue, surgical excision can be dangerously bloody; flowing or decreasing the blood flow prior to ligation is usually the safest way to approach these problems.

Reproductive Endocrinology

for Questions 1–30: Select the one best answer or completion.

1. **Ovaries are unable to synthesize mineralocorticoids because they lack**

   A. 3-β-ol-dehydrogenase
   B. 17-hydroxylase
   C. 21-hydroxylase
   D. 11-hydroxylase
   E. 19-hydroxylase

2. **The highest concentration of β-endorphin is found in the**

   A. arcuate nucleus
   B. median eminence
   C. pituitary
   D. serum
   E. ovary

3. **The reason gonadotrophin-releasing hormone analogues can be used to inhibit follicle-stimulating hormone (FSH) and luteinizing hormone (LH) is that**

   A. the unoccupied receptors become refractory to binding
   B. the receptors are all bound and therefore can no longer respond
   C. a change in the ratio of the bound to the unbound receptors is needed to stimulate FSH and LH
   D. the analogues are not similar enough to gonadotrophin-releasing hormone (GnRH) and therefore do not cause stimulation
   E. the analogues do not bind the receptors but shield them from being bound by GnRH

4. **Delta 5 (Δ5) steroid compounds have**

   A. a double bond between carbon atoms 5 and 6
   B. a double bond between carbon atoms 4 and 5
   C. five carbon atoms in the A ring
   D. five carbon atoms in the B ring
   E. a fifth benzene ring

5. **Tanycytes are cells in the third ventricle thought to be important in the transfer of**

   A. GnRH
   B. thyroxin
   C. cortisone
   D. FSH
   E. estrogens

6. **Of the following, the sex steroid present in the plasma in the greatest concentration during any part of the menstrual cycle is**

   A. androstenedione
   B. testosterone
   C. estrone sulfate
   D. estradiol
   E. progesterone

7. **FSH has the same beta subunit as**

   A. LH
   B. adrenocorticotropic hormone (ACTH)
   C. thyroid-stimulating hormone (TSH)
   D. human chorionic gonadotrophin (hCG)
   E. none of the above

8. **The hormone with the greatest affinity for sex hormone–binding globulin (SHBG) is**

   A. progesterone
   B. estrogen
   C. testosterone
   D. dehydrotestosterone
   E. cortisol

9. **If the preovulatory plasma concentration of estradiol is 250 pg/mL and the metabolic clearance rate is 1350 L/day, the daily production rate of estradiol is**

   A. 0.19 mg
   B. 0.338 mg
   C. 5.4 mg
   D. 0.338 g
   E. 5.4 g

10. **Compared with a female of normal weight, a grossly obese woman has increased conversion of**

    A. estradiol to estriol
    B. testosterone to progesterone
    C. progesterone to testosterone
    D. estradiol to androstenedione
    E. androstenedione to estrone

11. **The reason that the concentration of protein hormones in the blood is expressed in international units or milli-international units per milliliter (rather than milligrams per deciliter) is that**

    A. protein hormones metabolize so rapidly they cannot be measured by weight
    B. protein hormones are a combination of different molecules that constantly change
    C. protein hormones are hard to isolate in a pure form
    D. protein hormones exist in such small amounts that milligram weights would be meaningless
    E. measurement of protein hormones was developed by arbitrary convention, which is difficult to change

12. **Thromboxane differs from prostacyclin in that it**

    A. causes vasoconstriction
    B. causes platelet aggregation
    C. is not formed from arachidonic acid
    D. is not an eicosanoid
    E. has 20 carbons

13. **The structure of the ovum that prevents its fertilization by sperm of another species is the**

    A. granulosa
    B. theca interna
    C. zona pellucida
    D. vitelline membrane
    E. theca externa

14. **There is a direct correlation between the increase of serum estrogen during an ovulatory cycle and the**

    A. thickness of the theca externa
    B. size of the dominant follicle
    C. number of hilar cells in the ovary
    D. number of follicles in the ovary
    E. thickness of the ovarian cortex

15. **An ovulatory sequence is characterized by the following order of steps, starting with increased FSH secretion:**

    A. follicular growth, increased estradiol production, LH surge, ovulation, increased estradiol and progesterone production
    B. increased estradiol and estrogen production, follicular growth, increased progesterone production, LH surge, ovulation
    C. follicular growth, increased progesterone production, LH surge, ovulation, increased estradiol production
    D. increased progesterone production, follicular growth, LH surge, increased estradiol production, ovulation
    E. LH surge, follicular growth, increased estradiol production, increased progesterone production, ovulation

16. **In serum obtained from a peripheral vessel, the pulsatile nature of the secretion of LH is apparent, whereas the concentration of FSH is much less variable because**

    A. GnRH does not affect FSH secretion
    B. FSH is not secreted in response to GnRH pulses, but only in response to the steady state of GnRH
    C. FSH has a longer half-life than LH
    D. inhibin decreases the amount of FSH secreted by the pulsatile GnRH
    E. estrogen interferes with the measurement of FSH in immunoassays

17. **The sensitivity of a laboratory test refers to**

 A. the ability to measure only one substance
 B. the least amount of substance that can be measured
 C. the ability to measure the exact amount
 D. the variation between intraassays and interassays
 E. none of the above

18. **The sequence of events leading to menstruation is**

 A. coiling of arteries, vasoconstriction, decrease in endometrial thickness, vasodilation, menses
 B. coiling of arteries, vasodilation, vasoconstriction, decreased endometrial thickness, menses
 C. decrease in endometrial thickness, coiling of arteries, vasoconstriction, vasodilation, menses
 D. vasoconstriction, coiling of arteries, decrease in endometrial thickness, vasodilation, menses
 E. vasoconstriction, decrease in endometrial thickness, coiling of arteries, vasodilation, menses

19. **Ovulation in the human usually occurs**

 A. at the same time as the LH peak
 B. within 24 hours before the LH peak
 C. within 24 hours after the LH peak
 D. at the same time as the estradiol peak
 E. at the same time as the progesterone peak

20. **The primary target of FSH activity is the**

 A. adenohypophysis
 B. neurohypophysis
 C. ovarian theca
 D. ovarian hilum
 E. ovarian granulosa

21. **Which of the following directly stimulates ovarian steroidogenesis?**

 A. epidermal growth factor
 B. inhibin A and B
 C. follistatin
 D. transforming growth factor
 E. insulin-like growth factor (IGF)

22. **A main action of prostaglandin 2α (PGF$_{2\alpha}$) is**

 A. vasodilation
 B. platelet aggregation
 C. bronchoconstriction
 D. smooth muscle relaxation
 E. vascular permeability

23. **GnRH is most active in producing an LH surge when it is secreted**

 A. tonically
 B. in pulses every 2 to 4 minutes
 C. in pulses every 12 minutes
 D. in pulses every hour
 E. in pulses every 3 hours

24. **Inhibin, a substance produced in the ovary,**

 A. is a steroid hormone
 B. is produced mainly in the theca cells
 C. inhibits LH more strongly than it inhibits FSH
 D. is synonymous with follistatin
 E. stimulates thecal androgen production

25. **Activin is a glycoprotein that**

 A. stimulates FSH release
 B. has no structural relationship to inhibin
 C. promotes luteinization
 D. was called *follistatin*
 E. has no autocrine function

26. **Steroid receptors are found**

 A. on cellular surface membranes
 B. only in the cytoplasm
 C. in both the cytoplasm and the nucleus
 D. only in the cell nucleus
 E. on the nuclear membrane

27. **Which is shed during menstruation?**

 A. the entire functional layer of endometrium
 B. both the functional and the basal layers of endometrium
 C. the entire endometrium uniformly
 D. the myometrial matrix supporting the endometrium
 E. various amounts of various parts of the endometrium

28. **A 48-year-old woman asks you what her menstrual cycle will be like during perimenopause. You can accurately inform her that**

 A. the mean age of menopause is approximately 48 years
 B. periods are apt to be regular up until the actual cessation of menstrual flow
 C. the time between periods usually decreases toward menopause
 D. the follicular phase gets shorter as women get older

29. **Growth factors belong to which of the following groups of compounds?**

    A. glycoproteins
    B. peptides
    C. steroids
    D. fatty acids
    E. nucleic acids

30. **In which part of the menstrual cycle is the LH pulse the slowest?**

    A. early follicular
    B. midfollicular
    C. late follicular
    D. early luteal
    E. late luteal

DIRECTIONS:

for Questions 31–42: For each numbered item, select the one heading most closely associated with it. Each lettered heading may be used once, more than once, or not at all.

31–33. **Match the endometrium with the correct time of the cycle.**

    A. menstrual
    B. early follicular
    C. late follicular
    D. early luteal
    E. midluteal

31. Figure 4–1.

32. Figure 4–2.

33. Figure 4–3.

34–36. **Match the site of action of the following enzymes with the correct number on Figure 4–4.**

    A. 17-α-hydroxylase
    B. 17-β-hydroxysteroid dehydrogenase
    C. 17-20 lyase
    D. aromatase
    E. delta 5-4 isomerase

37–39. **Match the times of the cycle with the appropriate serum level of hormone.**

    A. early follicular phase
    B. late follicular phase
    C. ovulation
    D. midluteal phase
    E. late luteal phase

37. Estrogen 100–150 pg/mL, progesterone 10–15 g/mL

38. Estrogen > 200 pg/mL, progesterone 1–2 ng/mL

39. Estrogen < 50 pg/mL, progesterone < 1 ng/mL

40–42. **Match the listed substance with its action.**

    A. estrogen
    B. progestin
    C. glucocorticoids
    D. antiestrogens
    E. GnRH

40. **Inhibits synthesis of estrogen receptors.**

41. **Increases synthesis of estradiol dehydrogenase.**

42. **Binds estrogen receptors but initiates little transcription.**

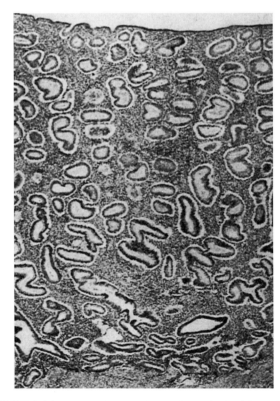

FIGURE 4–1 (From Novak E, Novak ER, eds: Textbook of Gynecology, 4th ed. Baltimore, Williams & Wilkins, 1952.)

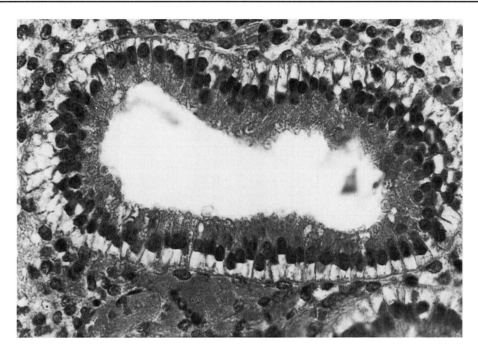

FIGURE 4–2 (From March CM: The endometrium in the menstrual cycle. In Stenchever DR Jr, Davajan V, eds: Infertility, Contraception and Reproductive Endocrinology, 2nd ed. Oradell, NJ, Medical Economics Books, 1986.)

FIGURE 4–3 (From March CM: The endometrium in the menstrual cycle. In Stenchever DR Jr, Davajan V, eds: Infertility, Contraception and Reproductive Endocrinology, 2nd ed. Oradell, NJ, Medical Economics Books, 1986.)

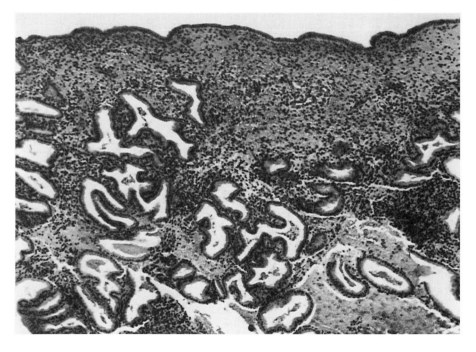

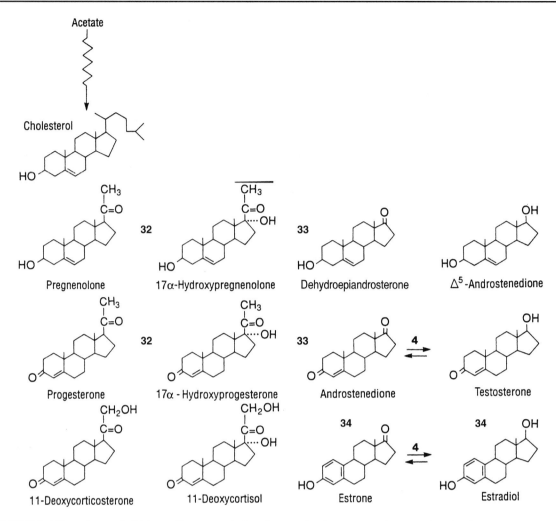

FIGURE 4–4 (From Stanczyk FZ: Steroid hormones. In Stenchever DR Jr, Davajan V, Lobo RA, eds: Infertility, Contraception and Reproductive Endocrinology, 3rd ed. Cambridge, MA, Blackwell Scientific, 1991.)

ANSWERS

1. **C,** Page 92, Figure 4–20 in Stenchever. 21-Hydroxylase is needed to hydroxylate carbon 21. This must be done before the steroids have a significant mineralocorticoid effect. 11-Hydroxylase is needed to confer the glucocorticoid effect by hydroxylation of the carbon in position 11.

2. **C,** Page 79. The reason for the high concentration of β-endorphins in the pituitary is unknown. The infusion of β-endorphins decreases LH by causing an inhibitory effect on GnRH neurons in the hypothalamus, probably by modulating synthesis of norepinephrine. This action is thought to contribute to anovulation in female athletes, who have high levels of β-endorphins.

3. **A,** Page 81. GnRH analogues function in a fashion similar to native GnRH—that is, they bind some of the target cell membrane receptors and stimulate them maximally. When the bound receptors are maximally stimulated, the unoccupied receptors become refractory to further binding. The already saturated receptors are not able to sustain the release of the second messenger, cyclic adenosine monophosphate (cAMP), which maintains the activation of protein kinase. Protein kinase is needed to supply energy for the protein substrate that produces FSH and LH. The decreased FSH and LH levels result in anovulation.

4. **A,** Page 91, Figure 4–19 in Stenchever. *Delta* stands for a double bond between carbon atoms in the steroid molecule. When steroids are synthesized by the ovary, the adrenal gland, or the placenta, they follow specific pathways. Those with a double bond between carbon atoms 5 and 6 are called *Δ5 steroids*. They have not yet been acted on by the enzyme 4-5 isomerase, which changes the position of the double bond. This step is necessary to produce progesterone from pregnenolone and androsterone from dehydroepian drosterone.

5. **A,** Page 75. Tanycytes line the third ventricle and have microvilli, which are postulated to absorb GnRH continuously and transport it into the portal system, thereby providing an alternative method for GnRH to reach the pituitary in a constant, low-grade continuous (tonic) manner. Peaks of GnRH are carried to the anterior pituitary directly by the portal system.

6. **E,** Page 94, Table 4–3 in Stenchever. Estrogens are present in picogram levels. The concentration of estrone sulfate is greater than that of estradiol or estrone. However, the estrone sulfate is conjugated and less potent than estradiol. Both androgens and progesterone are present in nanogram amounts. Although graphs often depict a higher curve for estrogen than for progesterone, the scales are different. Progesterone is present at levels of 4 to 19 ng/mL during the luteal phase. More important than concentration is the biologic potency of a compound.

7. **E,** Page 83. FSH, LH, TSH, and hCG have the same alpha subunit but different beta subunits. Although also a pituitary hormone, ACTH has a different structure. Sensitive radioimmunoassay techniques use the beta subunit to identify the specific compound.

8. **D,** Page 73. Dihydrotestosterone, testosterone, and estrogen are bound to SHBG in order of decreasing affinity. Cortisone and progesterone are bound to cortisone-binding globulin. Steroids are also bound to albumin, and approximately 5% of steroids circulate as free hormone. SHBG is increased by estrogen, obesity, and increased T_4. SHBG is decreased by androgens and hypothyroidism. Therefore, thyroid dysfunction may change the concentration of SHBG and may cause changes in the amount of free estrogen, which in turn may cause abnormal uterine bleeding.

9. **B,** Page 94. The production rate equals the metabolic clearance rate times the concentration. Therefore, 1350 L/day × 250 pg/mL × 1000 mL/L = 337,500,000 pg/day, or approximately 0.338 mg/day. Preovulatory estrogen levels are higher than at any other phase of the cycle. The dose of replacement estrogen should have a pharmacologic effect similar to approximately 0.3 mg/day of estradiol after systemic absorption.

10. **E,** Page 93. Androstenedione is converted to estrone in fatty tissue. In obese women, regardless of age, a greater percentage (up to 7% from 1.3%) of androstenedione is converted to estrone than in women of normal weight. This conversion can provide a constant pool of estrone, which inhibits ovulation and causes constant endometrial stimulation. This stimulation, in turn, can lead to the increased incidence of endometrial hyperplasia found in obese women.

11. **C,** Page 115. Because most protein hormones are of high molecular weight and circulate attached to numerous other molecules, they are extremely difficult to isolate in pure form. Therefore, a reference standard is agreed on and measurements are expressed in terms of that standard. If the standard is internationally agreed on, the results will be expressed as international units or milli-international units.

12. **A,** Pages 89–90. Both thromboxane and prostacyclin are formed from arachidonic acid; they are eicosanoids having 20 carbons. Thromboxane has an oxane ring rather than a cyclopentane ring. Both cause platelet aggregation; however, thromboxane causes vasoconstriction, whereas prostacyclin causes vasodilation. Both are inhibited by cortisol, which decreases phospholipid hydrolysis and release, and by type I (aspirin and indomethacin) nonsteroidal antiinflammatory drugs (NSAIDs), which inhibit endoperoxide formation.

13. **C,** Page 97. The zona pellucida is a mucopolysaccharide layer that allows only sperm of the same species to penetrate. When it is removed, as in a zona-free hamster egg penetration test, human sperm can penetrate the hamster egg. The sperm's ability (or inability) to penetrate the egg is used to determine the fertilizing potential of the sperm. The theca interna and theca externa do not accompany the ovulated egg. The vitelline membrane blocks repeated penetration by sperm after one sperm has successfully entered the egg.

14. **B,** Page 97. The dominant follicle produces approximately 80% of the estrogen synthesized before ovulation. Its mean diameter is about 2 cm, and its mean volume is approximately 3.8 mL. This increase in size, as monitored by ultrasonography, is used in the follow-up of women who are undergoing stimulation for in vitro fertilization. Follicular size is a criterion used to indicate maximum potential for ovulation.

15. **A,** Pages 97–101. Knowledge of the normal sequence of events in the menstrual cycle enables one to evaluate abnormalities and prescribe rational therapy. FSH stimulates the follicle, which in turn produces estradiol, which promotes the development of an LH-responsive dominant follicle and triggers the LH surge, resulting in ovulation. After ovulation, the follicle develops into a corpus luteum, which produces both estrogen and progesterone. The progesterone causes secretion by an estrogen-stimulated endometrium preparing for the implantation of a fertilized ovum.

16. **C,** Pages 85, 101. GnRH does affect secretion and release of FSH, but because FSH has a half-life of approximately 4 hours, short bursts of its secretion are not apparent. LH has a half-life of 30 minutes, so the episodic nature of its secretion is apparent.

Although inhibin, a nonsteroidal hormone produced in the granulosa cells, does inhibit FSH, it manifests only when the granulosa is large; therefore, inhibin is not a constant inhibitor of FSH. Estrogen does not interfere with immunoassays used to measure FSH.

17. **B,** Page 117. The ability to measure only one substance is *specificity.* The least amount of substance that can be measured is *sensitivity.* The ability to measure the exact amount is *accuracy.* The variation between intraassays and interassays is the *precision* of a test.

18. **C,** Page 106. According to Markee's studies, first there is regression in the thickness of the endometrium, with coiling of the spiral arteries and slowing of blood. This is followed by vasoconstriction, after which vasodilation occurs, leading to escape of blood and menses. The initial decreased blood flow is thought to cause tissue ischemia, which releases lysosomal enzymes, which in turn break down the endometrium. This degraded tissue and blood from the coiled arteries of the functional layer of the endometrium make up the menstrual flow.

19. **C,** Page 97. In a normal cycle, the rapid rise of estrogen from a growing follicle triggers a rise of LH at a time when the follicle is 18 to 25 mm in diameter and is ready to release an egg. The endometrium has been estrogen primed to respond to the progesterone, which will be produced by the postovulatory corpus luteum. Ovulation usually occurs within 24 hours after the LH peak, maintaining the exquisite timing needed to provide an egg at an optimum time for fertilization and subsequent implantation. The estradiol peak occurs before ovulation, and the progesterone peak takes place after ovulation.

20. **E,** Pages 96–97. FSH receptors exist primarily on the granulosa cell membrane. When androgens or theca cells (which produce androgens) are added to FSH-stimulated granulosa cells, large amounts of estrogen are produced; only small amounts are produced without the androgen precursor. According to the two-cell hypothesis of ovarian estrogen production, LH acts on theca cell receptors to stimulate production of androgens, which are transported to the granulosa cells. Granulosa cells, under the influence of FSH, aromatize androgens to estrogens. FSH and estrogen stimulate LH receptors on the granulosa cells, allowing LH to be bound and cause luteinization.

21. **E,** Pages 86–88, Table 4–1 in Stenchever. IGF-1 and IGF-2 are produced in the granulosa cells as well as in many other organs. They stimulate steroidogenesis in the ovaries and have autocrine and paracrine functions, including increased androgen production. High levels of insulin may mimic their action by binding IGF-I receptors in the ovary. Insulin is also responsible for regulating the circulating levels of the binding proteins of IGF-1 and IGF-2 and may be involved in the symptom complex of polycystic ovary syndrome. Inhibin is produced by granulosa cells and is used as a marker in granulosa cell tumors of the ovary. Follistatin binds activin, preventing its activity and thereby inhibits FSH. Transforming growth factor (TGF) and epidermal growth factor (EGF) both inhibit steroidogenesis.

22. **C,** Pages 89–90, Table 4–2 in Stenchever. Actions of $PGF_{2\alpha}$ include vasoconstriction, bronchoconstriction, and smooth muscle contraction. For these reasons, this agent is used to cause contraction of the uterine muscle in cases of uterine atony and is generally contraindicated in patients with asthma. $PGF_{2\alpha}$ is found in increased concentration during menses and may add to the uterine cramping common at that time. It also has an effect on menstrual flow. Nonsteroidal antiinflammatory drugs, which inhibit prostaglandin formation, are useful to decrease both menstrual cramps and flow.

23. **D,** Pages 75, 81–82. When GnRH is given tonically in high doses, gonadotrophins are inhibited. They are also inhibited if GnRH is given in pulses every 2 to 12 minutes. If LH is given in pulses every hour, a midcycle surge of LH occurs. However, if the pulses are as infrequent as every 3 hours, the LH decreases and the FSH secretion increases. Therefore the rate, the amount, and the spacing of GnRH doses affect the release of LH and FSH. GnRH agonists, which are more potent and have a longer half-life than GnRH, cause an initial gonadotrophin release (flare) lasting 1 to 3 weeks and then inhibit gonadotrophin release. GnRH antagonists have been synthesized and inhibit gonadotrophins without causing an initial increase. The newer antagonists do not cause an allergic reaction as the initial ones did.

24. **E,** Pages 87–88. Inhibin is a glycoprotein produced by granulosa cells, Sertoli cells, the corpus luteum, and the placenta. It inhibits oocyte maturation and FSH release. Inhibin is unrelated to follistatin, although both of them inhibit FSH release. However, follistatin inhibits FSH release by binding with activin and decreasing the bioactivity of activin. Inhibin decreases in the postmenopausal years and may allow the postmenopausal rise in FSH.

25. **A,** Page 88. Activin is similar in structure to inhibin in that it shares some of the subunits of inhibin. Activin has both paracrine and autocrine functions and promotes folliculogenesis while preventing premature luteinization. It is totally different from follistatin, which inhibits FSH release by binding activin, preventing the stimulation of FSH by activin.

26. **C,** Page 94. Steroid receptors are found intercellularly in both the cytoplasm and the nucleus. Binding of these receptors with steroid forms a steroid receptor complex that binds to a hormone responsive element in the nuclear DNA. This results in formation of messenger RNA, which then migrates into the cell cytoplasm and translates information to ribosomes, which in turn synthesize new protein. Protein hormone receptors, on the other hand, are found on the cellular membrane. Examples are those that bind with LH, FSH, and prolactin.

27. **E,** Pages 106–109. Because there is no basement membrane between the myometrium and the endometrium, the baseline endometrium is interdigitated between the muscle fibers of the myometrium. This produces the gritty sensation felt during dilation and curettage. During menses, many of the endometrial cells remain in both functional and basal layers. Shedding does not occur uniformly over the entire endometrium, and regeneration of cells begins even though bleeding is continuing. Although enzymes may destroy endometrial cells, muscle cells are generally unaffected.

28. **D,** Page 103. The irregularity of periods that is common both at the beginning and at the end of menstrual years is more worrisome in the older woman, since the risk of endometrial carcinoma is much higher than in the teenage years. A certain amount of irregularity is normal, but the most usual pattern is a shorter time between menses and a decreased flow. The follicular phase length decreases with age, from 14 days to approximately 10 days. The mean age of menopause is about 51.

29. **B,** Page 72. Growth factors are large or small peptides that usually enhance cell differentiation or proliferation, or both. Not all peptides are growth factors—for example, leptin is a peptide secreted by fatty tissue and may signal the amount of fat stores. Eicosanoids are fatty acids, and DNA is a nucleic acid.

30. **E,** Page 101. LH is released in an pulsatile fashion presumably because of GnRH pulses. Its frequency is the slowest in the late luteal phase (approximately 1 every 3 hours) and is fastest in the mid and late follicular phases (approximately 1 every hour). The rate of release is probably important in stimulating production of estradiol. In the luteal phase, progesterone is also secreted in pulses corresponding to the LH pulses.

31–33. 31, **C;** 32, **D;** 33,**E;** Pages 104–105, 112–113. The endometrium undergoes specific, recognizable histologic changes during the menstrual cycle. These changes can be dated accurately to correlate with the days of the menstrual cycle. Endometrial biopsy and dating can provide indirect evidence of ovulation. One should recognize that the cells lining the glands in Figure 4–1 are pseudostratified. In Figure 4–2 there is subnuclear vacuolization, and in Figure 4–3 the glands are tortuous, and the stroma vascular and edematous.

34–36. 34, **A;** 35, **B;** 36, **D;** Page 92, Figure 4–20 in Stenchever. Knowing where specific enzymes act in the process of steroid anabolism allows you to recognize the results of different enzyme deficiencies. The absence of an enzyme along the pathway causes the steroids formed before the point of loss to be present in large quantities because they are not used in further conversion. The steroids formed after the loss of the enzyme are reduced in amount, leading to a clinical symptom complex. Note that the same enzyme may act between different molecules.

37–39. 37, **D;** 38, **C;** 39, **A;** Page 102, Table 4–28 in Stenchever. The estrogen level rises throughout the follicular phase and peaks just before the LH surge. Progesterone is low until after ovulation, when it rises along with the secondary rise in estrogen. Because progesterone is secreted in a pulsable manner, finding a single low level of serum progesterone does not necessarily mean ovulation has not occurred. Both estrogen and progesterone levels fall just before menses. The 17-hydroxyprogesterone level rises slightly before the LH surge and falls again just before menses.

40–42. 40, **B;** 41, **B;** 42, **D;** Page 95. Estrogens stimulate the synthesis of estrogen receptors and progesterone receptors in target tissues such as the endometrium. Progestins inhibit the synthesis of both estrogen receptors and progesterone receptors. Progestins also increase the intracellular synthesis of estradiol dehydrogenase, which converts the more potent estradiol to the less potent estrone, further decreasing estrogenic activity in the target cell. Antiestrogens, such as clomiphene and tamoxifen, bind to estrogen receptors but do not initiate transcription; therefore, they decrease the usual effects of estrogen.

Evidence-Based Medicine and Clinical Epidemiology

for Questions 1–24: Select the one best answer or completion.

1. In an epidemiologic study, all of the following can be an exposure *except*

   A. a genetic factor
   B. a behavior
   C. a screening program
   D. a measure of functional status

2. A change in the course of an existing disease would be classified as a(n)

   A. exposure
   B. outcome
   C. random error
   D. attributable risk

3. Randomized controlled trials (RCTs) are examples of what kind of study?

   A. experimental analytical
   B. cross-sectional
   C. cohort
   D. case-controlled

4. In which type of study are all other factors that might influence the study outcome equalized by the nature of the study design?

   A. case-controlled
   B. cohort
   C. observational
   D. RCT

5. When a subject is recruited for a study, all of the following should be provided *except*

   A. cost of the study
   B. purpose of the study
   C. risks
   D. benefits
   E. available alternatives

6. Which of the following would be a clinical problem most readily studied with an RCT?

   A. causes of ovarian cancer
   B. best management of fibroid tumors
   C. cure rates in the treatment of pelvic infections
   D. factors contributing to domestic violence

7. Which of the following types of study provides the weakest evidence?

   A. RCT
   B. cohort
   C. cross-sectional
   D. case-controlled

8. Which type of study is always retrospective?

   A. cohort
   B. cross-sectional
   C. case-controlled
   D. RCT

9. Which of the following relative risks (RRs) and odds ratios (ORs) indicates protection from the outcome?

   A. 0.8
   B. 1.0
   C. 1.8
   D. 8.0

10. For both RR and OR, what is the implication for a value that is further away from 1.0?

    A. protection from outcome
    B. risk of outcome
    C. no association to outcome
    D. stronger relationship

11. **The precision of the point estimate is increased by which of the following combinations?**

    A. wide confidence interval, small study
    B. wide confidence interval, large study
    C. narrow confidence interval, small study
    D. narrow confidence interval, large study

12. **Systematic differences between study participants and nonparticipants is a description of what type of study bias?**

    A. recall bias
    B. selection bias
    C. testing bias
    D. observer bias

13. **Which type of study is the *least* likely to be affected by biases?**

    A. RCT
    B. cross-sectional
    C. case-controlled
    D. cohort

14. **In the Bradford-Hill criteria for causation, a strong RR fits which of the following?**

    A. >2.0
    B. <0.5
    C. >0.5
    D. <2.0
    E. >2.0 *or* <0.5

15. **The criterion of coherence in the Bradford-Hill set of criteria for causation refers to**

    A. precision of data
    B. temporal cause and effect
    C. homogeneity of study population
    D. other knowledge

16. **The Cochrane Collaboration is a source for**

    A. meta-analyses
    B. systematic reviews
    C. expert opinions
    D. RCTs

17. **The primary purpose of a meta-analysis is to**

    A. collect data
    B. identify bias
    C. improve precision
    D. settle controversy

18. **Systematic reviews can be shortened into shorter, clinically useful documents called**

    A. algorithms
    B. handbooks
    C. flow charts
    D. practice guidelines

19. **The grading system used to evaluate studies according to quality comes from the**

    A. Cochrane Collaboration
    B. U.S. Preventive Services Task Force
    C. Canadian Task Force on the Periodic Health Examination
    D. Agency for Healthcare Research and Quality

20. **Which term used in clinical epidemiology refers to the probability of correctly identifying a nondiseased person with a screening test?**

    A. sensitivity
    B. specificity
    C. relative risk
    D. positive predictive value

21. **What is the significance if the confidence interval overlaps 1.0?**

    A. The association is strong.
    B. The change in risk is statistically insignificant.
    C. The study design is flawed.
    D. No meaningful conclusions are available.

22. **Which of the following best describes the term *positive predictive value*?**

    A. proportion of people with a positive test result who have the target disorder
    B. ratio of risk measured in the treated group
    C. probability that any given case will be identified by the test
    D. frequency with which a true difference is identified

23. **In categorizing levels of evidence, what is a controlled trial without randomization?**

    A. I
    B. II-1
    C. II-2
    D. II-3
    E. III

24. **What term describes the size of the effect of any exposure in absolute terms?**

    A. attributable risk
    B. incidence
    C. power
    D. precision

ANSWERS

1. **D,** Page 127. The purpose of an epidemiologic study is to estimate the relationship between and exposure and an outcome. This determines whether or not there is a causal relationship. Examples of an exposure include a behavior, a genetic factor, a screening program, or any aspect of a treatment.

2. **B,** Pages 126–127. Outcomes are all the possible results that may stem from exposure to a causal factor or from preventive or therapeutic interventions; all identified changes in health status arising as a consequence of the handling of a health problem could be included. Examples include a symptom, a measure of functional status, a new-onset disease, or a change in the course of an existing disease.

3. **A,** Pages 127–128. In experimental studies, the investigator controls exposure to the factor of interest. These RCTs are characterized by the prospective assignment of study participants to a study group or a placebo/no treatment/standard care group. Cross-sectional studies examine the relationship between exposure and outcome in a defined population at a single point in time. In cohort studies, the exposure is selected by the individual subject, not the investigator. Case-controlled studies are always retrospective, and participants are selected on the basis of having the identified outcome (case group) or not (control group).

4. **D,** Page 127. By randomizing study participants, the RCT can equalize all other factors that might influence the study outcome and leave only the effect of the study treatment itself. RCTs usually provide the best evidence for making clinical decisions. The theoretical advantage of this type of study design only holds true if the study has been thoughtfully designed, implemented with care, and analyzed appropriately.

5. **A,** Page 127. Subjects recruited for a trial must receive information about the study purpose, its procedures, the likely risks and benefits, and available alternatives. For a clinician to recruit or refer a patient to a clinical trial, the study treatments need to be balanced in terms of benefits and harm.

6. **C,** Page 127. Practical considerations frequently determine whether or not a clinical question is appropriate to be addressed by a randomized clinical trial. RCTs to study long-term or rare outcomes are extremely difficult to carry out. The following are examples in which RCT data could be relied on: comparisons of short-term pain or febrile morbidity following different surgical approaches; comparisons of cure rates or side effects in the treatment of infections; pregnancy rates following different infertility treatment regimens. Acute clinical problems in which every patient has a relevant outcome in a short period of time are ideally suited to clinical trials.

7. **C,** Page 128. Observational studies in which the investigator does not control the exposure provide an alternative approach to the more powerful randomized clinical trial. Cross-sectional studies generate prevalence data by examining the relationship between exposure and the outcome in a defined population at a specific point in time. They do not provide strong causal evidence, but they can highlight associations that might deserve additional attention. Cohort and case-controlled studies provide stronger evidence.

8. **C,** Page 128. Study participants are selected on the basis of already having the outcome of interest (case group) or of not having the outcome (control group). After identifying the cases and controls, data are then gathered, usually by interview, concerning past exposures. The exposure information from cases and controls is then compared quantitatively to obtain an estimate of risk.

9. **A,** Page 129. *Risk* in study subjects is the number of cases or outcomes that occur over time. The *relative risk* is the risk of the outcome among the exposed subjects divided by the risk in the unexposed subjects. A case-controlled study calculates its results as an OR, generally equivalent to an RR in a cohort study. RRs and ORs less than 1.0 indicate a decreased risk of the outcome.

10. **D,** Page 129. For both RRs and ORs, the further away the value is from 1.0, the stronger the relationship between the exposure and the outcome. If there is no association at all between the exposure and the outcome, then the RR or OR is 1.0.

11. **D,** Page 130. Because the RR is based on results from just the people in a particular study and not the entire universe of subjects, sampling error is inherent. The quantitative description of a study results need to include a measure of this uncertainty. The confidence interval expresses the precision of the point estimate. A wide confidence interval indicates less precision, while a narrow confidence interval suggests greater precision. Generally, the larger the study, the narrower the confidence interval.

12. **B,** Pages 130–131. In any study, the process of data collection, analysis, and interpretation can lead to conclusions that are systematically different from truth. These deviations may occur through study bias or confounding variables. Selection bias is an error due to systematic differences in characteristics between those selected to participate in the study and those not selected.

13. **A,** Pages 130–131. When the available evidence comes from observational studies, it is generally necessary to apply additional criteria to decide whether the reported associations are likely to be causal. Biases are more likely in observational studies than in randomized trials.

14. **E,** Page 131. In the United States, the Bradford-Hill criteria have been used as one approach to differentiate causality and association. These criteria are also called the *surgeon general's criteria* because of their initial use in interpretation of evidence regarding cigarette smoking and lung cancer. According to these criteria, the RR should exceed 2.0 or be less than 0.5.

15. **D,** Page 131. Coherence of the evidence demands that the criteria be considered in conjunction with all of our other knowledge. Some of the other criteria consider the internal validity of the study, while others consider the external validity. We must also consider how the study results fit in with general biologic knowledge, including that gathered from animal and laboratory studies.

16. **B,** Page 132. The Cochrane Collaboration is the major source of systematic reviews. Systematic evidence reviews include a comprehensive review and evaluation of the literature and are reported using a standardized format, which includes a detailed description of the search strategy used to identify the relevant literature and the results of the search. These reviews also critically appraise the studies evaluated. The goal of systematic reviews is to synthesize the world literature in a specific area and to use an approach that minimizes bias and random error.

17. **C,** Page 132. The main purpose of any meta-analysis is to improve precision. Because individual studies often have imprecise results, statistical methods to combine the results sometimes proves helpful. Meta-analysis is a collection of techniques to produce a pooled effect estimate from several studies. At its best, it involves pooling an reanalyzing raw data from several similar randomized trials to produce a result with a tighter confidence interval.

18. **D,** Pages 132–133. The Cochrane Collaboration aims to help people make well-informed health care decisions by preparing, maintaining, and promoting accessibility of systematic reviews of the effects of health care interventions. The U.S. Preventive Services Task Force systematically reviews clinical preventive services. To help translate the lengthy reviews into shorter and clinically useful documents, many professional organizations now distribute practice guidelines to help clinicians make patient-care decisions.

19. **C,** Page 132. The Canadian Task Force on the Periodic Health Examination described three levels of evidence to make the assessment of studies more uniform. The highest level of evidence is the RCT. Opinion, whether that of an individual or an expert committee, is the least valuable source of information.

20. **B,** Page 126. Specificity is the proportion of truly nondiseased persons who are so identified by the screening test. It is a measure of the probability of correctly identifying a nondiseased person with a screening test.

21. **B,** Page 125. The confidence interval is a range of values determined by the degree of presumed random variability in the data, within which the point estimate is thought to lie, with the specified level of confidence. The confidence interval is symmetric around the point estimate. If the confidence interval overlaps 1.0, the change in risk is statistically insignificant.

22. **A,** Page 126. The positive predictive value is the proportion of people with a positive test result who have the target disorder.

23. **B,** Page 132. Level I evidence includes at least one properly controlled randomized trial. Level II-1 studies are controlled trials without randomization. Level II-2 evidence includes well-designed cohort and case-control studies.

24. **A,** Pages 125, 130. Also called the *population excess rate* or the *rate difference,* the attributable risk includes the excess cases or the fraction of a disease in the population that is due to a particular factor or exposure. The risk in the exposed minus the risk in the unexposed is the risk difference. The risk difference describes the size of the effect in absolute terms. This is also called *attributable risk.*

PART TWO

Comprehensive Evaluation of the Female

History and Physical

DIRECTIONS:

for Questions 1–8: Select the one best answer or completion.

1. Each of the following neoplasms can be screened during routine physical examination *except*

   A. carcinoma of the cervix
   B. carcinoma of the breast
   C. carcinoma of the ovary
   D. carcinoma of the endometrium
   E. carcinoma of the rectum

2. If the screening interval value is extended from 2 to 3 years, the increased risk of developing carcinoma of the cervix is approximately

   A. twofold
   B. threefold
   C. fourfold
   D. fivefold
   E. sixfold

3. The percentage of neoplastic bowel lesions that can be palpated on digital rectal examination is

   A. 30%
   B. 40%
   C. 50%
   D. 60%
   E. 70%

4. As the primary physician for postmenopausal women, a gynecologist should obtain which of the following annually?

   A. mammography
   B. thyroid-stimulating hormone (TSH)
   C. total cholesterol
   D. electrocardiogram
   E. Pap (Papanicolaou) smear

DIRECTIONS:

for Questions 5–17: For each numbered item, select the one heading most closely associated with it. Each lettered heading may be used once, more than once, or not at all.

5. An 8-year-old girl with a 2-month history of vaginal bleeding

   A. mammography
   B. colposcopy
   C. hysteroscopy
   D. endometrial sampling
   E. pelvic ultrasonography
   F. vaginoscopy

6. A 44-year-old nulligravida woman in clinic for an annual examination

   A. mammography
   B. colposcopy
   C. hysteroscopy
   D. endometrial sampling
   E. pelvic ultrasonography
   F. vaginoscopy

7. A 44-year-old woman with a problem of frequent "irregular periods"

   A. mammography
   B. colposcopy
   C. hysteroscopy
   D. endometrial sampling
   E. pelvic ultrasonography
   F. vaginoscopy

8. A 21-year-old nulligravida with an unusually large cervical "erosion" (cockscomb cervix)

   A. mammography
   B. colposcopy
   C. hysteroscopy
   D. endometrial sampling
   E. pelvic ultrasonography
   F. vaginoscopy

9–11. Match the diagnosis with the most appropriate patient findings listed.

   (A) cystocele
   (B) enterocele
   (C) total procidentia
   (D) rectocele

9. Prolapse of the cervix and uterus through the introitus

10. Bulging of the vaginal mucosa that can be seen at the vaginal introitus with Valsalva maneuver; it occurs from the anterior wall of the vagina

11. Cystic bulge from the area of the cul-de-sac contained in the rectovaginal septum

12–14. Bleeding manifestations of which of the following conditions are listed below?

   A. an anovulatory cycle
   B. cervical inflammation or neoplasm
   C. an ovulatory cycle
   D. ovulation breakthrough bleeding
   E. endometriosis

12. Consistent postcoital bleeding with regular menses

13. Irregular painless bleeding episodes with variable flow

14. Bleeding every 2 weeks alternating between 4 to 5 days of bleeding with some cramping and 1 to 2 days of painless spotting

15–17. Examination of the female reproductive organs involves many components. Match the goals listed with one of the following components:

   (A) abdominal examination
   (B) abdominal/vaginal (bimanual) examination
   (C) no component of the typical pelvic examination
   (D) rectovaginal examination
   (E) speculum examination

15. Identify the transformation zone

16. Appreciate the uterosacral ligament nodules

17. Identify a normal postmenopausal ovary

DIRECTIONS:

for Questions 18–27: Select the one best answer or completion.

18. A Pap smear is likely to identify all the following *except*

    A. cervical squamous cell carcinoma
    B. gonorrhea
    C. human papilloma virus
    D. inflammatory changes
    E. trichomoniasis

19. First-order relatives include all the following *except*

    A. brother
    B. children
    C. father
    D. maternal aunt
    E. mother

20. Abdominal palpation may elicit the following findings. All these represent intraabdominal pathologic conditions *except*

    A. fluid wave
    B. rebound
    C. referred pain
    D. rigidity
    E. trigger points

21. History regarding prior pregnancies should include all the following *except*

    A. gestational diabetes
    B. infant weight at delivery
    C. molar pregnancy
    D. number of prenatal care visits
    E. paternity

22. **Dermatologic findings of the vulvar and perineal skin of potential significance include all the following *except***

    A. cherry angioma
    B. diffuse alopecia
    C. hyperkeratosis
    D. pediculosis
    E. pigmented nevi

23. **Nonverbal clues given by patient behavior may be helpful in making the clinical diagnosis of all the following *except***

    A. anxiety neurosis
    B. apathetic patient
    C. endogenous depression
    D. hidden anger

24. **Characteristics of the normal squamocolumnar junction (transformation zone) include all the following *except***

    A. areas of squamous metaplasia
    B. nabothian cysts and ectropion
    C. typical visibility just inside the external os
    D. ulcerations
    E. shifts in location in response to infectious or hormonal influences

25. **Items in the sexual history that usually relate to the presence of an organic gynecologic pathologic condition include**

    A. anorgasmy
    B. decreased libido
    C. entrance dyspareunia (vaginismus)
    D. homosexuality
    E. postcoital bleeding

26. **Descriptions of appropriate Pap testing include all the following *except***

    A. Air dry before fixative is applied.
    B. Perform yearly in most patients.
    C. Contain an adequate sampling of endocervical cells.
    D. First perform regularly with onset of coitus or at age 18.
    E. Sample the transformation zone.

27. **Positive historical findings that help identify a 43-year-old patient at increased risk for endometrial neoplasia include all the following *except***

    A. chronic oligoovulation
    B. history of dysfunctional uterine bleeding
    C. infertility
    D. obesity
    E. use of oral contraceptive pills

28. **A 55-year-old woman presents for her annual examination and health maintenance visit. In a discussion of vaccinations, which of the following should be offered annually?**

    A. hepatitis A vaccine
    B. hepatitis B vaccine
    C. influenza vaccine
    D. pneumococcal vaccine
    E. tetanus-diphtheria booster

ANSWERS

1. **D,** Pages 151–152. Small endometrial tumors may not be appreciated by routine examination unless they are associated with a significant change in bleeding pattern. The others can be suspected by routine examination and diagnostic procedures such as the Pap smear and stool guaiac testing. Endometrial sampling is reserved for patients with abnormal menstrual histories or perimenopausal or postmenopausal bleeding. Some authors advocate such sampling as a routine procedure in postmenopausal estrogen users.

2. **C,** Page 147. Patients with later coital exposure who have had one sexual partner and who have had two successive negative annual Pap smears may be considered low-risk and should be screened by Pap testing every 1 to 3 years. A study by Shy and colleagues showed that although the risk of cervical cancer did not increase significantly in women screened every 2 years compared with women screened annually, the risk increased 3.9 times if the interval was 3 years and 12.3 times in women not screened for 10 years.

3. **E,** Page 150. The value of the rectal examination should not be underestimated. This is the most efficient way to assess the uterosacral ligaments and the size of the uterus in cases of retroflexion. Rectal examination should permit digital palpitation of as many as 70% of bowel lesions. Because bowel cancer is common in women, particularly after the age of 35, this part of the examination should not be overlooked.

4. **A,** Pages 151–152. Of the tests listed, the mammogram is mandatory on an annual basis, as recommended by the American Cancer Society and the American College of Obstetricians and Gynecologists. The other tests may be obtained when indicated but not as part of routine yearly screening. It is recommended that a TSH level be obtained every 3 years after the age of 60; a lipid profile, including total cholesterol, every 3 years after the age of 50; a Pap smear as indicated by patient risk factors but not necessarily each year; and an electrocardiogram as indicated by the patient's needs and symptoms after one baseline examination at the age of 50. Guidelines for primary and preventive health care in postmenopausal women are still not well defined in all medical specialties, but an aging population will require the gynecologist of the future to assume many roles in primary health care and preventive medicine.

5–8. 5, **E;** 6, **A;** 7, **D;** 8, **B;** Pages 151, 280–284. A prepubertal girl with vaginal bleeding is at greatest risk for vaginal foreign body. A less likely source for this problem is a functional ovarian neoplasm. Pelvic ultrasonography might be helpful in ruling out a neoplasm and possibly even a foreign body. Since ultrasound imaging is noninvasive and more easily available, it is a reasonable first step. If ultrasonography is unrevealing, one would consider vaginoscopy with the patient under anesthesia to rule out a vaginal foreign body or a rare lower tract neoplasm. Mammography is indicated as a routine screening examination in gynecologic perimenopausal patients, particularly patients with any risk factors. Perimenopausal patients (older than 35) with a change in bleeding (menstrual) patterns should be screened by office sampling of the endometrium. Further assessment by dilation and curettage or hysteroscopy should be dictated by other pertinent history or physical examination features. An unusual configuration of the glandular cervical epithelium should alert the clinician to the possibility of maternal diethylstilbestrol (DES) exposure. If previous colposcopic evaluation did not yield normal results or was not performed, the patient should undergo such evaluation as well as careful palpation of the vaginal fornices.

9–11. 9, **C;** 10, **A;** 11, **B;** Pages 143–146. When a physical examination is performed on patients with pelvic relaxation, a knowledge of potential herniations and loss of pelvic supporting structures is imperative. A cystocele and rectocele are usually apparent when present, but they are not always symptomatic. Both a cystocele and a rectocele represent a protrusion of the wall of a hollow viscus. In the true sense they are not

hernias. An enterocele is a herniated peritoneal surface and is often subtle, necessitating a thorough working knowledge of this defect. This is especially important with regard to planning surgical procedures designed to correct disorders of pelvic support. All three anomalies—herniation, cystocele, and rectocele—can protrude through the vaginal introitus, and all three can be repaired vaginally. Prolapse or procidentia involves the protrusion of the cervix and uterus into the barrel of the vagina. *First-degree* is slight descent. *Second-degree* has prolapse to or near the introitus. *Third-degree* or *total* prolapse is outside the vagina introitus with or without the Valsalva maneuver.

12–14. 12, **B;** 13, **A;** 14, **D;** Pages 138–139. Postcoital bleeding usually results from some inflammatory or neoplastic disorder of the cervix or endometrium. It is not a reflection of an ovulatory or an anovulatory endocrinologic milieu. Likewise, intermenstrual bleeding should be viewed as neoplastic or inflammatory until proven otherwise. Intermenstrual bleeding also can be associated with ovulation if it regularly occurs near midcycle. This association is due to the change in hormonal milieu at this time. Regular painful menstruation is usually associated with ovulation, presumably because of the association of progesterone production with enhanced activity of prostaglandin on the smooth musculature of the uterus. Therefore irregular, painless bleeding with variable flow is commonly anovulatory bleeding.

15–17. 15, **E;** 16, **D;** 17, **C;** Pages 142–150. The cervix is visualized with the speculum. Normally, the transformation zone is just barely visible inside the external os. Because the uterosacral ligaments insert onto the posterior cervicouterine junction and extend backward to the hollow of the sacrum, they are best appreciated by rectovaginal examination. An enlarged postmenopausal ovary is not necessarily better appreciated by either physical examination technique, depending on the anatomic relationships of the patient being examined. This finding suggests an ovarian neoplasm and needs further diagnostic assessment, regardless of how it is suspected. Adnexae are usually not palpable in postmenopausal women because of involution and retraction of the ovary to a position higher in the pelvis.

18. **B,** Pages 150–151. Neither chlamydia nor gonorrhea can be specifically identified by the cytologic techniques used in Pap screening. Koilocytosis, which is detectable by Pap smear, suggests an infection by the human papilloma virus. Both chlamydia and gonorrhea are best identified by endocervical culture. Recent preliminary data suggest that cytologic screening for chlamydia may have promise, but it is not yet generally

accepted as a reliable, sensitive screen for this organism. (Kiviat NB, Peterson M, Kinney TE, et al: Cytologic manifestations of cervical and vaginal infections. II. Confirmation of *Chlamydia trachomatis* infection by direct immunofluorescence using monoclonal antibodies. JAMA 253:997–1000, 1985.) Perform a Pap smear before obtaining endocervical cultures.

19. **D,** Page 140. A detailed family history of first-order relatives (mother, father, sisters, brothers, and children) should be taken, and a family tree should be constructed.

20. **E,** Page 142. Palpation of the abdomen affords the possibility of noting a fluid wave, which would suggest either ascites or hemoperitoneum. Palpation also yields evidence of rigidity of the abdomen secondary to intraabdominal irritation. When the irritation is caused by intraabdominal hemorrhage or infection, this rigidity is often evidence of an acute abdomen. Rebound signifies intraabdominal irritation and is demonstrated by gently pressing the abdomen and then releasing. The release may cause pain either under the spot *(direct rebound)* or in a different portion of the abdomen *(referred rebound).* Gentle pressure carried out systematically may elicit painful "trigger points" in the abdominal wall, which are myofascial in origin and do not represent an intraabdominal pathologic condition.

21. **D,** Page 139. Any pregnancy in the patient's history should be recorded, including nonviable and preterm pregnancies, metabolic pregnancy complications, and paternity. These events may help the clinician in predicting future reproductive outcomes and in offering a rationale for specific diagnostic or therapeutic measures, such as ultrasonography, testing for β-human chorionic gonadotrophin (β-hCG), testing for carbohydrate intolerance, and identification of potential chromosomal problems.

22. **A,** Page 143. Although skin findings such as hyperkeratosis and pigmented nevi may be normal variants, they warrant more careful follow-up. Usually, the diagnosis of intraepithelial neoplasia or atrophic dystrophy requires biopsy. Scattered cherry angiomata are not associated with a serious pathologic condition when they occur as an isolated incidental finding. The pubic hair overlying the mons pubis may thin as women enter their later postmenopausal years. However, total alopecia in a pre- or perimenopausal woman may represent a skin abnormality. Inspection of the skin should include looking for evidence of body lice (pediculosis), excoriation, and discoloration or loss of pigment.

23. **D,** Page 138. Anger and seductiveness are not clinical diagnoses, but they may be part of another pathologic process. Depression and anxiety are

diagnoses (DSM-IV) and may be detected by nonverbal patient behavior.

24. **D,** Page 147. The transformation zone, by definition, is the functional zone between the squamous epithelium of the ectocervix and the columnar epithelium of the endocervix. It contains elements of both surfaces. This zone is dynamic. It changes continually throughout the reproductive years in response to inflammation, trauma, pregnancy, and hormonal influences. These changes occur by the process of metaplasia, in which squamous epithelium covers the columnar epithelium. This process, however, may leave small areas of irregularities and inclusion cysts, called *nabothian cysts,* which are of no clinical significance.

25. **E,** Page 139. Although anorgasmy, vaginismus, and decreased libido are usually related to psychological dysfunction, postcoital bleeding is more likely related to potential nonsuppurative inflammation or neoplastic disorders. This finding from the history warrants further assessment to rule out a potential gynecologic pathologic condition.

26. **A,** Pages 147–148. The American College of Obstetricians and Gynecologists guidelines suggest that Pap testing begin at age 18 or when regular coital activity begins. In patients at higher risk—those with a history of early coital activity or multiple partners or those with other risk factors such as prior herpes or condylomatous changes—this examination should occur at least annually. In patients with two successive negative Pap smears and a single sexual partner, the interval between smears may safely be extended for up to 3 years. The Pap smear is inadequate and thus less diagnostic if it does not contain a sample of the endocervical canal. A number of fixatives are available, but it is important that they be applied immediately, before drying and distortion of the cell take place.

27. **E,** Pages 139, 920–921. Aspects of the gynecologic history that place the patient at risk are factors relating to her chronic anovulation, which is also suggested by the infertility. Of course, more history is necessary, but as isolated fragments of information, oligoovulation and infertility should alert you to the potential for endometrial neoplasia. Oral contraceptive pills are used to provide the progesterone influence that prevents endometrial hyperplasia by regular withdrawal bleeding.

28. **C,** Page 152. Hepatitis A and B vaccine series are administered once at any age. Tetanus-diphtheria booster is offered every 10 years. Pneumococcal vaccine is given to a 55-year-old woman only if she is at high risk. Otherwise, it is offered at age 65 and repeated every 5 years. The influenza vaccine should be offered yearly for women at risk or routinely starting at age 55.

Differential Diagnosis of Major Gynecologic Problems by Age Groups

DIRECTIONS:

for Questions 1–20: For each numbered item, select the one heading most closely associated with it. Each lettered heading may be used once, more than once, or not at all.

1–3. Match the ovarian neoplasm with the description.

A. malignant teratoma
B. serous cystadenocarcinoma
C. cystic teratoma
D. serous cystadenoma
E. granulosa cell tumor

1. Most common ovarian tumor in all age groups

2. Most common neoplasm of adolescence

3. Stromal cell tumor producing sex hormone

4–5. Match the adnexal mass with the description.

A. follicle cyst
B. corpus luteum cyst
C. cystic teratoma
D. serous cystadenoma
E. mucinous cystadenoma

4. Accounts for the majority of adnexal masses during the reproductive years

5. Most commonly mimics ectopic pregnancy

6–8. Assume that each of the following pregnancies has progressed to approximately 18 weeks according to the patient's stated last normal menstrual period. Given the stated diagnosis, which clinical finding is most likely?

A. quantitative human chorionic gonadotrophin (hCG) > 210,000 mIU
B. size/dates discrepancy
C. polyhydramnios or oligohydramnios
D. adnexal mass with cardiac activity
E. dilated cervical os

6. Complete molar pregnancy

7. Anomalous fetus

8. Normal intrauterine pregnancy

9–11. Although any bleeding abnormality may occur with the conditions listed below, the classic association is

A. menorrhagia
B. metrorrhagia
C. postmenopausal bleeding
D. amenorrhea

9. endometrial carcinoma

10. uterine leiomyomata

11. carcinoma of the cervix

12–13. Match the condition with the symptom.

A. atrophic vaginitis
B. endometrial carcinoma
C. cervical carcinoma
D. epithelial ovarian carcinoma
E. urethral caruncle

12. Most common cause of postmenopausal bleeding

13. Least likely to be associated with postmenopausal bleeding

14–17. Match the symptom with the inflammatory process.

    A. right upper quadrant pain
    B. right lower quadrant pain
    C. left upper quadrant pain
    D. left lower quadrant pain
    E. bilateral lower quadrant pain

14. Acute salpingitis

15. Tuboovarian abscess

16. Acute diverticulitis

17. Acute mesenteric adenitis

18–20. Listed below are several conditions that can be associated with pain. Match the characteristic with the condition.

    A. pelvic adhesions
    B. myofascial component
    C. major depressive disorder
    D. degenerating myoma
    E. ovarian torsion

18. Responds to local anesthetic.

19. Is associated with sexual abuse.

20. Is the most common finding in patients with chronic pelvic pain.

21–23. Match the following diagnosis with the most typical presentation in a 23-year-old woman with last period starting 5 days earlier.

    A. acute pelvic inflammatory disease
    B. appendicitis
    C. ectopic pregnancy
    D. renal stone

21. Presents with right low quadrant pain with rebound and afebrile.

22. Presents with acute right and left lower quadrant pain with rebound, high fever, and decreased appetite.

23. Presents with right lower quadrant cramping pain, rebound, fever, and nausea with emesis.

DIRECTIONS:

for Questions 24–30: Select the one best answer or completion.

---

24. Characteristics of dysfunctional uterine bleeding include all the following *except*

    A. association with polycystic ovarian syndrome
    B. irregular menstrual interval
    C. perimenopausal bleeding
    D. secretory endometrium
    E. varied flow from scanty to heavy

25. Hormonally functional ovarian neoplasms include all the following *except*

    A. mucinous cystadenoma
    B. granulosa cell tumor
    C. Sertoli-Leydig cell tumor
    D. struma ovarii
    E. thecoma

26. Most gynecologic processes signaled by acute abdominal pain

    A. start with periumbilical pain
    B. are associated with lower gastrointestinal symptoms
    C. are most often limited to the pelvic peritoneum (right or left lower quadrant)
    D. are commonly accompanied by dysuria
    E. can be blocked by lidocaine (Xylocaine) injections in trigger points

27. Causes of abdominal masses between birth and the onset of puberty include all the following *except*

    A. dysgerminoma
    B. follicle cyst
    C. hematometrium
    D. teratoma
    E. Wilms tumor

28. Malignant adnexal neoplasms in adolescence include all the following *except*

    A. malignant teratoma
    B. embryonal carcinoma
    C. dysgerminoma
    D. choriocarcinoma
    E. Meigs syndrome with ovarian fibroma

29. In women older than 50, predictors of ovarian malignancy include all the following *except*

    A. bilateral masses
    B. cell type
    C. menstrual status
    D. size of neoplasm
    E. presence of ascites

30. **The differential diagnosis of an adnexal mass in the postmenopausal patient should encompass all the following except**

    A. colon cancer
    B. corpus luteum cyst
    C. diverticular disease
    D. endometriosis
    E. lymphoma

ANSWERS

1–3. 1, **D**; 2, **C**; 3, **E**; Pages 165–173. Bennington's cross-sectional study of a general gynecologic population by age group revealed that the serous cystadenoma is the most common true neoplasm of the ovary in all age groups combined. The majority of patients with this tumor fell into the 20- to 44-year-old group. Of primary ovarian neoplasms occurring in all age groups, the serous cystadenocarcinoma is most often bilateral. In adolescence, a cystic teratoma is the most common type. It is important clinically because of the possibility of torsion or rupture. True ovarian neoplasms that produce sex steroids are called *functioning tumors*. An example is a granulosa cell tumor, which is associated with the production of estrogen. Functional enlargements, on the other hand, refer to variations of ovarian follicular or ovulatory apparatus that are in fact variants of normal reproductive anatomy.

4–5. 4, **A**; 5, **B**; Pages 165–167. In assessing patients with adnexal masses, it is important to differentiate between neoplasms and variations of normal functional ovarian anatomy. Cystic teratomas and serous and mucinous cystadenomas are true neoplasms of the ovary and occur less frequently than do either of the functional cysts. During the reproductive years, the majority of adnexal masses are follicle cysts. These may vary from 3 to 10 cm in diameter. They are often appreciated during the time of routine pelvic examination. They are unlikely to cause symptoms unless they become particularly large or rupture, releasing follicular fluid into the pelvic cavity. Even then, they usually cause only transient symptoms. Often, vaginal ultrasonography is useful in assessing these cysts. Their regression can be followed through one or two menstrual cycles. Characteristically, these cysts are unilocular and smooth without evidence of internal excrescences. Corpus luteum cysts are also common during the ovulatory years and usually do not enlarge significantly beyond 5 cm. They may be somewhat tender to palpation. On occasion, they bleed into the pelvic cavity and mimic an ectopic pregnancy. These cysts persist past the time of anticipated menses. They may delay the expected period, further suggesting ectopic pregnancy. Vaginal ultrasonography, coupled with a negative hCG result, is helpful in making this diagnosis and ruling out an ectopic pregnancy. The intent of these questions is to create an appreciation for the clinical presence of functional cysts.

6–8. 6, **A**; 7, **C**; 8, **B**; Pages 155–157. The unexplained enlarged uterus may create a diagnostic dilemma. This physical finding, when related to pregnancy, has a number of implications. Molar pregnancy is associated with massive proliferation of trophoblasts and therefore is generally associated with quantitative hCG levels of more than 100,000 mIU/mL. Although size/dates discrepancy can be cause by a number of potentially serious factors, the most common is poor menstrual history and thus the discrepancy is associated with normal pregnancy. Polyhydramnios or oligohydramnios at 18 weeks is very suspicious for significant fetal anomaly. Decreased fluid may represent a renal agenesis or urinary obstruction. Excessive fluid may represent a fetal swallowing problem (anencephaly) or gastrointestinal obstruction (duodenal atresia). Diagnostic studies should be instituted to rule out the presence of the anomalous fetus in the case of polyhydramnios or oligohydramnios.

9–11. 9, **C**; 10, **A**; 11, **B**; Pages 157–159. Endometrial carcinomas are most common in the postmenopausal age group, and thus the usual bleeding manifestations of this tumor are not associated with true menstruation; irregular perimenopausal bleeding or, more commonly, postmenopausal bleeding is more likely. *Menorrhagia* is the occurrence of regular, probably ovulatory bleeding of a greater amount than usual for 10 days or more and is most often associated with uterine myoma. *Metrorrhagia* is the occurrence of significant intermenstrual bleeding one or more times and is most commonly found with cervical carcinoma. Less commonly, it may present as postmenopausal bleeding.

TABLE 7–1
Conditions That May Cause Signs and Symptoms of Acute Abdomen and Abdominal Quadrants in Which They Most Often Occur

Conditions	Quadrant			
	Right Upper	**Right Lower**	**Left Upper**	**Left Lower**
Salpingitis	−	+	−	+
Tuboovarian abscess	±	+	±	+
Ectopic pregnancy	−	+	−	+
Torsive adnexa	−	+	−	+
Ruptured ovarian cyst	−	+	−	+
Acute appendicitis	−	+	−	−
Mesenteric lymphadenitis	−	+	−	−
Crohn's disease	−	+	−	−
Acute cholecystitis	+	±	−	−
Perforated peptic ulcer	+	±	+	±
Acute pancreatitis	+	−	+	−
Acute pyelitis	+	±	+	±
Renal calculus	+	+	+	+
Splenic infarct	−	−	+	−
Splenic rupture	−	−	+	−
Acute diverticulitis	−	−	−	+

+, More frequently; ±, may occur.

12–13. 12, **A**; 13, **D**; Pages 159–160. Although postmenopausal bleeding may be associated with a number of conditions, it must always be investigated because many causes are premalignant or malignant. The best way to rule out endometrial neoplasia is by outpatient endometrial sampling. This is possible in most patients. On occasion, technical difficulties require performance with the patient under anesthesia. The majority of women with postmenopausal bleeding have atrophic vaginitis, as documented in a study by Dewhurst of 249 women. More than half of these patients had atrophic vaginitis as a presenting condition. This should be compared with the approximately 15% to 20% of patients with postmenopausal bleeding who will have endometrial carcinoma. Unless the ovarian carcinoma is a granulosa cell tumor (and this is relatively uncommon), ovarian carcinoma is not associated with postmenopausal bleeding. A urethral caruncle may occur in postmenopausal women and represents an eversion of the urethral epithelium. The caruncle is recognizable by sight, is benign, and needs no treatment.

14–17. 14, **E**; 15, **E**; 16, **D**; 17, **B**; Pages 160–165, Table 7–1 (*above*). Abdominal and pelvic pain often occur together and may be caused by a variety of gynecologic and nongynecologic entities. Pain of significant organic origin usually involves sudden onset, tenderness to palpation, mild to significant degrees of rebound tenderness, and alteration in bowel sounds. Acute salpingitis and tuboovarian abscess are typically bilateral processes and thus elicit bilateral lower quadrant pain. Acute diverticulitis most often manifests in the rectosigmoid, thus appearing as acute left lower quadrant pain. Mesenteric adenitis often mimics appendicitis or right adnexal disease and thus occurs as acute right lower quadrant pain. A clinician is frequently called on to differentiate these and other entities based on the pain-related history and physical findings.

18–20. 18, **B**; 19, **C**; 20, **A**; Pages 160–165. Handling patients with pain presents the clinician with a number of diagnostic problems. Acute pain is associated with more objective findings. Usually, the differential diagnosis is more limited. With chronic pain, symptoms tend to be vague. The pain in affected patients frequently has a significant psychological component. Slocumb has called attention to the presence of "trigger points" that are discernible by palpation along the myofascial junctions of the abdominal wall. These are often treated successfully by injection of a local anesthetic, such as 0.25% bupivacaine, on one or several occasions. In analyzing the laparoscopic findings of 100 women who complained of constant pelvic pain in the same location for a minimum of 6 months, Kresch and associates reported that, overall, 83% of the group with chronic pain had abnormal pelvic findings, whereas only 29% of a control group had abnormal findings. Of these findings, pelvic adhesions were the most common, accounting for 38%. However, the role of adhesions in causing pain is still unclear. It is clear that in a significant number of patients who have otherwise unexplained chronic pelvic pain, major affective disorders may play a role. Among this group of patients suffering from past or current affective disorders, the likelihood of childhood or adult sexual abuse is greatly increased.

21–23. 21, **C**; 22, **A**; 23, **B**, Pages 160–163. A number of intraabdominal conditions can lead to the findings of an acute abdomen. These findings include acute pain, generally of sudden onset; tenderness to palpation; rebound tenderness; and diminished or absent bowel sounds. Appendicitis classically presents initially as periumbilical pain that localizes to the right lower quadrant and is accompanied by anorexia or nausea and vomiting and fever. Patients with salpingitis tend to have a higher fever than those with appendicitis; although their pain may be severe, they tend to be less ill than those with appendicitis. Pelvic inflammatory disease often flares as a menses is finishing. Ectopic pregnancy generally is associated with unilateral continuous crampy pain, although there may be some bilaterality to the presentation and minimal if any fever. Most ectopic pregnancies are associated with vaginal bleeding.

24. **D**, Pages 157–158. Dysfunctional uterine bleeding implies irregular bleeding secondary to the lack of regular ovulation. This is most common shortly after menarche, until regular ovulatory cycles are established, as well as at the other end of the reproductive spectrum. Women in the perimenopausal period with early evidence of ovarian failure experience irregular periods. When the endometrium is sampled, it usually is proliferative.

25. **A**, Page 173. Many neoplasms of the ovary are hormonally functional and may first appear as a result of the effects of the hormone produced rather than as a mass effect. Granulosa cell tumors and thecomas are feminizing tumors with estrogen production. Precocious puberty in the very young girl, menometrorrhagia in the woman of reproductive age, and bleeding in the postmenopausal woman may signal a granulosa cell tumor. Defeminization or masculinization of the patient may suggest a masculinizing tumor of the ovary (eg, Sertoli-Leydig tumor). In the prepubertal girl, the presenting symptom may be precocious heterosexual (opposite-sex) puberty.

In the postpubertal woman, the complaint may be hirsutism or virilization. *Struma ovarii* is a teratoma with thyroid elements; it may appear as hyperthyroidism. Cystadenomas are epithelial in origin and do not produce hormones.

26. **C**, Page 160. The common acute gynecologic entities listed in Table 7–1 share a common pattern: right or left lower quadrant pain. Some include bilateral pain, depending on the pathologic process. Visceral pain from most gastrointestinal tract disorders is usually more specifically related to the part of the viscus involved. Urinary tract disease may present more diffuse pain, depending on the part of the tract involved. Gastrointestinal symptoms and periumbilical pain are not characteristically associated with gynecologic disorders. Dysuria is more commonly related to cystitis and trigonitis. Trigger points are associated with musculoskeletal disorders of myofascial origin rather than with a true gynecologic pathologic condition.

27. **C**, Pages 168–169. Occasionally, infants are born with adnexal cysts that appear as abdominal masses. These are generally follicular cysts secondary to maternal hormone stimulation of the fetal ovaries. The cysts usually regress within the first few months of life. Of the true ovarian tumors that appear later in childhood, dysgerminomas and teratomas are the most common. Six to eight percent of these tumors are dysgerminomas. Although benign and malignant teratomas have been reported in childhood, they are rare before the age of 10. Abdominal masses found in the young child are more likely to be Wilms tumors or neuroblastomas. At the end of the normal sequence of puberty, a girl may have problems with primary amenorrhea and an imperforate hymen or vagina. This allows the buildup of menstrual flow, resulting in a hematometrium. This problem appears only late in puberty.

28. **E**, Pages 168–170. Solid or cystic adnexal tumors, although rare in adolescence, are usually dysgerminomas or malignant teratomas. These are germ cell in origin. In a study of tumors in women under the age of 21 by Diamond, all six malignant lesions were of germ cell origin. Likewise, in a study by Norris and Jensen, germ cell tumors accounted for 28% of the 353 primary ovarian neoplasms found in patients younger than 20. Of the remaining tumors that were not germ cell, 19% were of epithelial origin and 19% stromal. Meigs syndrome includes ascites and pleural effusion associated with benign fibroma of the ovary.

29. **C**, Page 172. In a study by Rulin and Preston that analyzed 150 adnexal tumors in women older than 50, 47 tumors were malignant. Of the 32 that were less than 5 cm, only one tumor proved to be malignant, whereas 40 of 63 tumors larger

than 10 cm were malignant. The majority of the larger tumors were of the epithelial cell type. Bilateral adnexal masses in a peri- or post-menopausal woman greatly increase the risk of malignancy over a unilateral mass. There was no apparent association with menstrual status. Thus, it would appear that size, bilateral involvement, and cell type are reasonable predictors of malignancy in this age group.

30. **B,** Page 172. Adnexal masses occurring in post-menopausal women may be benign, but the chance of malignancy increases with age. Although endometriosis occurs primarily in women of the reproductive years, as many as 5% of cases appear postmenopausally. Masses from other organ systems are common in this age group, including diverticulitis, accounting for painful left adnexal masses. Tumors such as lymphomas may appear as rapidly growing, firm masses, which at times are accompanied by ascites. Colon cancer may be appreciated as an adnexal mass. A corpus luteum cyst requires that ovulation occurs, which is inconsistent with the postmenopausal ovarian status.

CHAPTER 8

Emotional Aspects of Gynecology

1. **A 68-year-old woman is concerned because her 70-year-old spouse, since undergoing prostatic surgery, is no longer capable of an erection. Initially you should**

   A. recommend testosterone therapy for him
   B. recommend a penile prosthesis
   C. tell her that he should not be worried about this at his age
   D. refer both for sexual counseling
   E. discuss this with the spouse

2. **A 21-year-old woman who has been married for 2 years is referred by her family physician, who was unable to obtain a Pap smear. You find that you also are unable to insert a speculum; in fact, when you approach the woman, her levator muscles contract and she slides away from you on the examining table. From this information you can conclude that this woman**

   A. has a phobic avoidance to the insertion of the speculum
   B. has an unhappy marriage
   C. has a vaginal septum or intact hymen
   D. will never respond adequately to sexual stimulation
   E. has never had intercourse

3. **Acceptance of the inevitability of death proceeds in the following stages:**

   A. denial, anger, bargaining, depression, acceptance
   B. denial, bargaining, anger, depression, acceptance
   C. denial, depression, anger, bargaining, acceptance
   D. anger, denial, bargaining, depression, acceptance
   E. anger, denial, depression, bargaining, acceptance

4. **Which medication is most useful in the treatment of bipolar disorder?**

   A. monoamine oxidase inhibitor
   B. lithium salt
   C. selective serotonin-reuptake inhibitor
   D. estrogen replacement therapy

5–6. **A 15-year-old states that she began her menses at age 11 and that during her 13th year she had a regular 26- to 30-day cycle. She has not had a period in the last 6 months, and she has never had intercourse. The medical history is unremarkable except that she feels that she is 20 pounds overweight.**

   Physical Examination
BP:	100/70 T: 97.8 P: 55
Ht:	5 ft 4 in
Wt:	105 lb
Breast:	Tanner stage IV
Abdomen:	Unremarkable

   Pelvic:
Escutcheon:	Tanner stage IV
Outlet:	Unremarkable
Cervix:	Unremarkable
Corpus:	Normal size, smooth, firm
Adnexa:	Unremarkable

5. **Given the most likely diagnosis, you would expect all the following *except***

   A. She abuses laxatives.
   B. She has an increased likelihood of having a relative with the same problem.
   C. She vomits frequently.
   D. She is an average student.
   E. She has had an adverse sexual experience.

6. **The therapy that will most likely be of benefit is**

   A. injectable menotropins (Pergonal)
   B. insulin
   C. psychoanalysis
   D. cognitive behavioral therapy
   E. high-potency vitamins

7. Of the following gynecologic procedures, which is most likely to cause sexual dysfunction in a psychologically stable woman who is happily married?

   A. total abdominal hysterectomy
   B. total vaginal hysterectomy
   C. anterior colporrhaphy
   D. simple vulvectomy
   E. retropubic urethropexy

8. Three years ago, after a lengthy illness, a 65-year-old woman's husband died. Since that time she has been depressed. This has manifested itself in chronic fatigue, irritability, and anhedonia. The patient once stated that she wanted to commit suicide and in the same breath said that she could not do that because it was against her religion. In this case, which of the following is not considered part of the normal grief reaction?

   A. length of the reaction
   B. chronic fatigue
   C. irritability
   D. anhedonia
   E. lack of decisiveness

DIRECTIONS:

for Questions 9–11: For each numbered item, select the one heading most closely associated with it. Each lettered heading may be used once, more than once, or not at all.

9–11. A large-boned 27-year-old woman is overweight. You recommend dieting. In addition, you would suggest (Table 8–1)

   (A) Weight Watchers
   (B) medically supervised behavior modification
   (C) pharmacologic therapy
   (D) gastric restriction operation
   (E) none of the above

9. If she is 5 feet 7 inches tall and weighs 215 pounds

10. If she is 5 feet 9 inches tall and weighs 275 pounds

11. If she is 5 feet 11 inches tall and weighs 210 pounds

TABLE 8–1
Height and Weight Table for Women*

Height		Weight (lb)		
Feet	Inches	Small Frame	Medium Frame	Large Frame
4	10	102–111	109–121	118–131
4	11	103–113	111–123	120–134
5	0	104–115	113–126	122–137
5	1	106–118	115–129	125–140
5	2	108–121	118–132	128–143
5	3	111–124	121–135	131–147
5	4	114–127	124–138	134–151
5	5	117–130	127–141	137–155
5	6	120–133	130–144	140–159
5	7	123–136	133–147	143–163
5	8	126–139	136–150	146–167
5	9	129–142	139–153	149–170
5	10	132–145	142–156	152–173
5	11	135–148	145–159	155–176
6	0	138–151	148–162	158–179

*Weights at ages 25 to 29 based on lowest mortality. Weight in pounds according to frame (in indoor clothing weighing 3 pounds; shoes with 1-inch heels).
From 1983 Metropolitan Height & Weight Tables, Metropolitan Life Insurance Company, Health and Safety Division.

DIRECTIONS:

for Questions 12–25: Select the one best answer or completion.

12. **Which phase of the sexual response cycle is characterized by the full development of the orgasmic platform?**

    A. excitement
    B. plateau
    C. orgasm
    D. resolution

13. **A refractory period following the sexual response cycle is typical of**

    A. men only
    B. men and women
    C. women only
    D. premenopausal women

14. **Which of the following commonly used medications has not been shown to have the potential for decreasing libido?**

    A. alprazolam (Xanax)
    B. amitriptyline (Elavil)
    C. cimetidine (Tagamet)
    D. diazepam (Valium)
    E. fenfluramine (Pondimin)

15. **A 25-year-old gravida 3, para 0, abortus 3, factory worker is seen 6 weeks after delivery. Her last pregnancy ended at 20 weeks, and you think that she has an incompetent cervix. Today she has multiple complaints, including tightness in the throat and chest, frequent sighing, and muscle weakness. You attribute this to a grief reaction. The patient continued to work during her last pregnancy despite your warning that doing so might lead to another pregnancy loss. Appropriate comments at this encounter include all the following *except***

    A. mentioning that she is still young and will have another chance
    B. acknowledging her feelings of grief
    C. referring her to a self-help group
    D. acknowledging that she may feel guilty

16. **A woman taking oral contraceptives who is anorgasmic during coitus should**

    A. use another form of contraception
    B. have the estrogen component of her oral contraceptive increased
    C. have the progestin component of her oral contraceptive increased
    D. discuss this with her partner

17. **Services included in a hospital-based hospice program are**

    A. social work
    B. home care
    C. postdeath follow-up
    D. all the above

18. **Which of the following has the greatest amount of alcohol?**

    A. 12 ounces of beer
    B. a wine glass of wine
    C. 30 mL of whiskey
    D. they are all equal

19. **Childhood self-esteem is enhanced by all the following *except***

    A. praising
    B. setting limits
    C. intimidation
    D. gentle touching

20. **A 35-year-old stockbroker was to be married for the first time 6 months ago, but her fiancé was killed in an auto accident on the way to the church. When she saw your partner a month ago, your partner decided that she was severely depressed and prescribed amitriptyline. The patient returns with a list of new symptoms, which are listed below. These symptoms are frightening to the patient, but they do not prevent her from functioning as a normal human being. Those that are secondary to the medication and not her basic problem include**

    A. dry mouth
    B. constipation
    C. hesitancy of urination
    D. all the above

21. **In addition to these symptoms, the woman is still depressed. You would now**

    A. tell her to take a glass of wine at bedtime
    B. add another antidepressive medication
    C. offer her reassurance
    D. encourage her to "snap out of it" and stop feeling sorry for herself

22. **Which of the following antidepressant drugs does not have the potential to decrease libido?**

    A. bupropion (Wellbutrin)
    B. citalopram (Celexa)
    C. fluoxetine (Prozac)
    D. paroxetine (Paxil)
    E. sertraline (Zoloft)

23. **You are counseling a 16-year-old patient and her parents regarding anorexia nervosa. As part of this counseling, you provide the following facts** *except*

    A. Good to fair outcomes were observed in almost 60% of those not formally treated at all.
    B. Anorexia occurs in 1 of 1000 middle-class adolescent girls.
    C. Anorexia occurs in 5% to 20% of ballet dancers.
    D. Anorexia occurs six times more frequently in first-degree relatives than in the general population.
    E. In men, anorexia usually occurs in those training for competitive athletic events.

24. **Which of the following statements is an accurate statement regarding obesity in America?**

    A. Severely obese women treated nonsurgically have a 15% incidence of severe depression.
    B. Severe obesity carries a 12-fold increase in mortality for persons between 25 and 34 years old.
    C. Over 20% of American women are classified as obese.
    D. White women have a higher rate of obesity than black women.
    E. Women in the age range of 45–54 have the lowest obesity rate.

25. **You are teaching a college course on preventive health issues for women. The following are accurate statements regarding substance abuse in women** *except*

    A. In a cited study of pregnant women, fewer than 1% were noted to be heavy drinkers.
    B. In women ages 18–25, over one third have used marijuana in the past month.
    C. Over 50% of women are current alcohol consumers.
    D. Smoking during pregnancy is one of the most significant reversible causes of intrauterine growth restriction.
    E. The overall smoking incidence among women is approximately 20%.

ANSWERS

1. **E,** Page 187. The first step is to discuss this concern with both partners. The husband and his wife need to decide whether his lack of an erection is a problem. The husband may be concerned that he can no longer satisfy his wife. A physician can be useful in helping a couple sort out their needs and desire for sexual compatibility at this stage of life.

2. **A,** Pages 189–190. The question describes a woman who, according to Lamont's classification, has fourth-degree vaginismus, levator and perineal spasm, and retreat. This problem is generally due to a phobia to vaginal penetration based on a previous traumatic episode or a lack of appropriate knowledge about sex associated with cultural or familial teaching that sex is evil, painful, or undesirable. Sexual dysfunction is not necessarily incompatible with a happy marriage. This couple could be very happy. The history did not suggest amenorrhea, so a septum or an intact hymen was ruled out. Treatment for this problem has a high success rate. Thus, one cannot assert that the woman will have an unhappy sex life. One cannot assert that she has never had intercourse.

Traumatic intercourse, especially rape, could have been a precipitating factor.

3. **A,** Page 197. The stages, as suggested by Kübler-Ross, are denial, anger, bargaining, depression, and acceptance. Unfortunately, many people die before passing through all these stages.

4. **B,** Page 193. Lithium is the most useful agent for manic depression (bipolar disorder). It has also been used to treat depression, as have monoamine oxidase inhibitors and the new selective serotonin-reuptake inhibitors. Estrogen is used appropriately to treat symptoms of menopause.

5. **D,** Pages 181–183. These patients tend to be high achievers, usually A students. The occurrence of anorexia and bulimia is six times greater in first-degree relatives than in the general population. Vomiting and laxative abuse are common findings. The incidence of adverse sexual experiences among anorectics may be underreported. These events occur in childhood or adolescence and usually involve a person known to the subject.

6. **D,** Page 183. A number of medications have been tried in the treatment of anorexia nervosa with varying success. These medications have included

insulin, lithium, tricyclic antidepressants, and phenothiazides, as well as high-potency vitamins. In many cases, such drugs have not been found to be better than a placebo. Psychoanalysis is a long-term approach, and anorexia nervosa requires prompt intervention. More recently, however, cognitive behavior therapy has been used in the treatment of anorexia. This therapy is aimed at bringing to the attention of the patient the fact that her beliefs, assumptions, and style of thinking have brought about distorted body image, food aversion, phobias, and unreasonable fears of weight gain. In short, the therapy is aimed at reshaping patients' thinking processes with respect to themselves and their body images. Behavior modification and cognitive therapy have met with some success. Behavior modification is based on reward and punishment for a number of behaviors. Cognitive behavioral therapy is directed toward the specific thinking disorder rather than toward body image and food.

7. **D,** Pages 186–187. Recently, several lay publications have suggested a role for the cervix in sexual response, basing this theory on the fact that the cervix is richly innervated. To date, no scientific data support this theory. Sexual gratification and orgasmic behavior definitely seem to be associated with nerve endings in the clitoris, mons pubis, labia, and possibly pressure receptors in the pelvis. Loss or disruption of the clitoris seemed to be the single most important factor in the development of sexual dysfunction after surgery.

8. **A,** Page 194. Early symptoms of depression include chronic fatigue; anxiety and irritability; anhedonia (loss of feelings of joy and pleasure); decreased interest in usual pursuits, including sexual activity and personal appearance; and mental changes, including poor concentration and lack of decisiveness. The physician should determine whether the patient has suicidal thoughts and assess whether these thoughts are likely to be put into practice. A patient who seems to be seriously considering suicide should be promptly referred to a mental health worker or facility. The physician should be alert to patients who have suffered personal loss or grief but who are still deeply depressed after 6 to 18 months of grieving. Although depression is normal in a grief situation, it should not last for a prolonged period.

9–11. 9, **B;** 10, **D;** 11, **A;** Pages 184–185, Table 8–1. All three patients have a large frame. The patient in question 9 is 50 pounds overweight and therefore moderately obese. The patient in question 10 is 100 pounds overweight and therefore severely obese. The patient in question 11 is 35 pounds overweight, or mildly obese. Mild obesity can be successfully managed by diet and behavior modification under lay supervision. Most prescribe or sell foods low in fat in an attempt to achieve a diet containing about 20% fat. Moderate obesity is best managed under medical supervision. Good results have been obtained in the severely obese who have undergone gastric restriction surgery. In severely obese patients, surgery results in the greatest weight loss that is maintained over many years.

12. **B,** Pages 185–186. The plateau phase is the culmination of the excitement phase and is associated with a marked degree of vasocongestion throughout the body.

13. **A,** Page 186. A refractory period is that time after the sexual response cycle during which another sexual response cannot be initiated in spite of adequate stimulation. Although a refractory period is typical of the sexual response cycle in the male, no such refractory periods have been identified in women. Therefore, new sexual excitement cycles may be stimulated at any time after orgasm. During the resolution phase, the woman generally experiences a feeling of personal satisfaction and well-being.

14. **A,** Pages 188–189. Table 8–3 in Mishell identifies a large number of drugs that have demonstrable effects on sexual functioning. Health care providers for women must be cognizant that such commonly used medications as amitriptyline (antidepressant), cimetidine (antacid), diazepam (anxiolytic and muscle relaxant), and fenfluramine (appetite suppressant) can adversely affect libido. Of the medications listed, only alprazolam (anxiolytic) is not reported to decrease libido.

15. **A,** Pages 194–195. In the immediate grief period, the bereaved often feels guilt. Although you should acknowledge her shock, guilt, and grief, you should not add to it. It is counterproductive to talk to her about working during her recent pregnancy. Self-help groups have a great deal to offer patients who suffer a pregnancy loss. If the local group is appropriate for the needs of a given patient, a referral should be made. One investigator has found that grieving couples prefer to receive support and help in dealing with the reality of the loss rather than to focus on other life events, such as the next pregnancy.

16. **D,** Pages 187, 190. Couples should be encouraged to communicate their sexual needs to each other so that appropriate stimulation is offered during the arousal period and during intercourse. If the patient is anorgasmic during intercourse but has experienced orgasms, her partner may aid in bringing about an orgasm during intercourse by allowing her to stimulate her clitoral area or he

may do so. Anorgasmia is not known to be secondary to oral contraceptive use. As many as 10% to 15% of women have never experienced an orgasm through any form of sexual stimulation. The woman should not be made to feel abnormal. Sexuality is a question of pleasure or happiness, not of "normalcy."

17. **D,** Page 198. Hospice organizations offer psychosocial support to patients and their families. The service includes postdeath follow-up. Hospital-based hospice teams may include physicians, nurses, social workers, chaplains, and volunteers who may minister to any patient in any bed. Home care programs are often available.

18. **D,** Page 192. Alcoholic strength is often denoted by the percentage of alcohol present. Proof is twice the percentage volume of alcohol. A 12-ounce can of beer, a glass of wine, and 30 mL of either whiskey or a liqueur have the same quantity of alcohol.

19. **C,** Page 180. Self-esteem begins to develop in early childhood and is the result of positive efforts. Touching, talking to the child in gentle ways, and praising the child's actions are reasonable steps in reinforcing the child's self-worth. Punishment should be limited to reinforcing the need for setting limits. Intimidation by verbal or physical means should be avoided.

20. **D,** Page 193. Most tricyclic drugs, including amitriptyline, have a parasympathomimetic effect. Dryness of the mouth, blurred vision, hesitancy of urination or dribbling, some menstrual disorders, and a decrease in sexual arousal are common complaints associated with their use.

21. **C,** Page 193. Although patients may note a reduction in depressive symptoms after 1 or 2 weeks of drug use, real improvement may take as long as 1 month. It is unnecessary to add a second drug. A tricyclic may enhance the response to alcohol. This can increase the danger of a suicide attempt or overdose. It is best to reassure this patient and tell her it is too soon to expect improvement.

22. **A,** Pages 188–189. As seen in Table 8–3 in Mishell, all the new selective serotonin-reuptake inhibitors (SSRIs) that are used to treat depression may adversely affect libido. All the drugs listed are SSRIs except for bupropion. Because patients with depression may have decreased libido as a symptom, this drug side effect should be kept in mind as other symptoms resolve, especially when using an SSRI for treating depression.

23. **B,** Pages 182–183. Although anorexia nervosa is uncommon in the general population (~1:100,000), it is quite common among middle-class adolescent girls, occurring in about 1 in every 100. The occurrence in ballet dancers ranges from 5% to 20% depending on the level of competition. When discussing treatment, remember that there are good or fair outcomes in 88% of those treated with inpatient care. Outpatient treatment yields 77% good to fair outcomes. However, 59% of patients without treatment have good to fair outcomes. Relapse is a serious problem, with a calculated risk of death of 0.5% per year.

24. **C,** Pages 183–185. If obesity is described as a body mass index (BMI) > 25 kg/m^2, then 25% of Americans are obese, with black women at a higher rate (37.6%) than white women (23.5%). Women 45 to 54 years old have a rate of obesity of 32.4%, which is the highest of any other age group. Severe obesity increases the risk of mortality for persons 25 to 34 years old, typically because of complicating factors such as hypertension, diabetes, hyperlipidemia, arthritis, increased operative complications, and compromised pulmonary functioning. In the severely obese patient, the success of diet and behavior modification is limited, with a high rate of patients regaining the weight lost within 2 years. This finding may partially explain the 15% plus rate of severe depression in severely obese patients.

25. **A,** Pages 191–192. A study by Sokol found that pregnant women in Cleveland had an 11% incidence of heavy drinking based on a careful detailed questioning wherein only 1.2% would state that they had an alcohol problem.

Rape, Incest, and Domestic Violence

for Questions 1–20: Select the one best answer or completion.

1. A young woman was seen 2 weeks ago in the emergency department after a rape that occurred in her apartment. She was not injured physically. She now complains of difficulty sleeping, fear of being alone in her apartment, and withdrawal from her usual personal contacts. This behavior is

   A. paranoid and delusional
   B. part of the rape-trauma syndrome
   C. a manifestation of preexisting psychoses
   D. an unusual response in the absence of physical injury
   E. rapidly resolved by moving from the apartment

2. You see a 22-year-old woman who has come alone to the emergency department after an alleged rape. Examination reveals no physical injury. Although there is evidence of recent coital exposure, the woman is calm and well organized and answers all questions regarding the incident. She states that she is fine and wants to return to her apartment after all the information and appropriate tests are obtained. The most appropriate action at this time is to

   A. discharge her to return to the health care facility in 2 weeks
   B. give her an appointment to see a qualified social worker in the next week
   C. have her see a qualified social worker before she leaves
   D. refer her to a local minister for counseling if she needs it
   E. ask her to call a friend to take her home

3. You see an apparently healthy 28-year-old woman, who gives a history of recent loss of interest in men and demonstrates increasing anxiety as you question her about her feelings. She states that she has become fearful and has had a loss of self-esteem. She has numerous minor physical complaints; including pelvic pain, but there are no objective findings. Of the following, the most likely etiologic factor is

   A. recent loss of a loved family member
   B. low-grade pelvic inflammatory disease
   C. a drug reaction
   D. AIDS-related complex
   E. a recent history of sexual assault

4. A 14-year-old girl is referred to you from a youth center. Her school grades have suddenly dropped, and she has run away from home and become involved in prostitution. The girl appears intelligent and healthy. Of the following, the most plausible explanation for her behavior is

   A. the excitement of street life
   B. nymphomania
   C. psychoses
   D. incest
   E. disenchantment with school

5. A victim of a sexual assault sustained no injuries, did not acquire any sexually transmitted disease (STD), and did not become pregnant. She feels very guilty, however, and has lost self-esteem and confidence. Of the following, which is the most appropriate action?

   A. Assure her that over time all will be well.
   B. Reevaluate her for STDs and normalcy of the pelvis to assure her that everything is all right.
   C. Provide professional counseling that attaches no blame to her.
   D. Point out that rape happens to a lot of women and they usually do well.
   E. Tell her that most women who are raped are asking for it and she should feel guilty.

6. A victim of an alleged rape is examined. The incident occurred approximately 8 hours ago. The woman states that vaginal penetration occurred. She is calm, has no injury, and has no motile sperm in her cervical mucus on examination. You should record

   A. that no recent intercourse took place
   B. that no rape occurred
   C. that the assailant probably wore a condom or had a vasectomy
   D. that sperm "die" in 4 to 6 hours
   E. the findings as you discovered them

7. Studies of persons who have had long-term incestuous relationships in childhood have found that

   A. only a small percentage (<10%) of them have abnormal psychosocial sexual development
   B. anxiety and psychosomatic complaints tend to get worse with time
   C. incestuous relationships with siblings are more damaging than with parents
   D. the closer the family member, the more damaging the incestuous relationship
   E. most incestuous relationships continue for years

8. Which of the following history or physical findings would constitute sufficient evidence for you to make a diagnosis of rape on the patient's record when seeing her in the emergency department?

   A. a vaginal laceration
   B. a patient's statement that she was sexually assaulted
   C. nonmotile sperm in the vagina
   D. motile sperm in the cervical mucus
   E. none of the above

9. When seeing an injured female in the office or emergency department, you should remember that many such patients are there because of domestic violence. What percentage of injured women seen in emergency departments are victims of battering?

   A. <1%
   B. 5%
   C. 10%
   D. 25%
   E. >40%

10. When you discover a case of marital, family, or elder abuse, what is the most appropriate action?

    A. Notify the police.
    B. Have a stern talk with the abuser.
    C. Involve community social resources.
    D. Ignore the incident because it will probably be resolved by the participants.
    E. Refer the patient to a psychiatrist.

11. The most accurate method of ruling out an individual as the perpetrator of rape is by

    A. a lie detector test
    B. the individual's sworn statement
    C. finding no evidence of trauma to the alleged victim
    D. finding no sperm or acid phosphatase in the alleged victim's vagina
    E. DNA typing of specimens from the alleged victim

12. Sperm survive for the longest time in which anatomic site?

    A. rectum
    B. vulva
    C. pharynx
    D. vagina
    E. endocervix

13. Forensic evidence in a case of possible rape should be

    A. submitted to the general hospital laboratory
    B. given to the emergency department nurse
    C. left in the emergency department "out" basket for routine collection
    D. sent to the county police laboratory
    E. handled according to a specific protocol that ensures security

14. The risk of pregnancy from a single random, unprotected coital exposure is approximately

    A. 1 in 5
    B. 1 in 15
    C. 1 in 30
    D. 1 in 60
    E. 1 in 100

15. **The legal definition of rape varies from state to state, but it must include**

   A. force or threat of force
   B. lack of mutual consent
   C. penile penetration
   D. presence of semen
   E. none of the above

16. **How long does the reorganization phase of the rape-trauma syndrome usually last?**

   A. a few hours
   B. a few days
   C. a few weeks
   D. a few months
   E. many months

17. **Cases of forcible rape resulting in injury that requires surgery or hospitalization occur in what percentage of victims?**

   A. 1%
   B. 5%
   C. 20%
   D. 40%
   E. >50%

18. **What is the recommended prophylactic treatment for STDs after an alleged rape?**

   A. benzathine penicillin
   B. ampicillin
   C. ampicillin and probenecid
   D. ceftriaxone, followed by doxycycline
   E. gentamicin and clindamycin

19. **Prophylaxis against an unwanted pregnancy after rape is best achieved by**

   A. performing dilatation and curettage
   B. inserting a Progestasert intrauterine device (IUD)
   C. using diethylstilbestrol (DES), 25 mg twice a day for 5 days
   D. using ethinyl estradiol, 2.5 mg twice a day for 5 days
   E. using norgestrel/ethinyl estradiol (Ovral) 0.5 mg, 2 tablets every 12 hours for two doses

20. **The most likely abuser of an elderly woman living with her family is a(n)**

   A. adult son or daughter
   B. husband
   C. sibling
   D. social case worker
   E. stranger who enters the home

DIRECTIONS:

for Questions 21–23: For each numbered item, select the one heading most closely associated with it. Each lettered heading may be used once, more that once, or not at all.

21–23. **You see a suspected rape victim who is worried about several STDs. Match the disease with the appropriate test at the time of the initial examination.**

   (A) culture on living cells
   (B) serologic testing
   (C) culture in agar
   (D) saline preparation
   (E) none of the above

21. *Chlamydia* infection

22. syphilis

23. hepatitis

DIRECTIONS:

for Questions 24–33: Select the one best answer or completion.

24. The described phases of the rape-trauma syndrome are divided into acute (short term) and reorganization (long term). Manifestations of the acute phase include

    A. physical symptoms
    B. job change
    C. development of phobias
    D. moving from one residence to another

25. You have been asked to give an in-service talk on sexual assault to the emergency department nursing staff. A correct statement that you might include is that

    A. perpetrators of rape are commonly known to the victim
    B. the disabled and elderly are relatively immune to rape
    C. more than half of all rapes are reported
    D. rape fulfills a sexual urge

26. During an examination for alleged rape, no sperm are found on a vaginal wet mount. Further appropriate diagnostic tests include

    A. sampling the cervical mucus for sperm
    B. determining the acid phosphatase concentration of the vaginal contents
    C. ABO typing of vaginal secretions
    D. all the above

27. Initial evaluation of a sexual assault victim who is seen in the emergency department should include

    A. specific tests for common STDs
    B. examination for the possibility of an existing pregnancy
    C. collection of evidence for medicolegal purposes
    D. all the above

28. You suspect marital abuse when you see a woman with bizarre injuries. If your suspicion is correct, sympathetic questioning may reveal that abuse is occurring. What else might be revealed?

    A. The woman is afraid that she will not be able to support herself if she leaves the marriage.
    B. The abuse has been repetitive over a long period.
    C. More than one member of the family is regularly abused.
    D. all the above.

29. An 82-year-old woman, apparently healthy, is seen with multiple circular sores on both her lower legs that do not correspond to any physiologic pattern. You discover that she lives with her daughter and son-in-law and has recently become unable to control her urine. She seems confused and somewhat frightened in the strange emergency department surroundings. The most likely diagnosis is

    A. diabetic ulcers
    B. bed sores
    C. domestic violence
    D. ringworm

30. "Statutory rape" is defined by

    A. lack of the victim's consent
    B. age of the victim
    C. presence of physical signs of trauma
    D. age of the attacker

31. According to statistics from the Centers for Disease Control and Prevention, what is the likelihood that a rape victim will contract gonorrhea?

    A. <1%
    B. 6%–12%
    C. 15%–20%
    D. >30%

32. Female genital mutilation is least likely to occur in what area?

    A. Africa
    B. Southeast Asia
    C. Middle East
    D. South America

33. While giving an in-service talk to social workers at the local Department of Health, you would provide the following statistics *except*

    A. About 10% of all child abuse involves sexual abuse
    B. Approximately 80% of all cases of sexual abuse of a child involve a family member
    C. Brother-sister incest may be the most common
    D. Father-daughter incest accounts for about 50% of reported cases
    E. Incestuous activities may be experienced by up to 25% of all women and approximately 12% of all men

ANSWERS

1. **B,** Page 206. The rape-trauma syndrome is common in victims of rape, even in persons who are in good mental health. It may take a long time to resolve the fear and distrust engendered by the rape event, even if no significant physical injury occurred.

2. **C,** Page 209. Although some rape victims are extremely calm and controlled after the assault, they should always have the benefit of a knowledgeable person for counseling and support. Regardless of the victim's apparent calmness and control of the situation, no victim should leave the health care facility without learning of a known and accessible support system.

3. **E,** Page 206. The story is highly suggestive of the *silent rape reaction,* manifested by a victim of sexual assault who has been psychologically traumatized but who has not admitted, or resolved, the episode and is unwilling to tell you about it. She would probably tell you of a recent loss of a loved one because such an occurrence carries no social stigma. Pelvic inflammatory disease should not be diagnosed without some objective confirmation. AIDS-related complex is a rare diagnosis in a low-risk, apparently healthy woman, in whom a drug reaction is also unlikely. The latter can usually be resolved through the history.

4. **D,** Page 211. You should consider rape, incest, or drug abuse whenever you encounter a sudden change in the behavior of a teenager. Obviously, many other factors could be responsible, but you should always ask straightforward questions about rape, incest, or drug abuse without moralizing.

5. **C,** Pages 209–210. Many rape victims struggle with feelings that they are to blame and somehow caused the episode. They should be supported and counseled that they are the victim and that they are not responsible for the attacker's behavior. Many victims need time and consistent support to overcome feelings of guilt and self-blame.

6. **E,** Pages 208–209. In alleged rape cases, it is important to record the findings and not make judgments either for or against rape. The patient's record is a medicolegal one, and it should not include speculation, such as a reference to the possibility that the assailant used a condom or was azoospermic. Sperm can "live" in midcycle cervical mucus for 3 to 5 days, although they usually "die" rapidly in vaginal secretions. Therefore, it is important to get specimens from the cervical mucus.

7. **D,** Page 211. Most incestuous contacts appear to be of short duration, with only about 27% lasting more than 1 year. Approximately one third of the children who have an incestuous experience consider that it was detrimental. An equal number think that it was neither positive nor neutral. Generally, the more trusted the family member with whom the incestuous act occurred, the more damaging the experience, but in most cases the impact fades with time. In any individual case, however, the effect is difficult to predict.

8. **E,** Pages 208–209. When a patient is examined for alleged rape, the facts should be entered in the record, but the diagnosis of rape is a legal statement (rather than a medical term) that should be decided in the courts.

9. **D,** Page 212. Studies have documented that up to 25% of injured women seen in emergency departments are victims of domestic violence. However, physicians treating these injured women made a diagnosis of domestic battering in only 3% of cases. They were often treated with pain medications or given psychiatric referrals only.

10. **C,** Page 214. The physician should not only arrange for appropriate involvement of the community resources but also follow up on the family to be sure that appropriate action is taken and continues to be taken.

11. **E,** Page 209. No test can absolutely prove that a given individual committed a sexual assault, but DNA typing can prove that a given individual did not do it.

12. **E,** Page 209; Table 9–1. The presence of motile or nonmotile sperm documents ejaculation. If motile sperm are found in the vagina, the ejaculation occurred within hours. Motile sperm may survive for several days in the endocervix.

13. **E,** Page 209. A verifiable trail of responsible and secure transmission of forensic evidence is desirable for the evidence to be accepted in a court without question. Such material should not be left unattended in an accessible area. Receipts for delivery should be obtained. Many emergency departments have a protocol for the transmission of such material, and you should follow the specified procedures. If there is no protocol, it would be wise to suggest that one be developed after consulting the statutes of the state in which you reside.

14. **C,** Page 208. A single random, unprotected coital exposure by a healthy woman results in a 2% to 4% pregnancy rate. A major factor influencing the rate is the time of exposure during the menstrual cycle. Still, most women do not accept even a small possibility of pregnancy and desire prophylaxis to protect themselves from becoming pregnant.

TABLE 9–1
Survival Time of Sperm

Source	Motile Sperm	Sperm	Acid Phosphatase
Vagina	Up to 8 hr	Up to 7–9 days	Variable (up to 48 hr)
Pharynx	6 hr	Unknown	100 IU*
Rectum	Undetermined	20 to 24 hr	100 IU*
Cervix	Up to 5 days	Up to 17 days	Similar to vagina

*Minimum detectable.
From Anderson S: Sexual assault—medical-legal aspects, an unpublished training packet for pediatric house staff, Harborview Medical Center, Seattle, Wash, 1980.

15. **E,** Page 206. Rape is legally defined by the states, so you should be familiar with the specific definition in your locale. However, rape generally is defined as sexual intimacy without consent, with or without penetration, and with or without force. The inability to give appropriate consent by virtue of age or mental condition is deemed to be lack of appropriate consent. The presence of semen is not necessary.

16. **E,** Page 206. If rape victims experience rape-trauma syndrome, the resolution phase involves long-term adjustment and reorganization of their life. This usually takes several months. If these issues are not adequately addressed, the syndrome can persist for years. This possibility should be considered when patients manifest unexplained anxieties, particularly in sexual areas.

17. **A,** Page 207. Although up to 40% of rape victims have minor bruises, only a small number have serious injury. However, it is important to document any bruising, even though it is minor, because this evidence is fleeting and may not be present at a revisit in 1 or 2 weeks. To outline epithelial injury painlessly (injury that could not be easily noted otherwise), you can apply gentian violet to the vulva and remove the excess with K-Y jelly. Fissures or breaks in the epithelium retain the dye and become easily visible. Application and removal do not cause pain.

18. **D,** Pages 207–208. Prophylactic antibiotic treatment is given after an alleged rape in an attempt to avoid infection with gonorrhea, chlamydia, or *Treponema pallidum.* According to the 1989 sexually transmitted disease treatment guidelines, the prophylactic treatment recommended after rape is ceftriaxone, 250 mg IM, followed by doxycycline, 100 mg twice a day for 7 days, or tetracycline, 500 mg four times a day. Ampicillin, 3.5 g, and 1 g of probenecid can be given to patients who are allergic to tetracycline or to pregnant women. Either regimen may result in some antibiotic side effects. Often, an antifungal preparation helps prevent vaginal yeast infection. Benzathine penicillin should not be used.

19. **E,** Page 208. Women worry greatly about pregnancy and STDs after a rape. The efficacy of "morning after" therapy for pregnancy prevention is good. The side effects are least from norgestrel/ethinyl estradiol, two tablets 12 hours apart for two doses. This treatment has a high rate of efficacy. DES causes a great deal of nausea. DES has a known teratogenic effect if a pregnancy does occur and is not interrupted. There is no reason to traumatize a rape victim further by inserting an IUD or performing dilatation and curettage.

20. **A,** Page 215. Abuse of aging adults is becoming increasingly common. Such abuse may be physical or emotional. The most common abuser is an adult child with whom the elderly person lives, although it may be the spouse. If such a situation is suspected, community resources should be involved to remove the victim and to counsel the abuser.

21–23. 21, **A;** 22, **B;** 23, **B;** Page 208. *Chlamydia trachomatis* is an obligate intracellular bacterium that must be grown on cell culture. It lacks the energy system to survive on its own. Syphilis can be diagnosed by serologic study or dark-field examination. Immediately after rape, neither test will yield positive results; more than 10 days must elapse before a lesion will show *Treponema* infection on dark-field examination. Positive serologic findings develop in 4 to 6 weeks. However, it is best to document that the victim has a negative serologic finding at the time of the incident. Serologic testing should be repeated 6 to 12 weeks later. Hepatitis screening is done to document seronegativity. The development of positive serologic findings takes 1 to 3 months.

24. **A,** Page 206. Burgess and Holstrom (1974) described the rape-trauma syndrome. Their report was based on the response of 92 victims of forcible rape. Reactions were divided into two phases. The first is *acute,* or *immediate,* and lasts for hours or days. It is associated with disorganization of usual behavior patterns as well as emotional and somatic symptoms. Fear is common in both phases. The second phase is one of *reorganization,*

with a general decrease in symptoms and a return toward normal functioning. During this phase, nightmares and fears of normal situations are common and may be difficult to resolve. Major lifestyle changes may be instituted, such as a change of job or residence.

25. **A,** Page 206. Rape is primarily an assertion of power rather than a fulfillment of a sexual urge. People who are relatively helpless are therefore at higher risk. Rape occurs regardless of any provocation or inducement on the part of the victim. Although (and perhaps because) many victims know their assailants, rapes often are not reported because of shame, guilt, fear of reprisal, or uncertainty about how to proceed.

26. **D,** Page 209. Sperm die and disintegrate rapidly in vaginal secretions. Therefore, cervical mucous sampling should always be undertaken. Careful scrutiny of a Pap smear may reveal sperm if any are present. Men who have undergone vasectomy will not deposit sperm but will ejaculate acid phosphatase secretions from the prostate and seminal vesicles. ABO typing may be useful if an ABO type is found that is other than the victim's. Such a finding would prove exposure to a different antigen and may also be useful in determining the identity of the assailant. DNA typing can also be used.

27. **D,** Pages 207–209. A general history and physical examination should always be undertaken because they may reveal serious injury (in approximately 1% of rapes) and minor injuries (in up to 40% of rapes). Preexisting conditions should be determined and documented. Obtain cultures, a serologic test for syphilis, and a β-human chorionic gonadotrophin (β-hCG) level to rule out preexisting STDs or pregnancy. A review of evidence for coitus is important if the victim intends to prosecute the perpetrator. The recognition of trauma is also valuable.

28. **D,** Pages 213–214. Marital abuse is more common than is generally recognized. It frequently involves many family members, especially if it has gone on for a long time. Often, the woman stays in the relationship because she does not recognize how abnormal it is and she is more afraid of being alone than of remaining in the relationship. The spouse may need help in developing an exit plan, including matters such as clothing, money, identification, and financial records, as well as a specific place to go.

29. **C,** Pages 213–214. If the sores are bizarre and not located on pressure points or over areas of decreased blood supply or dermatomes, the possibility of self-inflicted trauma or domestic violence should be considered. In this situation, the 82-year-old woman may be receiving punishment for urinary soiling.

30. **B,** Page 206. Almost all states have statutes that criminalize coitus with a female under a specified age. This is called *statutory rape*. Consent is irrelevant because the female is defined by the statute as being incapable of consenting.

31. **C,** Pages 207–208. A study from the Centers for Disease Control and Prevention states that for adult rape victims, the risk of acquiring gonorrhea ranges up to 26% and the risk of acquiring syphilis up to 5%. We do not think that the risk of acquiring STDs can be quantified, but we note that the acquisition of viral STDs, including HIV, has been reported in both adults and children who are victims of rape.

32. **D,** Page 210. The World Health Organization estimates that 80 million women have undergone these procedures. Although they are often performed in parts of Africa, the Middle East, and Southeast Asia, they are rarely performed in the United States or the rest of the Western world. Physicians may see the results of these procedures, however, in patients who emigrate from countries where they are practiced.

33. **D,** Pages 210–211. All of these statements are accurate except for the occurrence of father-daughter incest, which accounts for up to 75% of all reported cases of incest. In actuality, brother-sister incest may be the most common form but may not be reported as often.

Diagnostic Procedures

for Questions 1–14: Select the one best answer or completion.

1. For optimal safety, how should the placement of secondary trocars during laparoscopy be made relative to the symphysis?

	Above symphysis (cm)	Lateral to midline (cm)
A.	2	2
B.	2	6
C.	5	3
D.	5	8
E.	8	5

2. On examination, a patient has moderately severe cervical stenosis. She is about to undergo endometrial biopsy as part of an infertility investigation. The anesthesia of choice is

   A. pudendal
   B. paracervical
   C. epidural
   D. spinal
   E. general

3. The complication of hysteroscopy that is unique to the use of dextran as a distending media is

   A. anaphylaxis
   B. bleeding
   C. pelvic infection
   D. circulatory overload
   E. cardiac arrest

4. The successful reversal of a previous sterilization procedure is most likely to follow

   A. Pomeroy tubal ligation
   B. Irving tubal ligation
   C. laparoscopic tubal fulguration.
   D. laparoscopic tubal application of Silastic bands
   E. laparoscopic tubal application of Hulka clips

5. Laparoscopy would be contraindicated in the presence of

   A. a 25-cm intraabdominal mass
   B. a history of endometriosis
   C. primary infertility
   D. a history of pelvic inflammatory disease
   E. an ectopic pregnancy

6. A patient being treated for infertility has a history of a 28-day cycle. She undergoes endometrial biopsy as part of the investigation 6 days after her basal body temperature rises. The narrative of the report states that one strip of endometrium is day 19 and the other is proliferative. The most appropriate conclusion from this information is that there is

   A. a luteal phase defect
   B. irregular shedding
   C. a normal ovulatory cycle
   D. evidence of multiple ovulations
   E. a laboratory error

7. The patient depicted in Figure 10–1 was referred for pelvic ultrasonography because of increasing girth. The diagnosis is

   A. early intrauterine pregnancy
   B. molar pregnancy
   C. ruptured tubal pregnancy
   D. ascites
   E. ovarian carcinoma

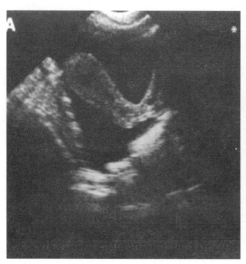 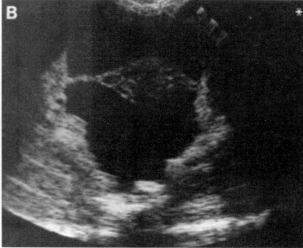

FIGURE 10–1   A, Longitudinal view of pelvis. **B,** Transverse view of pelvis.

8. A 48-year-old woman who underwent endometrial biopsy 6 months ago returns for a scheduled visit. The pathology report indicated proliferative endometrium. Since her biopsy, this patient has bled every 2 weeks for 8 to 12 days. She uses 10 to 15 pads a day but states that this is not a problem. You should advise

A. a repeat visit in 6 months
B. an endometrial biopsy
C. endometrial cytologic sampling
D. dilatation and curettage (D&C)
E. a hysterectomy

9. The failure rate of laparoscopic tubal interruption procedures is

A. < 1 in 1000
B. ~1 in 1000
C. ~4 in 1000
D. ~6 in 1000
E. >8 in 1000

10. Which of the following modalities uses beam attenuation that results from different densities of tissues?

A. ultrasonography
B. magnetic resonance imaging (MRI)
C. computed tomography (CT)
D. scintillation scanning
E. tomography

11. The most common complication of laparoscopy is

A. cardiac arrhythmia
B. gas embolism
C. laceration of the epigastric artery
D. intestinal perforation
E. hypercarbia

12. The patient is a 22-year-old gravida 0. Until 12 weeks ago, she was taking a low-dose oral contraceptive. Her last menstrual period was 9 weeks ago. For the last 6 weeks, the patient has had intermittent spotting. Ultrasonography performed at another facility reported that the patient had an empty gestational sac. Quantitative β-human chorionic gonadotropin (β-hCG) levels have been rising. The last β-hCG level, obtained 2 days ago, was 4000 mIU/mL. The patient is referred to you for care. The endovaginal sonogram you ordered is depicted in Figure 10–2. Vital signs are normal and stable. Proper management includes

A. quantitative β-hCG levels
B. culdocentesis
C. diagnostic laparoscopy
D. pelviscopy
E. laparotomy

13. Given the endovaginal ultrasound image depicted in Figure 10–3, one would conclude that the patient has

A. a benign cystic teratoma
B. a tubal ovarian complex
C. a ruptured ectopic pregnancy
D. an unruptured ectopic pregnancy
E. no evidence of pathology

14. The use of high-molecular-weight dextran to expand the endometrial cavity during hysteroscopy is preferred because it

A. is nonbiodegradable
B. is nonantigenic
C. is miscible with blood
D. is nonconductive
E. does not crystallize

FIGURE 10–2 Endovaginal scans. **A,** Coronal view. **B,** Enlargement of **A** taken slightly to patient's right. **C,** Enlargement of **A** taken to patient's left.

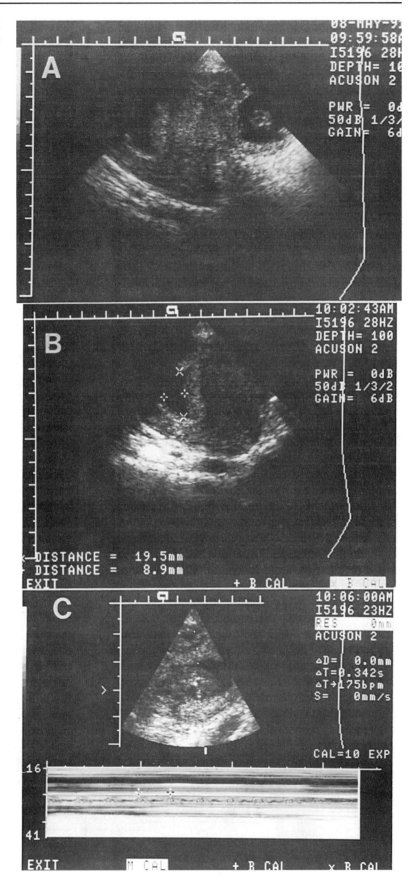

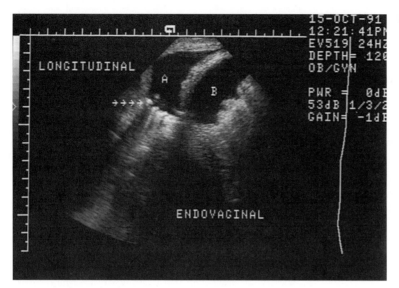

FIGURE 10–3

DIRECTIONS:

for Questions 15–22: For each numbered item, select the one heading most closely associated with it. Each lettered heading may be used once, more than once, or not at all.

15–17. Pick the procedure that is the most definitive and cost-effective in making the diagnosis.

A. hysteroscopy with or without biopsy
B. hysterosalpingogram
C. dilatation and curettage
D. laparoscopy
E. endovaginal ultrasound

15. submucous myoma

16. peritubal adhesions

17. unruptured tubal pregnancy at 6 weeks (menstrual dates)

18–21. Assume that your hospital is capable of supporting all the procedures listed below. Choose the appropriate initial procedure after a complete history and physical examination.

A. hysteroscopy
B. laparoscopy
C. CT
D. pelvic ultrasonography
E. MRI

18. A 28-year-old gravida 0 who is 5 feet 6 inches tall and weighs 134 pounds has been trying to become pregnant for 3 years. Her husband's semen analysis yields normal results. The woman ovulates and has good midcycle mucus.

19. A 30-year-old mentally retarded gravida 0 who is 5 feet 1 inches tall and weighs 190 pounds complains of pelvic pain. She is vague in her description of the pain and is impossible to examine.

20. A 25-year-old gravida 2, para 1 ab 1, had an induced abortion 1 year ago. Since then, she has had amenorrhea and intermittent pelvic pain.

21. A 30-year-old gravida 6, who is 5 feet 6 inches tall and weighs 130 pounds, has a 5-cm cervical lesion. This is histologically a squamous cell carcinoma.

DIRECTIONS:

for each numbered item 22–30, select the one best answer or completion.

22. Which of the following is a characteristic of the technique used to make the sonogram labeled *A* in Figure 10–4?

    A. Employs a fixed array of transducers to produce the image.
    B. Requires a rocking motion of the hand to make a full image.
    C. Provides a lower-resolution image than other techniques.
    D. Employs an acoustic mirror to form the image.
    E. Cannot be used to form images of moving or changing objects.

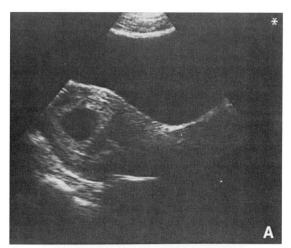

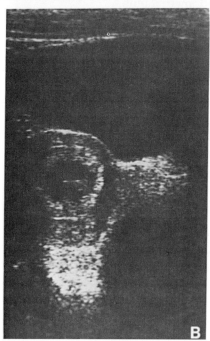

FIGURE 10–4

23. M.S. is a 25-year-old gravida 0. She has been trying to conceive for 5 years. Her history includes menses every 28 to 30 days with flow for 3 days and moderate dysmenorrhea the first 2 days. The patient experienced an acute pelvic infection at age 22 for which she had to be hospitalized. She has not had a clinical recurrence or reinfection. When M.S. was age 20, her gallbladder was removed because of stones. She is allergic to shellfish. M.S. smokes 1 pack of cigarettes a day and is a social drinker. Her physical examination, including a pelvic examination, is normal. This patient's investigation should include

    A. chromopertubation at laparoscopy
    B. pelvic ultrasonography
    C. hysterosalpingography
    D. endometrial biopsy
    E. CT of the pelvis

24. Which of the following conditions is most likely to result in a normal-appearing hysterosalpingogram?

    A. Asherman syndrome (endometrial sclerosis)
    B. cervical incompetence
    C. müllerian anomalies
    D. accessory ostia of the fallopian tubes
    E. endometrial polyposis

25. Figure 10–5 is a CT scan of a patient who is noted as having a pelvic mass on examination. The most appropriate interpretation is that

    A. there are metastases
    B. the patient is probably younger than 20 years
    C. the mass is thin-walled
    D. the uterus is enlarged
    E. there is evidence of distortion of the bladder by tumor

26. Figure 10–6 shows the uterus of a 25-year-old patient who wishes to have children. You would recommend

    A. insertion of a Foley catheter
    B. conjugated estrogen tablets (Premarin), 7.5 mg/day
    C. transabdominal metroplasty
    D. hysteroscopic metroplasty
    E. hysteroscopic resection

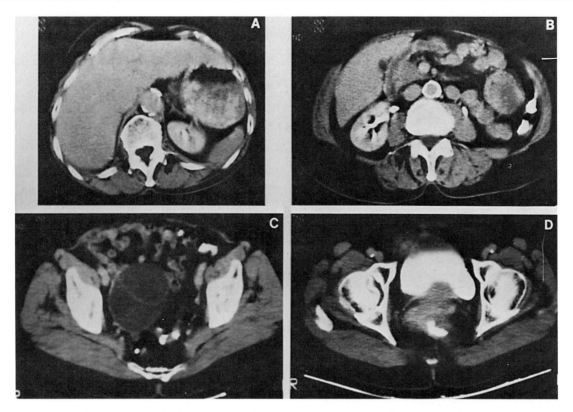

FIGURE 10–5   CT scan of pelvic mass. **A,** At level of liver. **B,** Below **A. C,** Above **D. D,** At level of bladder.

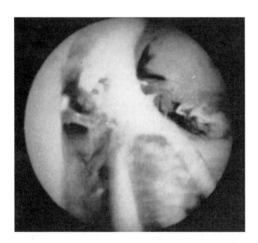

FIGURE 10–6   Hysteroscopic view of uterus. (From Mishell DR, Stenchever MA, Droegemueller W, Herbst AL: Comprehensive Gynecology, 3rd ed. St Louis, Mosby, 1997.)

27. **Based on recent experience, which of the following is a clinically accepted use for ultrasonography?**

    A. differentiation of benign and malignant adnexal conditions
    B. measurement of endometrial thickness to replace endometrial sampling in the evaluation of postmenopausal bleeding
    C. assessment of blood flow and vascular resistance in pelvic masses
    D. screening for ovarian cancer in patients with a family history of ovarian tumors

28. **On pelvic examination, a 40-year-old gravida 0 who is diabetic is thought to have 18-week-size myomata. Before performing a total abdominal hysterectomy, one should perform**

    A. pelvic ultrasonography
    B. endometrial biopsy
    C. a random blood glucose study
    D. chest radiography

29. **The most appropriate modality for the initial evaluation of a patient with ovarian carcinoma is**

    A. intravenous pyelography
    B. barium enema
    C. liver scintillation scan
    D. exploratory laparotomy
    E. CT

30. **Which of the following may be used to enhance MRI?**

    A. gadolinium
    B. glucagon
    C. iodine
    D. glucose
    E. water

ANSWERS

1. **D,** Page 242. To avoid the inferior epigastric vessels, secondary trocars should be placed approximately 5 cm above the symphysis and 8 cm lateral to the midline. Other placements risk subfacial hematomas, injury to the bladder, or damage to the great vessels.

2. **B,** Page 232. An endometrial biopsy is usually performed without anesthesia. In the presence of cervical stenosis, paracervical anesthesia blocks transmission from fibers in the cervical ganglion. Occasionally, the endocervical application of viscous lidocaine (2% to 4%) may decrease discomfort. Some authors have reported success with the transcervical introduction of 5 mL of mepivacaine 2%.

3. **A,** Pages 238–239. Complications of hysteroscopy include uterine perforation, pelvic infection, and bleeding. The potential complications of the distending media include circulatory overload with 5% dextrose and water. Anaphylaxis is a complication associated with the use of dextran. The potential of gas embolism exists with the use of carbon dioxide as the distending medium. Cardiac arrest has been reported with uterine insufflation when unmonitored amounts of carbon dioxide were used.

4. **E,** Page 240. The spring-loaded clip causes necrosis of less than 1 cm of the tube and is the easiest sterilization procedure to reverse successfully.

5. **A,** Page 241. An absolute contraindication to laparoscopy is a large intraperitoneal or pelvic mass. Laser ablation of an endometriotic implant, ovarian biopsy, lysis of adhesions, evaluation of infertility, and evacuation of a small ectopic pregnancy are recognized therapeutic laparoscopic procedures.

6. **C,** Page 232. The endometrium of the isthmus may be out of phase and give a false impression of lack of progesterone production. In this case, one of the strips probably came from the isthmus. The description is that of a normal ovulatory response. If there is a luteal phase defect, the endometrium should be more than 48 hours less than the 20 days expected, given this patient's menstrual history. With an endometrial biopsy as a part of an infertility investigation, however, one should perform the biopsy later in the cycle to be in a position to make the diagnosis of a luteal phase defect. Irregular shedding should be diagnosed on the fifth or sixth day of bleeding.

7. **D,** Page 220. Water, urine, and ascitic fluid are all extremely sonolucent. Blood is more complex and may give rise to faint echoes that can be detected by today's more sensitive equipment. In the longitudinal view, there is no evidence of a gestational sac, blood, or tissue inside the uterus. The ovaries are not visible in the transverse view shown in Figure 10–1. There is no mass in the pelvis. This patient is a woman with ascites caused by cirrhosis.

8. **D,** Page 233. The diagnostic accuracy of endometrial biopsy in determining malignancy is 90% to 98% when compared with subsequent findings at D&C or at hysterectomy. The gold standard is D&C. Therefore, if abnormal perimenopausal bleeding recurs after an endometrial biopsy, D&C should be performed to rule out carcinoma. In the future, hysteroscopy may replace many diagnostic D&C procedures. No matter how meticulous, surgeons may miss a focal lesion, particularly pedunculated structures. D&C is a blind hit-or-miss procedure.

9. **C,** Page 240. The failure rate of laparoscopic tubal sterilization is approximately 1 in 250 cases.

10. **C,** Page 225. Sonography uses sound waves that are reflected to the transducer from interfaces in the tissues. CT identifies local anatomy by using the difference in x-ray beam attenuation that results from different densities in adjacent tissues. MRI uses radiofrequency energy and a varying magnetic field. Before a scintillation scan is performed, a radioisotope is injected. The liquid or crystal radiation detector "records" the x-rays or gamma rays emitted from the subject. To perform tomography, objects out of the plane of interest are blurred during an x-ray study by simultaneously moving the x-ray tube and the recording plate.

11. **E,** Pages 242–243. The major complications of laparoscopy are laceration of vessels, intestinal injuries, and complications of the pneumoperitoneum, which include pneumothorax, diminished venous return, gas embolism, and cardiac arrhythmias. The most frequent complication of laparoscopy is hypercarbia, associated with hypoventilation.

12. **D,** Page 225. Figure 10–2, *A,* shows a uterus and a left adnexal mass that are compatible with a tubal pregnancy. The fluid within the uterine cavity has been measured in Figure 10–2, *B,* and cardiac activity is demonstrated by M mode in Figure 10–2, *C.* The latter is an endovaginal view of the left adnexal mass seen in Figure 10–2, *A.* With endovaginal ultrasonography, intrauterine pregnancies can be visualized as early as 4 weeks after the last menstrual period with a β-hCG titer of approximately 1000 mIU. A pregnancy should be routinely visualized by postmenstrual week 5, at which time the gestational sac is 4 mm in diameter. Since an ectopic pregnancy has been established, a quantitative β-hCG titer, diagnostic laparoscopy,

and a culdocentesis are unnecessary. Culdocentesis would yield negative results, since the scan suggests that the pregnancy is unruptured. If there were fluid in the cul-de-sac, on ultrasound imaging one would expect to see an echolucent area behind the uterus. The question is whether to treat by laparotomy or pelviscopy. This is a small gestation and could easily be removed through a laparoscope.

13. **E,** Pages 220–225. In Figure 10–3, labels *A* and *B* are within a cystic structure. Note that the contour of these structures is wavy. If real-time imaging were used, one would note movement. The arrows point to an echodense line beneath which there is shadowing. This represents gas within the bowel (labels *A* and *B*). Hence, there is no pathologic evidence. A disadvantage of ultrasonography is its poor penetration of bone and air. Thus, the symphysis pubis and the loops of the air-filled bowel often inhibit visualization.

14. **D,** Page 237. High-molecular-weight dextran is biodegradable, nontoxic, nonconductive, and immiscible with blood. It is antigenic, sometimes causing anaphylaxis. It also rapidly crystallizes; thus, endoscopic instruments must be cleaned shortly after the procedure.

15–17. 15, **A,** Page 238; 16, **D,** Page 241; 17, **E,** Page 225. Hysteroscopy is superior to hysterosalpingography for discovering and diagnosing an intrauterine pathologic condition. Likewise, laparoscopy is better than hysterosalpingography for discovering and diagnosing a peritubal pathologic condition. Comparative studies have documented that hysterosalpingography discovers only 50% of the peritubal disease diagnosed by direct visualization via the laparoscope. The only listed options to be considered in answering the question about the unruptured tubal pregnancy are laparoscopy and endopelvic ultrasound imaging. At 6 weeks, it is possible that an unruptured ectopic pregnancy would be missed at the time of laparoscopy. In addition, although the question indicates that the patient has this diagnosis, you would be approaching the patient not knowing that this was the problem. The differential diagnosis would be an intrauterine pregnancy, and this diagnosis should be ruled out before an operation such as laparoscopy is undertaken. This approach is probably the most cost-effective method of handling this case, although studies substantiating this point have not yet been reported. With an endovaginal probe, intrauterine pregnancies can be visualized as early as 4 weeks after the last menstrual period with a β-hCG titer of approximately 1000 mIU. A pregnancy should be routinely visualized by 5 postmenstrual weeks. In the case of an ectopic pregnancy, the gestational sac, fetal pole, and fetal heartbeat can be visualized outside the uterus by 6 weeks.

18. **B,** Page 241. In this hypothetical infertility patient, the male factor and the cervical factor appear to be normal. The patient is said to ovulate. As yet, the tubal factor has not been evaluated. This could be done with a hysterosalpingogram or by laparoscopy. Authorities differ in approach. Another option that was not given is an endometrial biopsy to evaluate the luteal phase.

19. **D,** Pages 220–225. The patient is unreliable in providing information. She will not permit a pelvic examination. The least expensive, least invasive procedure possible should be attempted first. This young patient may or may not have a pathologic condition. She is difficult or impossible to examine. Although the patient may not allow an endovaginal scan, she probably will cooperate for an abdominal pelvic evaluation. Ultrasonography may demonstrate disease. If disease is present, a specific diagnosis may be possible only if a more invasive procedure is used. If no pathologic condition is found, the best course to follow is observation, provided that the history given is complete and accurate. If ultrasound results are negative and symptoms continue, another consideration would be laparoscopic examination with the patient under anesthesia.

20. **A,** Page 238. It is likely that intrauterine synechiae (Asherman syndrome) developed after the therapeutic abortion. The patient's intermittent pain could be dysmenorrhea secondary to cervical stenosis, also a possible consequence of the induced abortion.

21. **C,** Pages 226–227. This is a patient with cervical carcinoma. CT often helps in the initial evaluation of a pelvic neoplasm, particularly with staging. CT is more accurate in diagnosing retroperitoneal metastases than intraperitoneal ones. CT is useful in detecting obstructed ureters and enlarged pelvic and paraaortic nodes that are suspected to have tumor involvement. MRI also has been used to evaluate local spread, but experience is limited.

22. **D,** Page 220. (Ziskin MC: Basic physics of ultrasound. In Fleischer AC, Romero R, Manning FA, et al, eds: *The Principles and Practice of Ultrasonography in Obstetrics and Gynecology*, 4th ed. New York, Appleton & Lange, 1991, p 7.) The picture obtained with a sector scan format is pie-shaped, as seen in Figure 10–4, *A*. Although the transducer is held stationary, incorporated within the transducer is an oscillating acoustic mirror for beam steering. The format of a linear array is rectangular, as demonstrated in Figure 10–4, *B*. The transducer of the sector scan is usually small, and thus it is easier to use to look at nonpregnant pelvic

structures. Most endovaginal probes employ sector technology. Because the transducer is closer to the pelvic organs than when a transabdominal approach is used, the resolution is often superior. In Figure 10–4, *A,* the bladder is full. An endovaginal scan is performed with an empty bladder, and the sound encounters the cervix, not the anterior abdominal wall, first. The piezoelectric effect is the generation of an electric voltage when a crystal is compressed. Ultrasound transducers are made up of piezoelectric crystals. When the crystals receive an electric charge, they vibrate and emit acoustic pulses. Acoustic echoes return from the tissues being scanned and cause the piezoelectric crystals to vibrate again and release an electric charge. The electric charges from the various crystals are then integrated by a computer in the machine to display a two-dimensional image. The transducer emits sound only 0.01% of the time. Most of the time it is receiving, not sending, sound pulses.

23. **A,** Pages 240–241. A pelvic sonogram or a CT scan is not indicated in the investigation of infertility if the physical examination is normal. Similarly, without reason to suspect either an endometrial or ovulatory problem, endometrial biopsy provides no useful information. The problem is this patient's previous infection and her allergy to fish. People who are allergic to shellfish often are allergic to iodine, which is found in the dye used for hysterosalpingography. The incidence of allergic reactions and the severity of these reactions, if they occur, are much less with the newer nonionic contrast media. (Katayama H, Yamaguchi K, Takashima T, et al: Adverse reactions to ionic and nonionic contrast media: a report from the Japanese Committee on the Safety of Contrast Media. Radiology 175 : 621–628, 1990.) Acute pelvic infection serious enough to require hospitalization develops in 0.3% to 3.1% of patients who undergo hysterosalpingography. This incidence of pelvic infection is directly related to the population studied, being more common in women with dilated tubes. For this reason, it is wise to observe the tubes directly. If they are grossly distorted, the diagnosis is confirmed. If the tubes appear relatively normal, chromopertubation at laparoscopy can be performed. Prophylactic antibiotics are appropriate.

24. **B,** Pages 236–239. Asherman syndrome (endometrial sclerosis) can be identified by slowly injecting a water-soluble medium under fluoroscopic control. Hysterosalpingography is a safe and rapid means of investigating abnormalities of the müllerian ducts. Tubal anomalies, including diverticula and accessory ostia, can be diagnosed by hysterosalpingography. During pregnancy,

ultrasonography can be used to detect funneling of the cervix, suggesting the diagnosis of an incompetent cervix; in the nonpregnant patient, hysterosalpingography cannot reliably demonstrate any abnormality, making it useless in the diagnosis of an incompetent cervix.

25. **C,** Pages 225–227. The scan depicted in Figure 10–5, *D,* is that of a bladder filled with contrast medium, indented by a uterus that appears normal in this view. In Figure 10–5, *A,* the scan shows a normal liver. None of the scans suggests lymph node involvement. The patient is probably older than 20, since her aorta is calcified (Figure 10–5, *B*). Figure 10–5, *C,* shows a thin-walled pelvic mass, probably benign and also ovarian.

26. **E,** Page 238. Figure 10–6 is a hysteroscopic view of uterine synechiae that can be cut with a pair of microscissors. After this resection, a large Foley catheter is placed in the cavity as a splint. For the next 2 months, the patient should receive 7.5 mg of conjugated estrogen per day. The use of the Foley catheter and hormonal therapy will be successful only if the synechiae have first been resected. This is most easily accomplished through the hysteroscope. This procedure and postoperative therapy avoid a transabdominal metroplasty. Because only synechiae are demonstrated, hysteroscopic metroplasty is not indicated.

27. **C,** Pages 220–225. Ultrasonographic studies can be used to document a number of factors that suggest benign or malignant disease, but only histopathologic evidence can establish the diagnosis. A growing body of literature investigates the role of endometrial thickness measurements in the management of clinical conditions. The experimental nature of these studies and a lack of consensus in the findings support the position that these measurements are an adjunct to clinical management and do not replace endometrial sampling at this time. The role of Doppler studies to evaluate blood flow and vascular resistance in the clinical management of suspected ectopic pregnancies and adnexal masses is growing. Ultrasonography has not been proved to be a cost-effective method of screening for ovarian cancer. It is helpful in the evaluation of patients if a pelvic mass is found, however.

28. **C,** Page 225. It is unnecessary and expensive to verify the obvious (Johnson HA: Diminishing returns on the road to diagnostic certainty. JAMA 265 : 2229, 1991.) Therefore, ultrasound imaging is not indicated. One can only condemn the practice of substituting pelvic ultrasonography for a pelvic examination. Routine preoperative endometrial biopsy in asymptomatic women undergoing hysterectomy has not been shown to be necessary. Since this patient has diabetes, the degree to

which this condition is controlled must be ascertained.

29. **E,** Page 227. One of the main advantages of CT in the evaluation of patients with ovarian cancer is the reduced need for multiple tests. Most studies indicate that the CT scan can replace the intravenous pyelogram, barium enema, and liver or spleen scans for identifying metastasis. Abdominal CT is superior to these other tests in differentiating between ovarian malignant disease and metastatic disease arising from the gastrointestinal tract or pancreas. As with other modalities, false-negative studies are possible.

Despite the information available through CT, exploratory laparotomy is still required for final histologic evaluation.

30. **A,** Page 230. While glucagon is often given before MRI to reduce bowel motility, glucagon does not enhance the images that result. Unlike ionizing radiation, the radiofrequency radiation used by MRI is not affected by the same material that affects the x-rays used in CT, such as calcium or iodine. As a result, the iodine-based contrast material used in CT does not affect the image produced by MRI. Only gadolinium may be used to increase tissue contrast for MRI imaging.

PART THREE

General Gynecology

Congenital Abnormalities of the Female Reproductive Tract

DIRECTIONS:

for Questions 1–26: Select the one best answer or completion.

1. **A 25-year-old female treated by another physician for congenital adrenal hyperplasia (CAH) is ready for a premarital examination. This patient is most likely to**

   A. be infertile
   B. be grossly overweight
   C. transmit the syndrome to all her offspring
   D. require cortisol replacement therapy
   E. have uterine anomalies

2. **Laparoscopy is useful during the surgical treatment of patients with**

   A. Rokitansky-Küster-Hauser syndrome
   B. hematocolpos
   C. uterine septum
   D. longitudinal vaginal septum
   E. CAH

3. **If an infant is born with ambiguous genitalia, the physician should**

   A. assign the sex as male and change it later if needed
   B. assign the sex as female and change it later if needed
   C. delay gender role assignment until an investigation is complete
   D. assign the sex as male with no subsequent change
   E. assign the sex as female with no subsequent change

4. **A newborn in the nursery has an enlarged clitoris and fusion of the labia. An older sister was diagnosed as having CAH. The most likely enzyme deficiency is**

   A. 5 α-reductase
   B. 21-hydroxylase
   C. 11-β-hydroxylase
   D. 20, 22-desmolase
   E. 3 β-ol-dehydrogenase

5. **A supernumerary ovary is the presence of**

   A. a third ovary separated from the normally situated ovaries
   B. one large ovary in the midline
   C. two ovaries, one normal in size and the other much larger, both situated on one side
   D. an ovary in a male with two testes
   E. excess ovarian tissue near a normally placed ovary and connected to it

6. **In patients with the Rokitansky-Küster-Hauser syndrome, vaginal reconstruction should be performed**

   A. when the patient is well motivated
   B. as soon as the condition is diagnosed
   C. in childhood
   D. only after marriage
   E. after coital attempts have been unsuccessful

7. **Enlargement of the clitoris is most frequently the result of**

   A. a müllerian duct defect
   B. an estrogen deficiency
   C. androgen stimulation
   D. masturbation
   E. early heterosexual activity

8. **CAH is an autosomal recessive disorder that usually**

   A. results in hematocolpos
   B. is due to a deficiency of 11-hydroxylase
   C. is caused by a deficiency of a gene on chromosome 8
   D. results in a person who is taller than normal
   E. may be diagnosed by an increase in 17-hydroxyprogesterone

9. **A newborn has the findings shown in Figure 11–1. The most likely diagnosis is**

   A. in utero exposure to 19 norprogestins
   B. CAH
   C. true hermaphrodite
   D. exposure to nonandrogen teratogens ingested by the mother
   E. XO chromosome pattern

10. **Infants born with CAH have a significant risk of**

    A. life-threatening salt loss
    B. abnormally tall growth
    C. hypothyroidism
    D. feminization
    E. hypotension

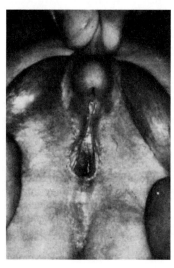

FIGURE 11–1 (From Jones HW Jr, Scott WW: Hermaphroditism, Genital Anomalies and Related Endocrine Disorders, 2nd ed. Baltimore, Williams & Wilkins, 1971.)

11. **Which of the following symptoms is *least* likely to occur in a 15-year-old female who has a complete transverse obstructive lesion of the vagina?**

    A. amenorrhea
    B. hematocolpos
    C. abdominal pain
    D. mucocolpos
    E. bulging at the introitus

12. **A 16-year-old feminized patient has a short blind vagina. She is most apt to have**

    A. Rokitansky-Küster-Hauser syndrome
    B. androgen resistance syndrome
    C. CAH
    D. gonadal dysgenesis
    E. polycystic ovaries

13. **A significant number of patients with the Rokitansky-Küster-Hauser syndrome have**

    A. secondary amenorrhea
    B. bowel malformation
    C. urinary tract malformation
    D. ovarian failure
    E. an abnormal karyotype

14. **A 15-year-old feminized patient with primary amenorrhea is seen in the clinic. On examination, she is found to have a short blind vagina and no uterus. Initial proper management includes**

    A. immediate vaginoplasty
    B. karyotype
    C. barium enema
    D. removal of gonads
    E. follicle-stimulating hormone (FSH) levels

15. **In cases of vaginal agenesis, the method of vaginal reconstruction most likely to result in a long vagina with the least chances of restricture is**

    A. coital pouch (Williams vulvovaginoplasty)
    B. McIndoe-Reed reconstruction
    C. graduated dilation (Frank's method)
    D. small bowel graft
    E. amniotic membrane graft

16. **A transverse vaginal septum is formed by**

    A. failure of fusion of the müllerian ducts
    B. persistent fusion of the wolffian ducts
    C. intact wall between the müllerian ducts and the sinovaginal bulb
    D. lack of canalization of the caudal wolffian duct
    E. loci of vaginal adenosis growing together

17. Which of the following would *not* result from failure of the complete or partial fusion of the müllerian ducts

    A. uterus didelphys
    B. longitudinal vaginal septum
    C. transverse vaginal septum
    D. septate uterus
    E. arcuate uterus

18. Pregnancy in a rudimentary uterine horn is most often associated with

    A. full-term birth
    B. multiple gestation
    C. rupture of the horn
    D. choriocarcinoma
    E. hydatidiform mole

19. An anomaly that should not be corrected surgically is a(n)

    A. uterus didelphys
    B. imperforate hymen
    C. rudimentary uterine horn
    D. transverse vaginal septum
    E. complete uterine septum

20. Findings helpful in determining whether a newborn infant with ambiguous genitalia is a male or female include palpation of the

    A. sacral curvature
    B. pelvis by rectal examination
    C. breasts
    D. thyroid gland
    E. phallus

21. Which of the following diagnostic tests is most apt to be helpful in the workup of a 15-year-old patient who complains of cyclic abdominal pain, a palpable abdominal mass, and primary amenorrhea?

    A. pelvic examination
    B. laparoscopy
    C. intravenous pyelography
    D. 17-hydroxyprogesterone
    E. FSH and luteinizing hormone (LH)

22. The condition that is most likely to be diagnosed before puberty or adolescence is

    A. CAH
    B. uterus didelphys
    C. rudimentary uterine horn
    D. polycystic ovary
    E. transverse septum

23. A patient with five repetitive first-trimester abortions underwent a hysterosalpingogram that showed a uterine septum. Which of the following diagnostic tests is most indicated?

    A. genetic studies on both partners
    B. laparoscopy
    C. endometrial biopsy
    D. FSH and LH levels
    E. Magnetic resonance imaging (MRI)

24. Absence of the uterus is found in women with

    A. Down syndrome
    B. Rokitansky-Küster-Hauser syndrome
    C. hematocolpos
    D. CAH
    E. Turner syndrome

25. A longitudinal vaginal septum is commonly associated with

    A. recurrent vaginal infection
    B. irregular menses
    C. uterus didelphys
    D. mucocolpos
    E. pyometra

26. If untreated, an imperforate hymen is *least* likely to cause

    A. endometriosis
    B. urinary obstruction
    C. abdominal pain
    D. difficult coitus
    E. urinary incontinence

DIRECTIONS:

for Questions 27–29: For each numbered item, select the one heading most closely associated with it. Each lettered heading may be used once, more than once, or not at all.

(A) Strassman procedure
(B) Tompkins procedure
(C) Williams procedure
(D) Ingram modification of the Frank procedure
(E) McIndoe procedure

27. **Vaginal construction by a progressive dilation**

28. **Vaginal construction by use of a split-thickness graft**

29. **Uterine reunification after wedge excision of the septum**

DIRECTIONS:

for Questions 30–32: For each numbered item, select the drawing in Figure 11–2 that corresponds with it.

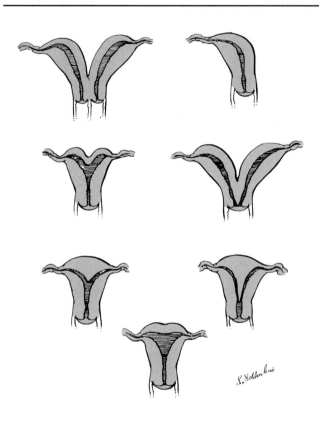

30. **Didelphic uterus**

31. **Bicornuate uterus**

32. **Septate uterus**

FIGURE 11–2 Nonobstructive maldevelopment of the müllerian system. (From Baramki TA: Treatment of congenital anomalies in girls and women. J Reprod Med 29:376–384, 1984.)

ANSWERS

1. **D,** Page 255. Patients with CAH have accelerated growth during childhood, but the epiphyseal plates close prematurely, reducing final adult height. With adequate cortisol replacement therapy, the growth pattern is expected to be normal. As with all autosomal recessive disorders, children are expected to inherit the syndrome only when both parents are affected. Infertility is not a predominant feature of the disorder since ovarian function is expected to be normal in patients who are adequately treated. However, some studies have shown that these patients suffer from relative infertility. These patients are not typically obese. Depending on the defect, masculinization of the external genitalia may occur.

2. **C,** Page 257. Hysteroscopic division of a uterine septum is the preferred method of surgical management. It is monitored by laparoscopy to ensure that the incision does not extend through the myometrium. Laparoscopy is rarely

indicated for patients with Rokitansky-Küster-Hauser syndrome, in whom the diagnosis is made clinically and supported by a pelvic sonogram. Laparoscopy has no role in the care of patients with hematocolpos or with a longitudinal vaginal septum, and CAH is managed medically.

3. **C,** Page 254. An infant born with ambiguous genitalia may present a neonatal emergency. The majority of the virilized females have CAH. Some are salt losers; unless treated with cortisol, they may die of an addisonian crisis. To avoid future change in gender assignment, it is recommended that the decision regarding a newborn's sex be deferred until the investigation is complete.

4. **B,** Page 255. The newborn described has ambiguous genitalia. Many female infants with ambiguous genitalia suffer from CAH. In addition, this child has an older sister with CAH, which is an autosomal recessive disorder. CAH is not associated with a 5 α-reductase deficiency. The remaining three enzymes listed as options are essential components in the production of cortisol. Deficiency of 20, 22-desmolase, which converts cholesterol to pregnenolone, is usually incompatible with life. Since the child has an older sister, this enzyme is not likely to be affected. The most commonly affected enzyme in patients with CAH is 21-hydroxylase. The second most common is 11-hydroxylase deficiency, accounting for about 5% of all CAH patients; 11-hydroxylase deficiency is associated with hypertension.

5. **A,** Pages 253, 265. A supernumerary ovary is defined as the presence of a third ovary separated from the normally situated ovaries, whereas an accessory ovary is defined as the presence of excess ovarian tissue near a normally placed ovary and connected to it. Supernumerary ovaries are rare and often associated with genetic urinary congenital defects.

6. **A,** Page 249. Patients with vaginal agenesis require vaginal reconstruction. Graduated dilation is probably the preferred method and should be delayed until the patient is cooperative and motivated to have a functional vagina. It should be performed after puberty, when the adolescent is contemplating sexual activity or marriage. Marriage should not be a precondition for vaginal reconstruction.

7. **C,** Page 254. Clitoral enlargement usually results from excessive androgen stimulation. Estrogen deficiency states or müllerian duct defects do not cause clitoral enlargement. The genital tubercle, from which the clitoris develops, is very sensitive to androgenic stimulation in utero. With age, the sensitivity diminishes, but even late in adult life prolonged exposure to androgens may cause clitoral enlargement. Masturbation and sexual activity do not increase the clitoral size.

8. **E,** Page 255. CAH is an autosomal recessive disorder caused by an enzyme deficiency in the pathway of cortisol production. As a result, cortisol levels are low, leading to increased adrenocorticotropic hormone (ACTH) production. Cortisol precursors, especially 17-hydroxyprogesterone, accumulate; the precursors can be measured easily as a diagnostic screening test. These precursors are converted to androgens that may virilize the female infant. In 90% to 95% of patients with CAH, the deficient enzyme is 21-hydroxylase, the gene for which is coded on chromosome 6. Hypertension occurs occasionally, especially if the defect is deficiency of 11-hydroxylase.

9. **B,** Pages 254–255. An infant with ambiguous genitalia may be a virilized female, which is most likely. It could also be a male lacking testosterone effect, such as occurs with androgen resistance syndrome, or a true hermaphrodite. Female infants may be virilized in utero when exposed to androgens ingested by the mother or androgens produced by the infant, most commonly because of CAH. Severe virilization caused by 19 norprogestins is extremely rare, and an infant with XO chromosomes would have female-appearing genitalia. Teratogens other than androgens ingested by the mother very rarely cause abnormalities of the genitalia.

10. **A,** Page 255. Infants born with CAH have a significant risk of life-threatening salt loss. This occurs frequently in patients with a virilizing adrenal hyperplasia and is usually evident within a few days of birth. Therefore, screening newborns with serial 17-hydroxyprogesterone measurements, especially in cases with ambiguous genitalia, and frequent determination of blood electrolytes in those found to have elevated levels are important for rapid diagnosis. Treatment involves restoring the electrolyte imbalance and starting glucocorticoids. Because of early bone growth and epiphyseal closure, these children—if they do not have severe illness and are untreated—grow rapidly initially and then stop growing, resulting in a much lower final height than normal. A growth chart is of value in documenting the rapidity of growth. Too much replacement cortisol retards the growth, whereas too little results in growth acceleration. Hypothyroidism is no more common than in the general population. Children with CAH become virilized, not feminized, and a small percentage become hypertensive because of an increase in mineralocorticoids, especially if the defect causes loss of 11-β-hydroxylase.

11. **E,** Page 259. A transverse obstruction is rare and usually high in the vagina, and therefore it does not cause bulging at the introitus. Such bulging is more common with an imperforate hymen. An obstructive transverse lesion of the vagina can cause accumulation of blood or fluid behind the obstructive membrane. The accumulation starts in the upper vagina, forming a mucocolpos in a child or a hematocolpos after menarche. As more fluid accumulates, it can back up into the uterus, causing a mucometra or hematometra and possibly retrograde menstruation through the tubes. This in turn may cause abdominal pain and increases the chances of endometriosis. The obstruction prevents egress of blood from the vagina. Therefore, primary amenorrhea is one of the diagnostic features.

12. **A,** Page 257. A short blind vagina indicates either no or little vaginal development or a transverse septum, which shortens the vagina and prevents one from seeing the cervix. Patients with CAH may have a narrow introitus, but the vagina is of normal length and the cervix is visible. A vagina is present in women with gonadal dysgenesis or with polycystic ovaries. Those with androgen resistance syndrome are males, and a vagina never develops; this syndrome is much less common than müllerian agenesis, which creates the Rokitansky-Küster-Hauser syndrome.

13. **C,** Page 257. Patients with Rokitansky-Küster-Hauser syndrome have vaginal agenesis and, in most cases, absence of the uterus. Because of this, they often have primary, not secondary, amenorrhea. In about 50% of patients, urinary tract malformation coexists. An intravenous pyelogram is indicated for all patients who have vaginal agenesis, who also have approximately 10% to 12% vertebral anomalies. Bowel development is normal, as is ovarian development. Secondary sexual characteristics are expected to develop normally. Patients with Rokitansky-Küster-Hauser syndrome usually have a normal (46,XX) karyotype.

14. **B,** Page 257. A karyotype should be ordered to identify those in whom the vagina did not develop because of müllerian-inhibiting factor produced by a testis (androgen resistance syndrome). A patient with vaginal agenesis will probably desire a functional vagina. This can be accomplished by gradual dilation or vaginoplasty. This procedure should be considered when the patient is contemplating intercourse, not necessarily when the patient is first seen. Intravenous pyelography should be requested at this visit to rule out the presence of a urinary tract or low vertebral anomaly, but a barium enema is not indicated.

Complete androgen resistance is a likely diagnosis, but the gonads would not be removed unless they were shown to be testes and then not until after puberty. Since feminization has occurred, you know clinically that the gonads are functioning and therefore that determining the FSH level is not necessary.

15. **C,** Page 259. There is a potential space, filled with loose areolar tissue, between the bladder and the rectum that can be developed to reconstruct a vagina. This can be achieved by graduated dilation (Frank's method): dilators of gradually increasing size are pressed against the location in which the vagina should be present, and with time a vagina is created. This method requires a well-motivated patient and is successful in about 60% of patients. Alternatively, this space can be created surgically and lined with a split-thickness skin graft (McIndoe-Reed), amnion graft, or small bowel graft. If such a space cannot be created, a coital pouch is created from the labia minor and perineal skin (Williams vulvovaginoplasty). All surgical procedures carry a risk of scarring, particularly if dilators are not used or if there is no regular coital activity to maintain vaginal diameter and depth.

16. **C,** Page 259. A lack of canalization of the junction between the sinovaginal bulb and the müllerian ducts causes a transverse vaginal septum. It is usually thin, and the other female organs are normal. Wolffian ducts are found in the male and have no role in normal vaginal formation.

17. **C,** Page 259. The uterus and the vagina are formed from paired müllerian ducts that fuse in the midline. When fusion fails to occur in the distal portion, the patient has a longitudinal vaginal septum. When fusion fails to occur in the proximal portion, a bicornuate septate or arcuate uterus is found. Complete failure of lateral (longitudinal) fusion results in genital tract duplication: a longitudinal vaginal septum and uterus didelphys. A transverse vaginal septum is an example of failure of vertical canalization between the müllerian tubercle and the sinovaginal bulb.

18. **C,** Page 261. Pregnancy in a rudimentary uterine horn is associated with missed abortion or fetal death and not with full-term or multiple gestations or gestational trophoblastic disease. The blood supply to a rudimentary horn is often compromised and insufficient to support pregnancy. On occasion, when the blood supply is adequate, the fetus grows and the horn ruptures, which may be catastrophic. Therefore, rudimentary uterine horns should be surgically removed at the time of diagnosis in most cases.

19. **A,** Pages 263–265. A uterus didelphys requires no surgical treatment. A rudimentary uterine horn exposes the patient to the risks of ectopic gestation, uterine rupture, endometriosis, and infertility. It needs to be removed as soon as the diagnosis is made, unless the woman is postmenopausal. An imperforate hymen and complete transverse septum lead to hematocolpos and should be incised. A complete uterine septum may be diagnosed by hysterosalpingography, hysteroscopy, and MRI. Many experts think that this condition should be treated in a patient with reproductive wastage, although the final efficacy of such treatment has been questioned.

20. **B,** Page 254. Certain physical findings may support an initial impression of the true sex of a newborn with ambiguous genitalia. When gonads are palpable in the labia or the inguinal canal, the infant is likely to be a male. Palpation of a uterus on rectal examination suggests that the newborn is a female. The presence or absence of breast tissue is a reflection of maternal hormones that crossed the placenta and not of infant gonadal sex. Sacral curvature develops as the child grows and is not present at birth. The size of the phallus is indicative of androgen exposure and can be large or small for either male or female. The thyroid gland is not involved.

21. **A,** Pages 255–256. The patient has an obstructed vagina that is trapping menstrual blood. A pelvic examination is the first test to perform. A sonogram may show the level of obstruction and provide useful information before surgical correction. Genitourinary abnormalities are not associated with either an imperforate hymen or a transverse vaginal septum. Laparoscopy is usually not helpful. 17-Hydroxyprogesterone is a test for CAH. Since the patient is feminized, FSH and LH levels are probably normal.

22. **A,** Pages 254–259. CAH, with its increased androgen production, is often diagnosed at birth in the virilized female. The male infant, even if not virilized at birth, may be diagnosed if he is a salt loser or when he undergoes virilization during childhood. Congenital anomalies of the genital tract are often not diagnosed until later in life, when they interfere with menstruation or fertility. The diagnosis of a uterus didelphys, a rudimentary uterine horn, or a transverse vaginal septum is rarely made in childhood. Polycystic ovary is usually not diagnosed before puberty.

23. **A,** Page 263. The patient has had five repetitive first-trimester abortions and, during her workup, is found to have a septate uterus. Division of the septum, which represents an unfavorable site for implantation, is indicated. A complete workup of both parents is indicated to exclude other causes of fetal wastage. Karyotypes of both parents should be obtained to identify chromosome abnormalities. Endometrial biopsy, laparoscopy, and FSH/LH levels are unnecessary, although they may be important steps in the evaluation of the infertile couple. The patient had no difficulty in conception but has had recurrent first-trimester abortions. Since the anatomic abnormality is known, little can be gained from MRI.

24. **B,** Page 257. Absence of the uterus is caused by a failure of the müllerian ducts to form properly, as in patients who have Rokitansky-Küster-Hauser syndrome or androgen insensitivity. Patients with testicular tissue (androgen insensitivity) produce müllerian-inhibiting factor, which causes regression of the müllerian ducts. These persons are born without a uterus. Patients with a hematocolpos have a uterus and obstruction of the vagina. Women with CAH or Turner syndrome (XO) have a uterus.

25. **C,** Page 264. A longitudinal vaginal septum is an example of failure of lateral fusion and is associated with uterus didelphys. The presence of a septum may interfere with sexual function, and the patient may complain of dyspareunia. Vaginal infections and irregular menses are unrelated to the presence of a longitudinal vaginal septum. Because there is usually drainage of the uterus and vagina, neither mucocolpos nor pyometra is likely, although in rare cases a longitudinal vaginal septum may be incomplete and closed at the distal end.

26. **E,** Page 257. Patients with imperforated hymen accumulate blood behind the obstructive membrane. As the blood accumulates, the pressure within the vagina increases and urethral obstruction may occur, causing urinary retention. As the blood flows from the uterus through the tubes into the peritoneal cavity, abdominal pain is a frequent symptom. Endometriosis may result. Because of the vaginal obstruction, coitus is difficult. There is no effect on urinary continence.

27. **D,** Page 259. The Frank procedure has been modified by Ingram. It is a progressive dilation of the vaginal dimple with progressively enlarging dilators.

28. **E,** Page 259. The McIndoe procedure uses a split-thickness skin graft superimposed on a stent and placed in an open space created between the urethra and the rectum. If regular postoperative coitus is maintained, the results are quite good. The Williams procedure uses labial skin and makes a vaginal pouch with a posteriorly directed axis. Through regular use, a more normal axis is created.

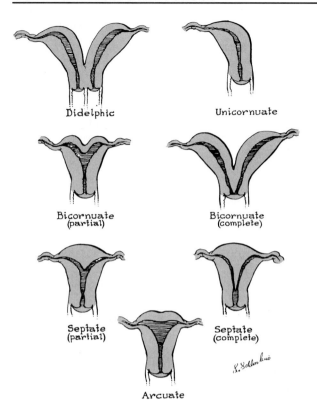

FIGURE 11–3 Nonobstructive maldevelopment of the müllerian system. (From Baramki TA: Treatment of congenital anomalies in girls and women. J Reprod Med 29:376–384, 1984.)

29. **A,** Page 265. A uterine septum should be removed if the patient is having repetitive fetal losses. It is assumed that the septum provides an unfavorable area for implantation and leads to abortion. There are many techniques for the removal of a uterine septum, including the Strassman procedure, in which a coronal incision is made through the fundus and the septum is excised. The Tompkins procedure is another choice: a sagittal incision is made through the fundus, and the septum is severed. In both methods, a laparotomy is performed and the full thickness of the myometrium is incised. The currently preferred method to remove the septum uses an operative hysteroscope, which is inserted through the cervical os. The procedure is monitored by laparoscopy. The advantages of this procedure are that (1) it does not require a laparotomy, (2) the risk of pelvic adhesions is reduced, and (3) the risk of future uterine rupture is less.

30–32. 30, **A;** 31, **E;** 32, **C;** Page 263 (Figure 11–3). A didelphic uterus has complete nonfusion of the müllerian ducts and two complete uterine horns, each with a cervix. The bicornuate uterus results from a greater degree of fusion and has two horns but only one cervix. A septate uterus results from even more fusion, leaving only a central septum of varying length. An arcuate uterus has only a slight bulging into the cavity at the fundus.

CHAPTER
12

Pediatric Gynecology

DIRECTIONS:

for Questions 1–30: Select the one best answer or completion.

1. **The most common ovarian neoplasm in premenarchal females is a(n)**

   A. dysgerminoma
   B. mature teratoma
   C. immature teratoma
   D. serous cystadenoma
   E. thecoma

2. **A neonate is found to have an ovarian mass. The most likely diagnosis is a(n)**

   A. mature teratoma
   B. immature teratoma
   C. dysgerminoma
   D. serous cystadenoma
   E. functional luteal cyst

3. **Which of the following would a physician usually *not* do when performing a complete gynecologic examination on an 8-year-old who has vaginal bleeding and pelvic pain?**

   A. history
   B. visualization of the cervix
   C. appropriate cultures of the vagina
   D. rectovaginal examination
   E. rectal examination

4. **A 4-year-old child has symptoms of dysuria and bloody discharge. Inspection of the external genitalia reveals a small hemorrhagic mass with a central aperture situated in the midline above the anterior aspect of the vaginal opening, as depicted in Figure 12–1. The most likely diagnosis is a(n)**

   A. endometrial polyp
   B. sarcoma botryoides
   C. urethral prolapse
   D. vaginal polyp
   E. clitoral tumor

5. **The ovarian tumor that most commonly causes GnRH-independent (pseudoprecocious) puberty is a**

   A. thecoma
   B. granulosa cell
   C. luteoma
   D. Sertoli-Leydig cell tumor
   E. teratoma

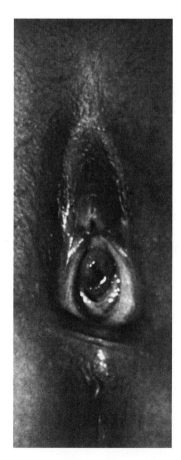

FIGURE 12–1

6. **In a child, the neutral pH obtained from vaginal fluid is the result of**

   A. a higher-than-usual vaginal sodium content
   B. the predominance of anaerobic bacteria
   C. a lack of glycogen in the epithelial cells
   D. poor perineal hygiene
   E. contamination of the vagina with urine

7. **The classic symptom of a pinworm infection is**

   A. vulvar pain
   B. nocturnal vulvar itching
   C. dysuria
   D. vaginal bleeding
   E. fever

8. **The most universal factor in the treatment of childhood vulvovaginitis is**

   A. application of topical estrogen
   B. application of topical corticosteroids
   C. application of topical antibiotics
   D. use of oral broad-spectrum antibiotics
   E. improvement in local perineal hygiene

9. **The most common foreign body found in the vagina of a young child is**

   A. toilet paper
   B. a toy
   C. a hair pin
   D. a crayon
   E. sand

10. **The patient with GnRH-dependent precocious puberty characteristically experiences**

    A. premature menopause
    B. abnormal intellectual development
    C. an infantile uterus
    D. elevated vaginal pH
    E. ultimately short stature

11. **A 5-year-old female had a small amount of bloody vaginal discharge 3 days ago. The discharge subsided, and she is now free of symptoms. General physical examination and inspection of the external genitalia are normal for age. Which of the following is the *least* likely cause of her bloody discharge?**

    A. foreign body
    B. infection
    C. sexual assault
    D. urethral prolapse
    E. GnRH-dependent precocious puberty

12. **A 9-year-old girl is brought to the emergency department after a straddle injury on a bicycle bar. A large nonexpanding vulvar hematoma is noted. There are no lacerations or bleeding. One should**

    A. obtain an intravenous pyelogram
    B. incise and drain the hematoma
    C. prescribe an ice pack and observe the child
    D. examine the child under anesthesia
    E. give the child a blood transfusion

13. **In a premenarchal child, which of the following organisms in the vagina is most indicative of possible sexual molestation?**

    A. *Neisseria gonorrhoeae*
    B. *Chlamydia trachomatis*
    C. *Shigella*
    D. human papilloma virus (HPV)
    E. *Candida*

14. **Examination of a 3-year-old reveals labial adhesions. The child is able to void without difficulty. One should initially recommend**

    A. topical estrogen
    B. surgical separation
    C. a workup for sexual abuse
    D. manual separation in the clinic
    E. no treatment

15. **Figure 12–2 is a photograph of a 7-year-old girl. It would be appropriate to tell this girl's family that**

    A. without proper treatment, hirsutism is likely
    B. this child should undergo laparoscopic examination
    C. without proper treatment, this child will likely be less than 5 feet tall
    D. this child needs surgical removal of the gonads

16. **A 7-year-old girl has accelerated growth and breast enlargement. The least appropriate initial study is**

    A. radiograph for bone age
    B. abdominal ultrasonography
    C. follicle-stimulating hormone (FSH) level
    D. laparoscopy
    E. androgen levels

17. **An 11-year-old girl underwent abdominal ultrasonography for abdominal pain. A 3-cm, unilocular, smooth-walled left ovarian cyst was seen. It is most likely a(n)**

    A. cystic teratoma
    B. ovarian epithelial carcinoma
    C. follicular cyst
    D. corpus luteum cyst
    E. benign neoplasm

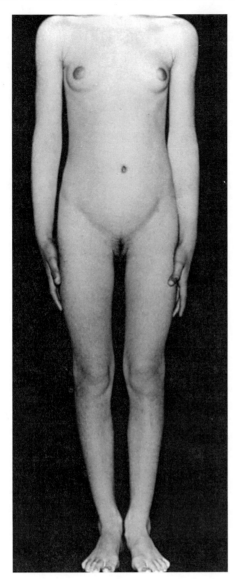

FIGURE 12–2

18. **The best management of genital trauma resulting in a nonexpanding vulvar hematoma without lacerations would be**

   A. surgical incision and removal of the clot
   B. application of an ice pack, after careful assessment
   C. cystoscopy and vaginoscopy
   D. suture of pudendal vessels
   E. abdominal incision with ligation of the epigastric arteries bilaterally

19. **Which of the following is the most common reason for vaginal bleeding in the prepubertal female?**

   A. bacterial infection
   B. foreign body
   C. precocious puberty
   D. urethral prolapse
   E. genital tumors

20. **The normal vagina of a prepubertal female**

   A. is sterile
   B. contains more species of aerobes than anaerobes
   C. has many lactobacilli
   D. is protected by labial fat pads
   E. has a neutral pH

21. **The most frequently recorded symptom of an ovarian tumor in children is**

   A. an abdominal pelvic mass
   B. vaginal bleeding
   C. abdominal pain
   D. constipation
   E. frequency of urination

22. **An 11-year-old girl underwent abdominal ultrasonography for upper abdominal pain, which then resolved. A 3-cm left ovarian unilocular cyst was seen incidentally. The best management of this condition is**

   A. laparotomy with cystectomy
   B. cycling on birth control pills
   C. thyroid hormone, bilateral salpingo-oophorectomy, and chemotherapy
   D. ultrasound-guided aspiration of the cyst
   E. watchful waiting

23. **The technique most likely to do more harm than good during the gynecologic examination of a child is**

   A. mother's assistance
   B. use of the child's own hand on her abdomen
   C. mild sedation
   D. allowing the child to see the examination instruments
   E. restraint

24. **An example of heterosexual precocious puberty would be a 7-year-old**

   A. virilized female
   B. female with breast development
   C. female with feminization and periods
   D. female with pubic hair
   E. virilized male

25. A 6-year-old girl with precocious puberty has a bone age of 5.5 years. Which of the following is the most likely cause of her precocious puberty?

 A. central nervous system hematoma
 B. congenital adrenal hyperplasia
 C. hypothyroidism
 D. ovarian estrogen-producing tumor
 E. factitious precocious puberty

26. The most common cause of GnRH-independent precocious puberty is

 A. central nervous system tumor
 B. granulosa tumor
 C. polyostotic fibrous dysplasia (McCune-Albright syndrome)
 D. central nervous system infection
 E. cranial irradiation

27. Precocious puberty in Caucasian females in North America is defined as an initiation of the signs of sexual maturity occurring before what age?

 A. 6 years
 B. 7 years
 C. 8 years
 D. 10 years
 E. 12 years

28. An 8-year-old girl is brought to you because of perineal warts. The most common reason for this condition is

 A. sexual abuse by manual manipulation
 B. consensual sexual activity
 C. nonsexual indirect transmission
 D. penile insertion
 E. transmission of infection via toilet seat

29. If a 3-year-old child is found to have pinworms, which family member should not be treated?

 A. father
 B. younger sister
 C. mother
 D. older sister
 E. older brother

30. A 6-year-old female has an area of thin white epithelium with an hourglass configuration surrounding the vaginal orifice and anus. Her major symptom is itching. This presentation is typical for

 A. sexual abuse
 B. HPV
 C. lichen sclerosis
 D. seborrheic dermatitis
 E. pinworms

DIRECTIONS:

for Questions 31–40: For each numbered item, select the one heading most closely associated with it. Each lettered heading may be used once, more than once, or not at all.

31–33. Match the most closely correct diagnosis with the clinical scenario.

 A. premature thelarche
 B. heterosexual premature puberty
 C. factitious premature puberty
 D. GnRH-dependent premature puberty
 E. GnRH-independent premature puberty

31. Vaginal bleeding develops in a 6-year-old girl, who is found to be regularly eating her mother's birth control pills.

32. A 6-year-old girl has an abdominal mass and vaginal bleeding with early breast development.

33. A 6-year-old girl has unilateral breast development. She has no bleeding, no growth changes, and no axillary or pubic hair.

34–36. Match the specific therapy with the abnormality resulting in precocious puberty.

 A. danazol
 B. surgery
 C. GnRH agonists
 D. injectable contraception (Depo-Provera)
 E. testolactone

34. Polyostotic fibrous dysplasia

35. GnRH-dependent precocious puberty

36. Ovarian tumor

37–40. Match the appropriate first diagnostic method with the problem in a pediatric patient.

 A. vaginoscopy
 B. pelvic ultrasonography
 C. computed tomography (CT)
 D. Pap smear
 E. rectal examination

37. Suspicion of a vaginal foreign object

38. Pelvic pain

39. Recurrent vulvovaginitis

40. Persistent abnormal vaginal bleeding

ANSWERS

1. **B,** Page 280. Approximately three of every four ovarian neoplasms in a premenarchal female are benign cystic teratomas. In one series, the dysgerminoma was the most common malignant neoplasm, but the benign teratoma was the most common neoplastic tumor overall. Both are germ cell tumors. In preoperative workup, obtain serum tumor markers including α-fetoprotein, human chorionic gonadotrophin (hCG), CA-125, inhibin, carcinoembryonic antigen, lactate dehydrogenase, estradiol, and testosterone.

2. **E,** Page 280. Functional luteal cysts of the ovary are not uncommon in neonates because of maternal levels of gonadotrophins. These cysts regress spontaneously and therefore do not require operative intervention.

3. **D,** Page 270. The successful gynecologic examination of a child requires a slow pace on the part of both the physician and the staff, with ample time taken to be gentle and patient. All instruments should be of a size appropriate for the individual. In an infant, attempts to visualize the cervix may be ill advised unless the child is sedated or anesthetized. A bimanual rectal-vaginal examination is not recommended. Instead, a rectal examination should be performed if the patient has vaginal bleeding or abdominal or pelvic pain. It is even sometimes best to defer the pelvic examination to a second visit to allay the child's anxiety. In pediatric gynecology, however, clinical errors tend to be those of omission rather than commission.

4. **C,** Page 277. Careful physical examination aids this differential diagnosis. A series from the Chelsea Hospital for Women showed that the four identifiable leading causes of vaginal bleeding in girls younger than 10 years were genital tumors, precocious puberty, vulvar lesions, and urethral prolapse.

5. **B,** Page 284. Granulosa cell tumors account for approximately 60% of cases of GnRH-independent (pseudoprecocious) puberty. GnRH-independent puberty is premature female sexual maturation and uterine bleeding without associated ovulation.

6. **C,** Page 275. The thin vaginal epithelium of a prepubertal child has a neutral pH, thus providing a better medium for bacterial growth than that of a woman of reproductive age. This higher pH is due to a lack of glycogen in the vaginal epithelium. Lactobacilli produce acid from the glycogen in the vagina of a woman of reproductive age.

7. **B,** Page 276. The classic symptom of a pinworm infestation is nocturnal perianal and vulvar itching. At night, the pin-size adult worms migrate from the rectum to the skin of the vulva to deposit eggs. They may be discovered by using a flashlight or by dabbing the vulvar skin with clear-cellophane adhesive tape and then examining the tape under the microscope.

8. **E,** Pages 276–277. The foundation of treating childhood vulvovaginitis is the improvement of local perineal hygiene. Approximately one in four cases is cured by improved local hygiene alone. Most nonspecific cases also respond to a combination of topical estrogen cream and oral antibiotics given for 10 to 14 days. The estrogen cream is applied to the vulvar area at night. The cream should not be used longer than 3 to 4 weeks because of systemic absorption.

9. **A,** Page 277. Symptoms related to a vaginal foreign body constitute 4% of all pediatric gynecologic outpatient visits. Neither the mother nor the child typically remembers inserting a foreign body, most often pieces of toilet paper. Large objects may be removed with bayonet forceps, and small objects such as sand may be washed out by irrigation.

10. **E,** Page 282. The cause of premature maturation of the hypothalamic pituitary axis is unknown in most cases. Idiopathic development accounts for 70% of these cases of gonadotrophin-dependent precocious puberty. Often, emotional problems arise in young girls with this condition because they are under extreme social pressure. They may be exposed to sexual exploitation and ridiculed by peers. Such children need extensive help in anticipating these difficulties. Their intellectual development is usually normal, as is their genital development. However, they almost always attain a less-than-normal height because of premature epiphyseal closure. They do not necessarily experience premature menopause.

11. **E,** Pages 278–281. Although GnRH-dependent precocious puberty is discussed in many texts, it is rare. Bloody discharge is most commonly due to a foreign body. Infection with specific bacteria, such as β-hemolytic *Streptococcus* or *Shigella*, must be considered. Sexual assault is another possibility, but in this case the absence of trauma makes it less likely. Urethral prolapse is also uncommon, but it can cause a bloody vaginal discharge, as can

vaginal neoplasms. GnRH-dependent precocious puberty, because of its rarity, is probably the least likely causative factor among those listed. GnRH-independent precocious puberty is even more rare but is not listed.

12. **C,** Page 289. The usual causes of genital trauma during childhood are accidental falls, the majority of which involve straddle injuries. If a sharp object is involved, a laceration with potential deep damage may occur. In most cases, the hematoma stops growing when the pressure from the expanding hematoma exceeds venous pressure. If an artery has been traumatized, bleeding may continue until the artery is surgically ligated. The treatment of a nonexpanding vulvar hematoma involves application of an ice pack. Only rarely are surgical evacuation and ligation of bleeding vessels necessary. Extensive lacerations require general anesthesia for diagnosis and management. Children with vulvar trauma should have a booster injection of tetanus toxoid if the last immunization was given more than 5 years before the event. In the absence of bleeding, an examination with the child under anesthesia is not required, nor is a blood transfusion or an IVP.

13. **A,** Page 275. Vulvovaginitis is the most common gynecologic problem in the premenarchal patient. Approximately 80% to 90% of children's visits to gynecologists involve introital irritation and discharge. When cultures of the vagina are taken, it must be remembered that the normal vagina is colonized by an average of nine different species of bacteria. The most likely of the above bacteria to be spread by sexual molestation is *Neisseria gonorrhoeae*. *Chlamydia* can be contracted during the birth process and remain for years. HPV is a common contaminant, and *Shigella* is unusual but not indicative of sexual molestation. *Candida* can be found at any age without indicating sexual activity.

14. **A,** Page 278. Adhesive vulvitis is a self-limiting consequence of chronic vulvitis. Denuded epithelium agglutinates and grows together. This occurs most commonly in girls 2 to 6 years old. Most infants are asymptomatic. Early stages in the process reveal posterior labial fusion. In more advanced cases, fusion over both urethral and vaginal orifices may occur. Although treatment is not absolutely necessary unless the child has difficulty voiding, use of topical estrogen cream results in spontaneous separation within 2 to 4 weeks. Forceful separation, done either with anesthesia or in the clinic, should be avoided. Although labial agglutination may be associated with sexual abuse, it usually is not.

15. **C,** Pages 283–284. Precocious puberty is arbitrarily defined as the appearance of any signs of secondary sexual maturation at an age that is more than 2.5 standard deviations below the mean. The principal concerns of the parents of these children are the social stigma and the diminished height caused by the premature closure of the epiphyseal growth centers. Without therapy, approximately 50% of patients will be less than 5 feet tall. Early in the course of this disease, the girls are taller and heavier than their chronologic peers, who have not yet experienced their growth spurt. All forms of precocious puberty are rare. GnRH-dependent precocious puberty occurs five to six times more frequently than GnRH-independent precocious puberty. Thus, it is unlikely that this child has an estrogen-producing ovarian tumor. Besides, before laparoscopy one would most likely perform an imaging procedure such as pelvic ultrasonography. If the secondary sex characteristics are discordant with the genetic and phenotypic sex, the condition is called *heterosexual precocious puberty.* Figure 12–2 does not raise suspicion of heterosexual precocious puberty.

16. **D,** Page 286. Initial evaluation of patients with possible precocious puberty emphasizes exclusion of neoplasms of the central nervous system, ovaries, or adrenal glands, which may be life-threatening. Bone films, usually of the hands and wrists, are typically repeated at 6-month intervals to evaluate the rate of skeletal maturation. If the skeletal maturation is rapid, treatment is more urgent. Advancement of bone age more than 95% of the norm for a child's chronologic age provides documentation of a peripheral estrogen effect. Ultrasound imaging or CT of the abdomen should be performed to discover enlargement of the ovaries, uterus, or adrenal glands. Laparoscopy is not needed. Additionally, serum levels of FSH, luteinizing hormone (LH), prolactin, thyroid-stimulating hormone (TSH), estradiol, testosterone, dehydroepiandrosterone sulfate, or a combination thereof may be of value in establishing the diagnosis. (Androgens are measured for androgen insensitivity.)

17. **C,** Page 279. Of asymptomatic adolescent females, 2% to 5% have small follicle cysts less than 4 cm in diameter that are discovered incidentally by ultrasonography. These cysts are clinically unimportant and usually disappear spontaneously. In this case, the abdominal pain is probably due to some other entity. Although another ovarian tumor is possible—a germ cell tumor such as cystic teratoma, a benign neoplasm, or an ovarian epithelial cancer—all of these are quite rare. A corpus luteum in a young woman of this age would be extremely unusual, although possible; however, it should not have a unilocular smooth-wall appearance.

18. **B,** Page 279. In this case, which involves no expansion of the vulvar hematoma and no bleeding lacerations, the best treatment would be application of ice and pressure. Cystoscopy or vaginoscopy to assess hidden injury should be performed if there is blood in the urine or blood coming from the vagina. Ligation of the pudendal vessels would require a major surgical procedure, which was not indicated in this patient. With a stable hematoma, ligation of the epigastric arteries would serve no purpose.

19. **B,** Page 277. Foreign body, with resultant infection, probably leads the list of causes of bloody vaginal discharge. However, all the other options, including infection, precocious puberty (which is extremely rare), urethral prolapse, and genital tumors, may cause a similar symptom. Sexual abuse should also be included in the differential diagnosis. Infections that are most likely to cause vaginal bleeding are group A β-hemolytic *Streptococcus* and *Shigella* species. These bacteria should be checked by culture if an infection is obvious.

20. **E,** Page 275. The prepubertal vagina is susceptible to infection because it has a neutral pH and a thin mucosa that is not protected by lactobacilli and because the vagina is not protected by swollen labial fat pads. The prepubertal vagina has many species of bacteria with more anaerobes than aerobes and few, if any, lactobacilli.

21. **C,** Page 280. In several large series, pain has been the most common symptom leading to the diagnosis of ovarian mass. Palpation of an abdominal mass is the most common sign, and the mass often causes an increase in abdominal girth. An ovarian mass rarely causes bleeding, although some (eg, granulosa cell tumors) may cause bleeding because they produce estrogen. However, such tumors are rare. Constipation is a common and not-at-all specific symptom, as is frequency of urination. Ovarian neoplasms in children are usually derived from germ cells, and most are benign teratomas. However, approximately 25% of ovarian neoplasms in children are malignant. Most of these are dysgerminomas.

22. **E,** Page 279. Most of the cysts in young women are physiologic, such as follicular cysts, which resolve spontaneously. Therefore, watchful waiting is the management of choice. Surgery is not indicated, and birth control pills are unnecessary. A solid tumor or a multiloculated cyst with solid areas requires further evaluation.

23. **E,** Page 270. Placing a child on the mother's lap and allowing the child to see and play with the instruments are reassuring measures in most instances. If the child is ticklish, placing the child's own hand on his or her abdomen stops the sensation. Mild sedation may be all right, but general anesthesia should be used only in urgent situations. The child should never be restrained because this may lead to both long- and short-term detrimental effects.

24. **A,** Page 282. If the secondary sex characteristics are discordant with the genetic and phenotypic sex, the condition is called *heterosexual precocious puberty.* An example is premature virilization in a female child with masculine secondary sex characteristics. Premature breast development exemplifies *premature thelarche.* A 6-year-old with feminization and periods shows *premature isosexual precocious puberty.* A 6-year-old with pubic hair has *premature adrenarche,* and a 6-year-old virilized male has *premature isosexual precocious puberty.*

25. **C,** Page 285. Hypothyroidism is the only cause of precocious puberty in which bone age is retarded. It is an unusual cause of precocious puberty because hypothyroidism most commonly is associated with delayed pubertal development. When hypothyroidism occurs, it is usually due to primary thyroid insufficiency caused by Hashimoto thyroiditis. Increased production of TSH is associated with an increase in production of gonadotrophins. Central nervous system lesions usually produce a GnRH-dependent precocious puberty. Congenital adrenal hyperplasia causes heterosexual precocious puberty in females. Estrogen-producing tumors cause non-GnRH-dependent precocious puberty. Factitious precocious puberty is due to ingestion of estrogen-containing medications. The symptoms usually regress on discontinuation of the estrogen.

26. **B,** Page 284. Although all types of GnRH-independent precocious puberty are rare, the most common cause is an estrogen-secreting tumor of the ovary, most likely a granulosa cell. All the other lesions usually cause GnRH-dependent precocious puberty if they manifest by causing premature puberty. Polyostotic fibrous dysplasia with café au lait spots, bone cysts, facial asymmetry, and precocious puberty is very rare.

27. **C,** Page 281. In North America, 7 years of age is more than 2.5 standard deviations below the mean age for secondary sexual maturation of Caucasian girls. For African American girls, the comparable age is 6 years. These ages define precocious puberty. The defined age of precocious puberty has decreased in the past 5 years because puberty occurs earlier now than it did 5 to 10 years ago.

28. **C,** Page 275. Although sexual abuse, either with genital or manual contact, is a possible means of spread of HPV, it is not the most common form of transmission. An 8-year-old is not able to consent to sexual activity. HPV may be indirectly transmitted by touching or by sharing clothing

or perhaps by the birth process itself. Toilet seat transmission is extremely unlikely.

29. **B,** Page 277. The most common symptom of pinworms is severe itching, particularly in the morning. All members of the family should be treated, except for a pregnant mother or a child younger than 2 years. The drug of choice is mebendazole (Vermox), given as one chewable tablet for each nonpregnant family member older than 2 years. Approximately 20% of female children infected with pinworms experience vulvovaginitis.

30. **C,** Page 276. Lichen sclerosis can be found at any age. It is important to recognize it and to reassure the parents that it is not due to a sexually transmitted disease or poor hygiene, nor is it evidence of sexual abuse. Warts (HPV) are usually not due to sexual abuse either because HPV is most commonly transferred vertically or by fomites. However, one must consider sexual abuse if gonorrhea, chlamydia, or trichinosis is found.

31–33. 31, **C;** 32, **E;** 33, **A;** Pages 282–285. Factitious precocious puberty is due to ingestion of or exposure to exogenous estrogen, such as through an estrogen hormone supply. The signs and symptoms usually regress when the estrogen source is removed. Although factitious precocious puberty is GnRH-independent, the factitious diagnosis is most closely related to these cases. GnRH-independent precocious puberty is due to increased circulating estrogens from a source other than the normal development of the hypothalamic pituitary axis. Premature thelarche refers to early development of the breasts; it can be either unilateral or bilateral. When premature thelarche is the only sign of sexual maturation, it is usually a benign, self-limited condition that does not require treatment and often spontaneously regresses. However, the child should be followed at regular intervals to ensure that true precocious puberty does not occur.

34–36. 34, **E;** 35, **C;** 36, **B;** Pages 287–288. It is important to rule out life-threatening diseases that may cause precocious puberty. Precocious puberty of any type is rare, and the treatment should be tailored to the cause of the precocity. If the precocity is due to tumor, removal is the treatment of choice and the symptoms often regress. If it is idiopathic (constitutional) and GnRH-dependent, GnRH agonists will reduce the increased steroid levels within 1 to 2 weeks and the symptoms will respond over time. Patients with polyostotic fibrous dysplasia may be treated with testolactone, which is an aromatase inhibitor that prevents conversion of estrogen precursors to biologically active estrogens.

37–40. 37, **A;** 38, **E;** 39, **A;** 40, **A;** Pages 272–275. Both vaginoscopy and bimanual rectoabdominal examination provide important information in evaluating various problems in the young child. Depending on the symptoms, different evaluation techniques must be used. Recurrent vulvovaginitis, persistent bleeding, suspected presence of a foreign body or neoplasm, and congenital anomalies are indications for vaginoscopy. Introduction of any instrument into the vagina of a young child takes patience and time. The prepubertal vagina is narrower, thinner, and lacking in the distensibility of the vagina of a woman in her reproductive years. Many narrow-diameter endoscopes suffice, including the Kelly air cystoscope, contact hysteroscopes, pediatric cystoscopes, small-diameter laparoscopes, plastic vaginoscopes, and special virginal speculums. A nasal speculum or otoscope is usually too short. The last step in the pelvic examination is a rectal examination. This aspect of the examination may sometimes be omitted, depending on the child's symptoms. Common reasons to perform a rectal examination include genital tract bleeding, pelvic pain, and suspicion of a foreign body or pelvic mass. The child should be warned that the rectal examination feels similar to the pressure of a bowel movement. Pelvic ultrasonography and CT, although useful for pelvic pain, should not be used before bimanual rectal examination.

Family Planning

for Questions 1–36: Select the one best answer or completion.

1. **The most common undesirable effect of depo-medroxyprogesterone acetate (DMPA) when used as a contraceptive is**

   A. hot flashes because of lower follicle-stimulating hormone (FSH) levels
   B. a disruption of the menstrual cycle
   C. an increase in body weight
   D. an increase in facial hair
   E. a lowering of total cholesterol

2. **The major mechanism of action of DMPA, which accounts for its contraceptive effect, is the**

   A. inhibition of the midcycle gonadotrophin surge
   B. production of an unfavorable endometrial environment
   C. alteration of tubal motility
   D. alteration of cervical mucus
   E. development of long-standing amenorrhea

3. **When compared with coitally nonrelated methods, coitally related methods of contraception have a much lower**

   A. method effectiveness
   B. use effectiveness
   C. continuation rate
   D. complication rate

4. **Of the 6.2 million pregnancies in 1994,**

   A. 2.9 million ended in a birth and 2.4 million ended by elective abortion
   B. 3.9 million ended in a birth and 1.4 million ended by elective abortion
   C. 4.9 million ended in a birth and 1.0 million ended by elective abortion
   D. 2.9 million ended in a birth and 1.0 million ended in a spontaneous abortion or ectopic pregnancy
   E. 3.9 million ended in a birth and 1.4 million ended in a spontaneous abortion or ectopic pregnancy

5. **Per the 1995 National Survey of Family Growth, of the 60 million women of reproductive age what percentage were using contraception?**

   A. 34%
   B. 44%
   C. 54%
   D. 64%
   E. 74%

6. **When factored over 5 years of use and adding the costs of the method, unintended births and complications of the methods, what is the most cost-effective form of contraception?**

   A. copper-based intrauterine device (IUD)
   B. male condom
   C. oral contraceptives
   D. tubal ligation
   E. vasectomy

7. **When compared with the male condom, the female condom**

   A. must be fitted to the individual before use
   B. provides less protection from sexually transmissible infections
   C. has a higher incidence of latex allergy
   D. may be reused
   E. has a higher failure (pregnancy) rate

8. **Evidence suggests that the use of latex condoms reduced the rate of the transmission of**

   A. herpesvirus
   B. human immunodeficiency virus (HIV)
   C. *Chlamydia trachomatis*
   D. human papilloma virus
   E. all the above

9. The rationale for developing the multiphasic combination oral contraceptives is to

    A. decrease the total dose of steroid administered
    B. increase the contraceptive effectiveness
    C. decrease the incidence of breakthrough bleeding
    D. decrease the incidence of fluid retention
    E. increase compliance

10. Which of the following 19-nortestosterone progestins has the least androgenic activity?

    A. norethindrone
    B. norethindrone acetate
    C. ethynodiol diacetate
    D. gestodene

11. Ovulation inhibition, by combination contraceptive steroids, occurs primarily by

    A. direct FSH suppression
    B. direct luteinizing hormone (LH) suppression
    C. alteration of ovarian responsiveness to gonadotrophin stimulation
    D. interfering with release of gonadotrophin-releasing hormone (GnRH)
    E. inhibition of endogenous estradiol production by the ovary

12. All the following are considered noncontraceptive benefits of oral contraceptives *except*

    A. decrease in endometrial proliferation
    B. reduction in the incidence of benign breast disease
    C. reduction in the occurrence of functional ovarian cysts
    D. reduction in ovarian cancer
    E. reduction in the incidence of cholelithiasis

13. The active progestin contained in Norplant is

    A. gestodene
    B. DMPA
    C. norethindrone acetate
    D. levonorgestrel
    E. norethindrone enanthate (NET-EN)

14. Risk factors associated with the development of pelvic inflammatory disease (PID) among IUD users include all the following *except*

    A. use of the IUD for 4 months or less
    B. nulliparity
    C. being a woman younger than 25 years
    D. use of copper-bearing devices
    E. previous history of PID

15. The lowest failure (pregnancy) rate is found for users of

    A. oral contraceptives
    B. implantable contraceptive rods (Norplant)
    C. DMPA
    D. female sterilization
    E. progesterone IUD

16. The Pearl Index reflects

    A. method effectiveness
    B. use effectiveness
    C. number of conceptions per year per user
    D. number of deliveries per year per user

17. Which of the following is associated with an increase in globulin factor precursors of angiotensinogen responsible for blood pressure elevations and an increase in factors VII and X associated with hypercoagulability?

    A. ethinyl estradiol
    B. norethindrone acetate
    C. ethynodiol diacetate
    D. gestodene
    E. norethindrone

18. The main mechanism of action of Norplant is

    A. increase in mean estradiol levels
    B. inhibition of ovulation
    C. inhibition of sperm capacitation
    D. formation of an atrophic endometrium

19. Side effects of Norplant include

    A. breast atrophy
    B. lower mean hemoglobin levels in long-term users
    C. irregular uterine bleeding
    D. weight gain

20. Effective postcoital contraception can be achieved by use of all of the following *except*

    A. ethinyl estradiol
    B. diethylstilbestrol
    C. danazol
    D. IUD
    E. douching with an alkaline solution

21. The main mechanism of action of the copper IUD is the

    A. alteration in tubal motility
    B. alteration in cervical mucus
    C. localized sterile inflammatory reaction that it causes within the uterine cavity
    D. direct spermicidal action

22. **The majority of women discontinuing the use of IUDs for contraception do so because of**

    A. excessive uterine cramping during menstruation
    B. fear of pelvic infection
    C. development of abnormal uterine bleeding
    D. displacement of the device

23. **Complications related to pregnancy and IUD use include an increase in**

    A. congenital anomalies
    B. septic abortion
    C. spontaneous abortion
    D. postmaturity

24. **Regarding the performance of elective abortion in the United States,**

    A. 25% of terminations occur with gestations of greater than 12 weeks' menstrual age
    B. complication rates are similar for first- and second-trimester pregnancy terminations
    C. 50% of abortions are obtained by married women
    D. two thirds of abortions are performed on women younger than 25
    E. the number of abortions performed annually has continued to increase gradually

25. **In comparing methods of second-trimester legal abortion, which of the following carries the least risk?**

    A. dilatation and evacuation (D&E)
    B. prostaglandin induction of labor
    C. instillation of hypertonic saline
    D. use of osmotic dilators, such as Laminaria, to induce labor

26. **Demographic characteristics most commonly associated with the use of sterilization in the United States include**

    A. a female younger than 30
    B. a couple married for more than 10 years
    C. upper-middle-class socioeconomic status
    D. couples with more than four children

27. **Approximately what proportion of unintended pregnancies occurs in women who are using a contraceptive method of birth control?**

    A. 10%
    B. 20%
    C. 30%
    D. 40%
    E. 50%

28. **Approximately what proportion of women whose partners use condoms use another method of contraception?**

    A. 10%
    B. 20%
    C. 30%
    D. 40%
    E. 50%

29. **Which of the following is a correct statement regarding the contraceptive diaphragm?**

    A. The use of a spermicide significantly increases the efficacy of the diaphragm.
    B. The diaphragm must be removed within 6 hours after use.
    C. The incidence of urinary tract infection is unchanged by the use of the diaphragm.
    D. Pregnancy rates are lower for older women.
    E. Pregnancy rates increase with duration of use.

30. **The female condom**

    A. must be fitted to the individual
    B. may be reused up to five times
    C. may be inserted well in advance of sexual activity
    D. provides greater pregnancy protection than the male condom
    E. is more likely to rupture during vigorous sexual intercourse

31. **In the United States, what percentage of reproductive-age women have taken oral contraceptives at some time in their lives?**

    A. 30%
    B. 45%
    C. 60%
    D. 75%
    E. 90%

32. **Over the years, many studies have evaluated the role of oral contraceptive pills in the occurrence of malignant neoplasms. Which of the following is the most accurate statement regarding oral contraceptives and malignancies?**

    A. Current users have a slightly increase risk of breast cancer.
    B. Decreased risk for ovarian cancer applies only to current users.
    C. The greatest decrease of endometrial cancer is among multiparous users.
    D. Risk of metastatic breast cancer is greater in current users.
    E. Women who have used oral contraceptives for more than 5 years need Pap smears every 6 months because of an increased risk of abnormal cervical cytology.

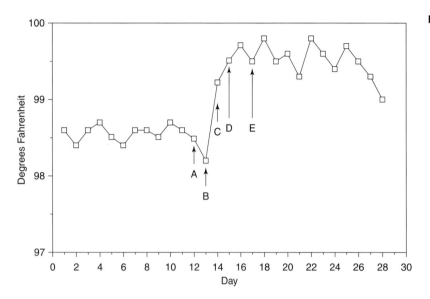

FIGURE 13–1

33. Which of the following precludes the use of an IUD?

A. diabetes mellitus
B. valvular heart disease
C. cervical dysplasia
D. genital bleeding of unknown etiology
E. all of the above

34. According to recent studies, which of the following has the highest rate of continuing use at 1 year?

A. male condom
B. diaphragm
C. oral contraceptives
D. copper IUD
E. implantable contraceptive rods

35. A couple wishes to use "natural family planning" for contraception. The woman's periods are regular, occurring every 28 to 30 days. This patient's "fertile" period would be days

A. 7–14
B. 7–17
C. 7–20
D. 10–17
E. 10–19

36. A couple is using "natural family planning" for contraception. Figure 13–1 shows the basal temperature graph made by the couple the previous month. Which letter (A–E) most closely identifies when unprotected intercourse may resume?

ANSWERS

1. **B,** Pages 329–330. DMPA has mechanisms of action similar to those of oral combination contraceptives. They include suppression of midcycle LH and maintenance of FSH in the follicular phase range. A major side effect of DMPA is the complete disruption of the menstrual cycle. As the duration of therapy increases, the incidence of frequent bleeding steadily declines. By the end of 2 years, 70% of women are amenorrheic. Levels of triglycerides and high-density-lipoprotein (HDL) cholesterol (but not total cholesterol) are significantly lower in long-term users. DMPA is extremely effective, with failure rates ranging from 0 to 1.2 per 100 woman-years. DMPA has little effect on facial hair. Although some studies have indicated that users of DMPA gain between 1.5 and 4 kg in their first year of use, the absence of controls and the absence of a similar effect in a retrospective comparative longitudinal study make unclear the true effect of DMPA on weight gain. For patients who are concerned about weight or weight gain, counseling about caloric intake and exercise should be offered.

2. **A,** Page 327. DMPA acts by inhibiting the midcycle gonadotrophin surge. Mean estradiol levels remain fairly constant (at about 40 mg/mL) for up to 5 years of treatment. These estradiol levels are higher than menopausal levels. Although the endometrium becomes atrophic as a result of the high progestin level, this is not the major

mechanism of action. Likewise, cervical mucus changes because of decreased estrogen production, but it is not the primary mechanism of action. The influence on tubal motility is assumed to be similar to that of oral contraceptives. As a result of endometrial atrophy, patients become amenorrheic after long-term treatment. This effect is secondary to the high progestin–induced changes.

3. **B,** Pages 296–298. Although the actual effectiveness of a contraceptive method is difficult to ascertain, method effectiveness and use effectiveness have been used to determine whether conception occurred while the contraceptive was being used correctly or incorrectly. In general, contraceptive methods used at the time of coitus, such as diaphragm, condom, or spermicide, have a much greater method effectiveness than use effectiveness. The overall value of a contraceptive method as used by a couple is determined by a calculation of the actual effectiveness and the continuation rate. Continuation rates for the barrier methods are lowest for the diaphragm, condom, and spermicide and highest for an IUD, which necessitates a visit to a health care facility to discontinue use. Complication rates for the barrier rates are also quite low.

4. **B,** Page 296. In 1994, there were about 6.2 million pregnancies in the United States. About two thirds of these pregnancies (3.9 million) ended in births of children, and about one fourth (1.4 million) were terminated by elective abortions. The remainder ended in spontaneous abortion or ectopic pregnancy. According to Henshaw's review of the 1995 National Survey of Growth, about half of the 6 million pregnancies were unintended and 54% of these unintended pregnancies were terminated by elective abortion.

5. **D,** Page 296. According to the 1995 National Survey of Family Growth, of the 60 million women of reproductive age in the United States in 1995, 64% (39 million) were using a method of contraception. Among the group using no method of contraception, about half had undergone prior hysterectomy or were pregnant, infertile, or trying to conceive. The other half either were not sexually active or were having infrequent episodes of coitus or otherwise did not think there was a need for contraception. A total of 5% of women of reproductive age were sexually active and not using a method of contraception.

6. **A,** Page 299. The calculations included the failure rate of the method with the resultant cost of an unintended pregnancy, direct costs of the method, and costs due to incurred or avoided events due to the adverse and beneficial side effects of the contraceptive method. The most cost-effective method over 5 years of use is with the copper IUD,

followed by vasectomy, implant, injectable contraceptives, oral contraceptives, and progesterone IUD.

7. **E,** Pages 298, 300–301; Table 13–2 in Mishell. Initial experience with the female condom suggests that it has "typical use" and "perfect use" failure rates almost twice those of the male condom. The female condom does provide increased protection from sexually transmissible infections because of the larger surface covered, including portions of the vulva. Because the female condom is made from polyurethane, it is stronger, transmits heat faster, and is not a source of latex allergy. Like the male condom, the female condom requires no fitting or intervention by a health care professional and should be used for only one act of sexual intercourse before it is discarded.

8. **E,** Pages 300–301. Several epidemiologic studies have shown that condoms reduce the frequency of clinical infection with sexually transmitted diseases, both bacterial and viral. Specifically, transmission of the herpesvirus, the human papilloma virus, and HIV, as well as *Chlamydia trachomatis* and *Neisseria gonorrhoeae,* is inhibited by condom use.

9. **A,** Pages 303–305. Biphasic and triphasic oral contraceptive formulations are generally called *multiphasic.* The rationale for this type of formulation is that a lower total dose of steroid is administered without increasing the incidence of breakthrough bleeding. Other side effects of oral contraceptives and compliance rates appear to be unchanged.

10. **D,** Pages 304–305. Of the progestins listed in the question, gestodene has the greatest progestational activity but is less androgenic than the other progestins.

11. **D,** Pages 307–308. Contraceptive steroids prevent ovulation mainly by interfering with the release of GnRH from the hypothalamus. In animal studies and a few human studies, this inhibitory action of contraception steroids has been overcome by the administration of GnRH. In addition, some studies suggest that despite administration of GnRH, there is residual suppression of LH and FSH, suggesting a direct pituitary effect as well. This effect is thought to be less important than the effect on GnRH secretion by the hypothalamus. Although suppression of hormone production by the ovary does occur, this is the result of the suppression of GnRH and not a direct effect.

12. **E,** Pages 323–325. The antiestrogenic action of progestins contained in oral contraceptives confer a number of noncontraceptive benefits. These include endometrial atrophy and inhibition of the synthesis of estrogen and receptors in breast tissue, exerting an antiestrogenic action on the breast and decreasing benign breast disease.

Symptomatic functional ovarian cysts are significantly decreased because of gonadotrophin inhibition. Future ovarian cancer secondary to incessant ovulation is also decreased. The likelihood of cholelithiasis increases slightly in oral contraceptive users.

13. **D,** Pages 333–334. Subdermal implants made of Silastic capsules containing levonorgestrel have been available in the United States for several years. Clinical trials of this long-acting, effective, reversible method of contraception were initiated in 1975. Currently, this method has been studied in more than 0.5 million subjects in 45 countries. The other progestins mentioned here are contained in other contraception delivery systems in both the United States and Europe (gestodene). NET-EN is another form of a long-acting injectable progestational agent.

14. **D,** Pages 342–343. Detailed analyses are available from Centers for Disease Control and Prevention data published in 1988 outlining risk factors for the occurrence of PID among IUD users. In a group of married or cohabitating women who had only one sexual partner and who had an IUD inserted more than 4 months earlier, the relative risk for developing PID compared with no method used was 1.0. Other populations at high risk for PID include those with a prior history of PID, nulliparous women younger than 25, and women with multiple sexual partners. No increased risk for PID associated with the use of currently available devices, including copper-bearing devices, has been shown in other groups.

15. **B,** Pages 297–299; Table 13–2 in Mishell. The rate of contraceptive failure is lowest among users of implantable contraceptive rods. It is estimated to be 0.09% of women using the method in the first year. Surprisingly, this rate is lower than that found for female sterilization, which carries a first-year failure rate of 0.4%. A similar failure rate (0.3%) is found for users of DMPA. Oral contraceptives have failure rates that approximate 0.1%. The IUD has a failure rate that varies with type; the progesterone-containing IUD has a failure rate of 1.5% to 2%, whereas the copper IUD has a rate estimated to be 0.6% to 0.8%.

16. **C,** Page 295. The Pearl Index is a nonactuarial method used to determine the pregnancy (failure) rate associated with any contraceptive method. Although contraceptive methods may fail because of imperfect use (use effectiveness) or factors inherent in the method itself (method effectiveness), the Pearl Index does not differentiate between the two. The Pearl Index is the number of pregnancies divided by total woman-months of contraceptives used. This figure is then multiplied by 1200. Note that this figure does not account for the outcome of the pregnancy.

17. **A,** Pages 307–312; Tables 13–4 and 13–5 in Mishell. Synthetic estrogens have been associated with an increase in globulins for which one, angiotensinogen, may cause increased angiotensin II, resulting in hypertension, whereas other globulins, such as factor VII and factor X, may be associated with the development of hypercoagulable states, which may lead to the development of thrombosis in susceptible oral contraceptive users.

18. **B,** Page 333. Through analysis of daily ultrasonographic scans of the ovaries of Norplant users with regular cycles and elevated luteal phase progesterone levels, it has been noted that about one third of these cycles include ovarian change consistent with an anovulatory pattern. Since only about one half of the cycles of Norplant users have a fairly regular menstrual pattern, probably less than 20% of these cycles are ovulatory. A number of these are progesterone-deficient. Thus inhibition of ovulation is the mechanism of action of this method of contraception. Cervical mucus remains scanty and viscid, and normal sperm penetration does not take place, as demonstrated in both in vivo and in vitro studies. Although this factor and the atrophic endometrium associated with progestin treament contribute to contraceptive efficacy, the major mechanism remains the suppression of ovulation.

19. **C,** Pages 334–335. The major side effect of Norplant use is irregular uterine bleeding. Bleeding episodes tend to be prolonged and irregular during the first year of use, although the mean number of days of bleeding declines steadily with time. Mean total blood loss in Norplant users is about 25 mL/month, which is slightly less than average. Several studies have shown that the mean hemoglobin concentration in the first 3 years of Norplant use tends to rise slightly. Although mastalgia is a complication of Norplant use, no evidence shows that breast atrophy occurs. Weight gain has been associated only with the use of long-acting injectable progestins (eg, DMPA), but even that link has been questioned.

20. **E,** Pages 336–337. Various preparations have been used effectively as a postcoital contraceptive (the "morning-after pill"). The most commonly used estrogen compounds include diethylstilbestrol (DES), ethinyl estradiol, and conjugated estrogens. The overall mean effectiveness of the estrogen compounds is greater than 99%. Danazol has also been administered in two separate doses of 400 to 600 mg separated by 12 hours. The effectiveness of this method is slightly less (about 98%). When placed within 48 hours of intercourse, an IUD often is effective in preventing

implantation and the continuation of pregnancy. Douching shows little effectiveness in preventing pregnancy.

21. **C,** Pages 338–339. The main mechanism of contraceptive action of the IUD is spermicidal. This mechanism is produced by a local sterile inflammatory reaction caused by the presence of the foreign body in the uterus. Moyer and Mishell found a nearly 1000% increase in the number of leukocytes in washings of the human endometrial cavity 18 weeks after the insertion of an IUD compared with the washings obtained before insertion. Tissue breakdown products of these leukocytes are toxic to all cells, including sperm and the blastocyst. There is no evidence of a direct spermicidal effect by the IUD per se, but only as a consequence of the more generalized inflammatory process.

22. **C,** Pages 339–341. Increased cramping is noted by IUD users, but it usually decreases significantly by the third cycle. Nearly all the medical reasons accounting for IUD removal involve one or more types of abnormal bleeding. These include heavy or prolonged menses or intermenstrual bleeding. The amount of blood loss that occurs during each menstrual cycle is significantly greater in IUD users than in nonusers. The mean blood loss per cycle more than doubles, increasing from approximately 35 mL to 80 mL. The exact mechanism causing an increased mean blood loss is not completely understood, although histologic studies of endometrium obtained by biopsy and hysterectomy demonstrate both vascular erosions and increased vascular permeability. Mefenamic acid ingested in a dosage of 500 mg three times per day during menstruation has been shown to reduce mean blood loss significantly in IUD users. After the initial placement, displacement of the IUD is unlikely.

23. **C,** Pages 341–342. All reported series of pregnancies with any type of IUD in situ include an increase in incidence of spontaneous abortion. This rate is approximately three times the rate that would be expected without IUD use. There is no increase in the rate of congenital anomalies. Since removal of the Dalkon Shield from the market, there is no conclusive evidence of an increased incidence of sepsis with currently available designs. Patients who carry a pregnancy with an IUD in place are at increased risk of premature delivery.

24. **D,** Page 347. Since 1980, the number of legal abortions performed has gradually declined. In 1988, an estimated 1.6 million elective abortions were performed in the United States, but by 1992 this number had dropped to 1.55 million, approximately one fourth of which were obtained by

married women. Ninety percent of abortions are performed within the first 12 weeks of pregnancy. After 10 weeks of menstrual age, abortion complication rates increase progressively with gestational age. Roughly one third of abortions are performed on women younger than 20, one third on women 20 to 24, and one third on women older than 25.

25. **A,** Page 347. Studies suggest that D&E is substantially safer than induction of labor (by any method) for abortions between 13 and 16 weeks from the last menstrual period. Dilation of the cervix for second-trimester abortions can be facilitated by osmotic dilators, but this method does not generally result in the induction of labor. Mechanically dilating the cervix decreases the risk of uterine trauma such as perforation and cervical injury.

26. **B,** Pages 345–347. In the United States in 1988, sterilization of one member of a couple was the most widely used method of preventing pregnancy. The popularity of sterilization is greatest if (1) the wife is older than 30 and (2) the couple has been married longer than 10 years. No information suggests that couples of more advantaged socioeconomic status choose this method. The decision to undergo sterilization is based on the desire to limit future pregnancies and is not limited to a specific family size.

27. **E,** Page 296. Roughly 50% of unintended pregnancies in the United States occur in women who are using a contraception method that failed to prevent pregnancy. The remaining 50% of unintended pregnancies occur in the roughly 10% of sexually active women who use no method of contraception.

28. **E,** Pages 296–297. Roughly 50% of women have partners who use a condom as an additional method of contraception. Of these women, half use oral contraceptives.

29. **D,** Page 300. The diaphragm provides contraception with approximately 95% efficacy when used perfectly and 85% during the first year of average use. The lowest rates are found in married motivated women and decline with age and duration of use. Although most diaphragm users use a spermicide in addition to the diaphragm, no conclusive studies have indicated a higher failure rate when the diaphragm is used alone. The diaphragm should be left in place for 8 hours after intercourse. If repeated intercourse occurs, a spermicide should be applied and the time for removal should be adjusted accordingly. The incidence of urinary tract infections is slightly higher than normal in diaphragm users.

30. **C,** Pages 300–301. The disposable single-use female condom provides contraception that is

thought to be comparable to that provided by the male condom while possibly providing enhanced protection from some forms of sexually transmissible infections such as herpesvirus or HIV. The female condom is made from polyurethane, which makes it stronger than the male condom and provides rapid transfer of heat, making it less noticeable in use. The female condom does not require any fitting and may be inserted in advance of sexual activity.

31. **D,** Page 297; Table 13–1 in Mishell. Roughly 75% of American women have used oral contraceptives at some time in their lives. Oral contraceptives are the choice of about one third of women who begin contraceptive use and are currently used by roughly 25% of all women of reproductive age.

32. **A,** Pages 316–319. In a collaborative group review of 54 studies, the analysis indicated that while women took oral contraceptives (OCs) they had a slightly increased risk of having breast cancer diagnosed (relative risk, 1.24). The magnitude of the risk declined steadily after OCs were stopped, so there was no longer a significantly increased risk by 10 or more years after stopping. It was noted that the cancers diagnosed in women taking OCs were less advanced clinically than those that occurred in nonusers. The risk of having breast cancer that had spread beyond the breast compared with a localized tumor was significantly reduced (relative risk, 0.88) in OC users compared to nonusers. Although it is uncertain whether OCs themselves increase the risk of cervical cancer or have no effect, users of OCs are at high risk for cervical neoplasia and require at least annual screening of cervical cytology. The protective effect of OCs relative to endometrial cancer is related to duration of use. The great protective effect is in nulliparous women or women of low parity. The magnitude of the decrease of risk in ovarian cancer is directly related to the duration of OC use. The protective effect begins within 10 years of first use and continues for at least 20 years after the use of OCs ends.

33. **D,** Page 344. Contraindications to IUD use include pregnancy, acute PID, postpartum endometritis within the last 3 months, known or suspected uterine or cervical malignancy, genital bleeding of unknown cause, untreated acute cervicitis, and a previously inserted IUD that has not been removed. Conditions previously thought to preclude IUD use but that are no longer considered to be contraindications include diabetes mellitus, valvular heart disease (including mitral valve prolapse), a history of ectopic pregnancy (excluding progesterone-containing IUDs), nulliparity, treated cervical dysplasia, irregular menses due to anovulation, breast-feeding, corticosteroid use, and age less than 25.

34. **E,** Page 298; Table 13–2 in Mishell. Recent studies show the highest rate of continuing use to be among users of implantable contraceptive rods (Norplant). Of the methods listed, the lowest rate of continuance is among users of the diaphragm, with only 58% of patients continuing their use at 1 year.

35. **E,** Pages 301–302. The use of periodic abstinence for contraception is based on three assumptions: (1) the ovum may be fertilized only during the first 24 hours after ovulation, (2) spermatozoa are capable of fertilizing the ovum for only about 48 hours after ejaculation, and (3) ovulation usually occurs 12 to 16 days before the onset of the next menses. Based on these assumptions, a woman's fertile period is calculated by subtracting 18 days from her shortest cycle length and 11 days from her longest cycle length. Given this woman's pattern of periods, every 28 to 30 days, abstinence from day 10 to 19 of the cycle would be required.

36. **E,** Pages 301–302. Although body temperature alone is less commonly used for natural family planning, it is often used to complement other methods, such as assessment of cervical mucus or of symptoms. When temperature is used to determine when sexual intercourse may be resumed, the third day of consistent temperature elevation is used.

CHAPTER
14

Breast Diseases

for Questions 1–12: Select the one best answer or completion.

1. Which factor associated with benign breast disease is more closely associated with an increased risk of developing breast cancer?

    A. degree of pain
    B. amount of nipple discharge
    C. size of the mass
    D. degree of epithelial hyperplasia
    E. presence of a palpable axillary node

2. The most commonly encountered cancer of the breast is

    A. lobular carcinoma in situ
    B. lobular infiltrating carcinoma
    C. ductal carcinoma in situ
    D. ductal infiltrating carcinoma
    E. inflammatory carcinoma

3. The clearest indication for open breast biopsy in a woman with known fibrocystic breast disease occurs when there is

    A. a persistent, dominant three-dimensional mass on breast examination
    B. blood-tinged fluid on cyst aspiration
    C. lack of pain relief in response to premenstrual diuretic therapy
    D. spontaneous unilateral nipple discharge
    E. multiple cystic areas seen on ultrasonography

4. A 52-year-old woman has persistent, unilateral, spontaneous bloody nipple discharge and a cluster of microcalcifications identified by xeroradiography to be 3 cm deep under the nipple of the left breast. The next step in her management should be

    A. needle aspiration under ultrasound guidance
    B. repeat mammography in 3 months
    C. submission of the bloody discharge for cytologic examination
    D. open biopsy of the left breast on an outpatient basis
    E. computed tomography (CT) examination of the breast and ipsilateral axillary nodes

5. The drug showing the most efficacy in treating severe symptomatic fibrocystic disease is

    A. tamoxifen
    B. danazol
    C. bromocriptine
    D. hydrochlorothiazide
    E. medroxyprogesterone acetate

6. The factor most predictive of an adverse outcome from therapy for invasive breast cancer is

    A. microscopic involvement of axillary nodes
    B. histologic type
    C. receptor status
    D. patient age
    E. extent of disease on mammography

7. **The lifetime risk of breast carcinoma in the future in a woman who has had a subcutaneous mastectomy for severe symptomatic fibrocystic breast disease is**

   A. increased fivefold
   B. increased twofold
   C. unchanged
   D. decreased twofold
   E. decreased fivefold

8. **A twofold to fourfold greater risk of breast carcinoma is associated with carcinoma of the**

   A. pancreas
   B. stomach
   C. breast
   D. cervix
   E. colon

9. **The greatest lifetime risk of breast cancer is associated with a(n)**

   A. early menarche
   B. late menopause
   C. history of oral contraceptive use longer than 10 years
   D. history of postmenopausal estrogen use longer than 10 years
   E. first-degree relative with breast cancer

10. **The main advantage of a fine-needle aspiration of a breast mass over open biopsy is**

    A. reduced cost
    B. a lower false-negative rate
    C. better documentation of invasive disease
    D. better documentation of in situ disease
    E. reduced distortion of the surrounding tissue

11. **The single best treatment for a 52-year-old woman with a unilateral 2-cm infiltrating carcinoma of the right breast is**

    A. a right radical mastectomy
    B. a right modified radical mastectomy
    C. a bilateral modified mastectomy
    D. a right lumpectomy plus radiation
    E. unknown

12. **The most significant factor in the prediction of systemic disease in a patient with breast carcinoma is**

    A. an initial tumor greater than 2 cm
    B. a high mitotic index
    C. a low thymidine labeling index
    D. the DNA content
    E. the absence of estrogen receptors

DIRECTIONS:

for Questions 13–22: For each numbered item, select the one heading most closely associated with it. Each lettered heading may be used once, more than once, or not at all.

13–16. Match the diagnostic procedure with the statement.

   A. digital radiography
   B. ultrasonography
   C. thermography
   D. CT
   E. magnetic resonance imaging

13. **Is best used in differentiating a cystic breast mass from a solid mass.**

14. **Can best differentiate benign from malignant tissue.**

15. **Radiation exposure is one-tenth that of conventional mammographic equipment.**

16. **Published clinical studies suggest low sensitivity and poor specificity.**

17–19. Match the disease with the description.

   A. fibrocystic breast disease
   B. fibroadenoma
   C. cystosarcoma phyllodes
   D. intraductal papilloma

17. **Rapidly growing breast tumor that occurs primarily in the fifth decade and accounts for 1% of breast malignancies.**

18. **Predominant symptom is spontaneous unilateral nipple discharge in perimenopausal women.**

19. **Most common breast tumor in adolescents.**

20–22. Match the phases of fibrocystic breast disease with the description.

A. hyperplastic
B. mazoplastic
C. adenosis
D. cystic

20. Usually occurs in women in their 40s and includes cysts up to 5 cm in size.

21. Usually occurs in women in their 20s and is characterized by pain in the axillary tails.

22. Usually occurs in women in their 30s with a histologic picture of marked ductal hyperplasia.

DIRECTIONS:

for Questions 23–32: Select the one best answer or completion.

23. On breast examination, you find a 3-cm cystic mass in the upper outer quadrant of the left breast of a 38-year-old woman. You plan to aspirate this cyst in the office. You should also plan to

A. perform an open biopsy to remove the cyst wall
B. submit the fluid for cytologic examination
C. recheck the site of the cyst in 2 to 4 weeks
D. perform a mammogram within 48 hours after the aspiration

24. Breast self-examination is recommended because it is associated with

A. earlier detection of cancer
B. predominately stage I disease
C. improved survival rates for malignant disease
D. fewer false-negative examination results

25. Fibrocystic breast change is characterized by

A. cyclic enlargement of the axillary nodes
B. diffuse bilateral findings
C. blunted response to cyclic ovarian hormones
D. uniform histologic changes
E. uniform clinical findings

26. A 48-year-old woman has undergone a screening mammogram (xeroradiography). The report states that there is an area of microcalcification. The characteristic of this microcalcification that conveys the most ominous prognosis is

A. a spherical distribution
B. a stellate (star-shaped) distribution
C. linear cords of calcification
D. the findings should be confirmed by ultrasonography
E. a negative fine-needle aspiration of the area would be reassuring

27. Identifiable risk factors predict what percentage of women who will experience the disease?

A. 25%
B. 35%
C. 50%
D. 65%
E. 75%

28. The American Cancer Society guidelines regarding screening mammograms for patients with a family history of breast cancer suggest that these patients should

A. undergo mammography twice annually
B. undergo mammography at 1-year intervals between the ages of 40 and 49 years
C. undergo annual mammography after the age of 35
D. undergo mammography beginning 10 years before the age of detection of cancer in a first-degree relative
E. (no guidelines are available)

29. Cyclic changes in breast tissue include

A. parenchymal ductal ectasia without proliferation
B. an increase in breast volume
C. differentiation of secretory cells into alveolar cells
D. increased prolactin production by the breast

30. Which of the following is true of fibroadenomas?

A. Fibroadenomas are characterized by pain.
B. They undergo cyclic change in response to the menstrual cycle.
C. Spontaneous resolution occurs in 30% of cases.
D. The risk of breast cancer is reduced.
E. They are solitary.

31. The most common symptom of an intraductal papilloma is

A. a unilateral nipple discharge
B. a bilateral nipple discharge
C. pain
D. skin change
E. a palpable mass

32. Mutations in the BRCA1 and BRCA2 genes are associated with a lifetime risk of breast cancer of approximately

A. 25%
B. 45%
C. 60%
D. 85%
E. 100%

ANSWERS

1. **D,** Page 363. The symptom complex and physical findings may be similar in benign breast disease and breast cancer. Pain and tenderness, a mass, and nipple discharge are characteristics of both. Numerous epidemiologic studies have found that the risk of breast cancer is increased in women with benign breast disease and associated epithelial hyperplasia. Although the presence of a palpable axillary node in a patient with breast cancer worsens the prognosis, this finding alone, with no known malignant disease of the breast, does not indicate an increased risk of breast cancer.

2. **D,** Page 383. There are numerous classifications of breast cancer that contain both clinical and pathologic subgroups. In general, this tumor is similar to other adenocarcinomas found in other female reproductive organs. It originates most often in the epithelium of the collecting ducts and less often in the terminal lobular ducts. Ductal infiltrating carcinoma is by far the most common cancer (80%), with infiltrating lobular carcinoma occurring in approximately 9% of patients. In situ ductal carcinoma is limited to the surface of the ductal epithelium, with invasive cancer developing from this disease within 10 years of diagnosis in 35% of patients. Both variants of lobular carcinoma occur in a young age group, are less virulent, and have a longer latency period. Inflammatory carcinomas account for approximately 2% of breast cancers. This type is recognized clinically as a rapidly growing, highly malignant carcinoma. Infiltration of malignant cells into the lymphatics of the skin produces a clinical picture that simulates a skin infection. There is not a specific histologic type.

3. **A,** Pages 382–383. Although most symptomatic patients with fibrocystic breast disease respond to medical treatment, the presence of a dominant three-dimensional mass that does not change mandates biopsy. When blood-tinged fluid is aspirated, it should be sent for histologic analysis. Biopsy is indicated if the histologic finding is positive or if the mass does not disappear with aspiration. The approach would be similar for

cysts seen on breast ultrasonography. Spontaneous discharge alone does not necessarily warrant biopsy until further diagnostic assessments (eg, mammography) are made. Likewise, lack of response to diuretic treatment of premenstrual pain symptoms does not by itself warrant biopsy.

4. **D,** Pages 382–383. This patient has two indications for open breast biopsy: the presence of a spontaneous bloody nipple discharge and the presence of microcalcification (cluster) on xeroradiography. The cluster itself creates an approximately 25% chance of cancer, which should be evaluated by thorough tissue evaluation. A positive needle biopsy alone is acceptable in certain centers, but open biopsy is still the procedure of choice in most centers in the United States because needle biopsy has a false-negative rate of approximately 20%. Additional imaging studies would not be useful in this patient before histologic evaluation.

5. **B,** Page 365. Danazol relieves breast symptoms and reduces nodularity in approximately 90% of patients. Depending on the age of the patient, this effect may last for several months after discontinuation of danazol, although symptoms eventually reappear. Tamoxifen, synthetic progestins, or bromocriptine may be beneficial in patients who are not responding to danazol. Diuretic therapy is often used for symptomatic treatment of women with mild to moderate premenstrual complaints associated with water retention. Some data indicate efficacy when tamoxifen is used as adjunctive treatment for breast cancer. This medication may be used in situations wherein positive estrogen receptors are identified in malignant breast tissue.

6. **C,** Page 383. Cure rates for breast cancer have steadily improved since 1989, and the majority of women with breast cancer survive their disease. The three most important variables to consider when planning breast cancer treatment are the inherent histologic aggressiveness of the tumor, the presence of histologically positive nodes, and the receptor status (as another indicator of cell maturation). Microscopic metastatic disease

occurs early via both hematogenous and lymphatic routes, with approximately one third of women having positive histologic involvement of the nodes without gross adenopathy. It should be understood that breast cancer is to be considered a systemic disease at the time of diagnosis regardless of the initial clinical presentation. In general, hormone receptor–positive tumors are better differentiated and exhibit less aggressive clinical behavior (with a 60% to 80% response rate to adjunctive hormonal manipulation) when both estrogen and progesterone receptors are positive, making receptor status the best predictor of outcome. Older women are likely to be in poorer health and thus less likely to be candidates for some of the treatment options, but this does not alter the efficacy of tumor therapy. Because breast cancer should be considered a systemic disease, findings on mammography generally do not predict the type of treatment that patients should receive or their prognosis.

7. **C,** Page 365. On rare occasions, a woman with severe fibrocystic change is treated surgically either by total mastectomy, which involves removal of all the breast tissue, or by subcutaneous mastectomy, which produces a better cosmetic result. The operative procedure is usually followed by insertion of prosthetics. However, subcutaneous mastectomy does not remove all the breast tissue; therefore, if surgery is being performed prophylactically, the patient should understand that the risk of breast cancer remains about the same. These risk factors are contingent primarily on other risk factors for the development of carcinoma—in particular, family history.

8. **E,** Pages 365, 368–369. Women with ovarian, endometrial, or colon carcinoma have a twofold to fourfold greater risk of breast carcinoma. Once the patient has carcinoma in one breast, the risk in the other breast is approximately 1% per year. The extent of epithelial hyperplasia and atypia in women with benign breast disease determines the magnitude of risk for carcinoma.

9. **E,** Page 368; Table 14–3 in Stenchever. Of the risk factors described, a first-degree relative with breast cancer confers the greatest risk. Early menarche and late menopause are less important but still increase the risk slightly. Estrogens are considered tumor promoters in respect to the pathophysiology of breast carcinoma rather than as inducers or initiators of carcinoma. Thus, any adverse effects should be increased with duration of use, and a dose-response curve should be recognized. Recently reported epidemiologic studies have found an elevated risk for subsets of women under the age of 45. However, there was no consistent evidence of an increase in breast cancer risk in middle-aged women, even long-term oral contraceptive users.

10. **A,** Pages 381–382. Fine-needle biopsy of suspicious breast lesions is an inexpensive way to provide rapid diagnosis in the ambulatory setting. When a fine-needle aspiration or biopsy is positive, this technique reduces the incidence of open biopsy. However, a negative result is nondiagnostic, and an open biopsy must be performed subsequently because of the high false-negative rate. Fine-needle aspiration does not differentiate noninvasive from invasive carcinoma, and it does not delineate the extent of an in situ ductal carcinoma. While fine-needle biopsy causes minimal distortion of both the tumor and the surrounding tissue, both open and needle biopsies cause enough tissue reaction that mammography must be delayed by at least a month to avoid the confounding effects of the induced artifacts.

11. **E,** Pages 387–388. Until the early 1980s, radical mastectomy was the standard operation for carcinoma of the breast. With a better understanding of cancer of the breast as a systemic disease, there has been a change in therapeutic emphasis toward less radical surgery and an increase in the use of radiotherapy and chemotherapy. Recently concluded randomized prospective studies have found no difference in the therapeutic results in terms of conservative surgery and postoperative radiation versus radical surgery for stage I or stage II breast carcinoma. It is important to offer every woman alternatives in the treatment of this disease, including a discussion of cosmetic results and patient concerns regarding body image.

12. **A,** Pages 385–387. The two major factors in predicting the likelihood of systemic spread in a patient with breast carcinoma are the diameter of the primary tumor and the number of positive axillary nodes. Women whose initial tumor is less than 2 cm in diameter with negative axillary tumors have a 5-year survival rate of over 90%. Other factors, such as mitotic index, the thymidine-labeling index, DNA content, and presence or absence of estrogen and progesterone receptors, are also predictors of an extended disease-free interval, but they are less important than the size of the initial lesion.

13–16. 13, **B;** 14, **E;** 17, **A;** 16, **C;** Pages 373–383. Certain characteristics of numerous screening and diagnostic tests available limit their usefulness and application to large-scale use. Ultrasound imaging may be useful when a cystic mass must be differentiated from a solid mass, especially when an attempt to aspirate the mass has failed. However, this method is limited by not being able to identify microcalcifications reliably or to detect lesions smaller than 2 mm. Thermography is both insensitive and nonspecific, so it is not recommended. Digital radiography is the technique by which x-ray photons are detected after passing through the breast tissue. It will probably be the screening modality of the future because it reduces radiation exposure to one tenth that of other radiographic techniques. Magnetic resonance imaging is too cumbersome to be considered an effective screening measure, but it can differentiate benign from malignant tissue. It may prove effective as a diagnostic test in certain cases, such as predicting the extent of disease and recurrence.

17–19. 17, **C**; 18, **D**; 19, **B**; Pages 362–367. Cystosarcoma phyllodes is a fibroepithelial tumor that usually arises from fibroadenomas. These tumors are rare, but since they are malignant approximately 25% of the time, they constitute the most common type of breast sarcoma. They contrast with fibroadenoma of the breast, which is often found in teenagers as an isolated painless lump. The treatment of a fibroadenoma is simple excision. An intraductal papilloma is usually small, and treatment is not necessary if malignancy has been ruled out by excisional biopsy.

20–22. 20, **D**; 21, **B**; 22, **C**; Pages 363–365. The three phases of clinical fibrocystic breast disease are mazoplastic, adenosis, and cystic. These phases correlate well with changes found in women in the third, fourth, and fifth decades of life. Each stage has associated histologic characteristics and a symptom complex. In general, the history of fibrocystic breast disease is characterized by proliferation and hyperplasia of the lobular, ductal, and acinar epithelium with accompanying fibrous tissue proliferation.

23. **C**, Page 364. Needle aspiration of pathologic breast tissue is a useful test that lies between palpation of the breast and open biopsy. Mammography, if warranted, should be performed first because needle aspiration might cause hematoma formation that would obscure mammographic detail. Aspirated fluid need not be sent for cytologic examination. Bloody fluid most often indicates a traumatic aspiration rather than the rare cystic carcinoma. In this event, if the mass concomitantly disappears, the aspiration completes the workup. All patients should be rechecked in 2 to 4 weeks to confirm complete resolution of the mass. If the mass has not disappeared, an open biopsy is required.

24. **C**, Pages 372–373. The kinetics of growth in breast carcinoma suggest that it doubles in volume every 3 months and doubles in diameter every year. It usually takes 6 to 8 years to reach a diameter of 1 cm. It takes another year before reaching 2 cm, which is the mean diameter of a breast cancer found through regular monthly breast self-examination (BSE). When the cancer is found by this technique, it is clinical stage I 38% of the time. The use of BSE has been shown to increase the woman's chance of survival from roughly 60% to about 75% and should be encouraged for all patients. While the majority of masses found by BSE are benign, all masses require further evaluation.

25. **B**, Page 364. Fibrocystic breast changes represent an exaggerated response of the breast tissue to cyclic ovarian hormone production, and clinical evidence of this entity can be found in approximately one third of American women. Characteristic findings in these patients do not include demonstrable cyclic changes in the axillary nodes, although some women complain of pain radiating toward the axilla along the axillary tail of Spence. It has been postulated that fibrocystic changes occur in response to increased daily prolactin production, although there is no documentation that fibrocystic change is more common in women with elevated serum prolactin levels. Both the histologic and the clinical findings in this condition are highly variable, though they tend to involve both breasts equally.

26. **B**, Page 376. The presence of five calcifications within a volume of 1 mL is called a *cluster*. Subsequent breast biopsies find 25% of these to be associated with cancer and 75% with benign disease. Therefore, this finding should be more vigorously pursued through tissue confirmation. Because of better edge enhancement with xeromammography, microcalcifications are generally better seen with this technique. Microcalcifications are not seen well through ultrasonography because of poor resolution of masses smaller than 2 mm. A negative fine-needle aspiration is never sufficient to rule out the possibility of carcinoma and should be followed by an open biopsy. Because of the increased risk of cancer with the findings stated, many authors advocate proceeding directly to open biopsy. Microcalcifications in a spherical pattern suggest a lesion that is pushing the surrounding tissue rather than infiltrating. Linear calcifications are most often associated with ductal processes but are not good predictors of histopathology.

27. **A**, Page 368. Although there are a number of known risk factors for the development of breast cancer, the long latency period of the disease before clinical presentation makes the importance of identifying risk factors less helpful. Although there are limits in the clinical applicability of risk factors, women at increased risk should be screened more frequently than persons at normal risk. Many risk factors are additive. At best,

knowledge of risk factors can be used to identify only 25% of women who experience the disease. In the United States, approximately 1 in 11 (9%) women can be expected to contract breast cancer. Although familial tendencies have been noted, no specific genetic inheritance pattern has been identified. Both the BRCA1 and BRCA2 genes have been implicated in the inheritance of breast cancer. Unfortunately, a large number of specific mutations of these genes have been identified, and no single gene has been identified that carries greater diagnostic implications. In general, women with mutations of these genes carry an 85% lifetime risk of breast cancer and are also at increased risk for ovarian cancer.

28. **D,** Pages 375, 378; Table 14–4 in Stenchever. Based on large-scale studies regarding the efficacy of mammographic screening programs (Health Insurance Plan of New York; Breast Cancer Detection Demonstration Project) and the development of sensitive low-dose radiation techniques, the American Cancer Society suggests a baseline mammographic examination between ages 35 and 40; mammography at least every other year between the ages of 40 and 50; and annual mammography for women age 50 and older. No specific guidelines were made for more frequent mammographic examinations with available techniques because an analysis of the rate of tumor growth versus sensitivity of current techniques did not support such recommendations. The current guidelines do not address screening for patients with a family history of breast cancer. It is generally accepted that these patients should begin regular screening studies 5 years before the youngest age of diagnosis of breast cancer in the family.

29. **A,** Page 361. Breast tissue responds to the cyclic hormonal changes of estrogen and progesterone production. During the follicular phase, parenchymal proliferation of the ducts occurs. This is followed by dilation of the ductal system and differentiation of the alveolar cells into secretory cells during the luteal phase. Premenstrual breast symptoms are thought to be secondary to increased blood flow, vascular engorgement, and water retention that results in increased breast volume. Although the breast secretory cells are sensitive to prolactin, none of this hormone is thought to be produced locally in the breast tissue.

30. **C,** Pages 365–366. Fibroadenomas are characteristically found serendipitously because they neither change with the menstrual cycle nor produce pain. Although 30% of fibroadenomas regress and an additional 10% to 12% become smaller with time, affected patients must be carefully followed up because their risk of breast cancer is increased twofold. Multiple fibroadenomas are present in 15% to 20% of patients.

31. **A,** Page 366. The most common symptom of an intraductal papilloma is unilateral nipple discharge.

32. **D,** Page 369. Mutations of the BRCA1 and BRCA2 genes are associated with an 85% lifetime risk of breast cancer. Patients with mutation of the BRCA1 gene have a lifetime risk of ovarian cancer that is approximately 40% to 50%, while mutations of the BRCA2 gene carry a 15% to 20% risk of ovarian cancer.

Adult Sequelae of Fetal Exposure to Diethylstilbestrol (DES)

for Questions 1–14: Select the one best answer or completion.

1. Clear cell adenocarcinoma appears to originate in a specific cell type within vaginal adenosis. This cell type is the

   A. endocervical cell
   B. tuboendometrial cell
   C. reserve cell
   D. underlying vaginal stroma cell
   E. underlying cervical stroma cell

2. The origin of vaginal adenosis is thought to be columnar epithelium derived from the

   A. metanephros
   B. yolk sac
   C. wolffian ducts
   D. vaginal plate
   E. müllerian ducts

3. A woman is known to have had an in utero exposure to DES. A cervical biopsy is taken from the most abnormal portion of the cervix as determined by colposcopic evaluation. Histologically, the area is reported as either active immature squamous cell metaplasia or dysplasia. Analysis of the DNA content of the lesion indicates aneuploidy. From these results, you would assume the chromosomal number and histologic diagnosis to be

   A. Chromosomal number—triple the haploid number; histologic diagnosis: dysplasia
   B. Chromosomal number—not an exact multiple of the diploid number; histologic diagnosis: dysplasia
   C. Chromosomal number—double the haploid number; histologic diagnosis: dysplasia
   D. Chromosomal number—less than the haploid number; histologic diagnosis: active immature squamous metaplasia
   E. Chromosomal number—not an exact multiple of the diploid number; histologic diagnosis: active immature squamous metaplasia

4. With a normal initial pelvic examination in a DES-exposed woman, follow-up examinations should be scheduled every

   A. month for a year, then every 3 months for a year, then every 6 months
   B. 3 months for 2 years, then every 6 months
   C. 6 months for 2 years, then every year
   D. 6 months
   E. year

5. The cervicovaginal abnormalities associated with exposure to DES, such as vaginal adenosis, over time are likely to

   A. remain stable
   B. become dysplastic
   C. develop into a clear cell adenocarcinoma
   D. develop into a squamous cell carcinoma
   E. regress

6. DES-associated clear cell adenocarcinoma is a time-limited disease because the FDA placed limitations on its use in

   A. 1941
   B. 1951
   C. 1961
   D. 1971
   E. 1981

7. While following up a 30-year-old patient with vaginal adenosis associated with in utero DES exposure, you learn that she is planning to conceive. Before she becomes pregnant, she should undergo

   A. cerclage
   B. hysterosalpingography
   C. adenosis ablation
   D. laparoscopic examination
   E. routine preconception counseling

8. In a DES-exposed woman, the risk of clear cell adenocarcinoma of the vagina or cervix is

   A. 1 in 100
   B. 1 in 200
   C. 1 in 400
   D. 1 in 500
   E. 1 in 1000

9. A 32-year-old gravida 0 was examined by you for the first time 4 weeks ago. Because of the appearance of her cervix, you asked her to find out whether her mother had taken DES while "carrying her." Her mother's physician forwarded all the medical records. They indicate that 50 mg of DES per day had been prescribed from the 10th to the 20th week of pregnancy because your patient's mother experienced vaginal bleeding during early pregnancy. The Pap smear obtained 4 weeks ago is normal. The patient states that she has had a Pap test every year for more than 5 years and she has never had abnormal results. Today you use a colposcope and see the cervix as pictured in Figure 15–1. You would recommend

   A. a hysterectomy
   B. a large loop excision of the transformation zone (LLETZ)
   C. a laser conization
   D. four-quadrant biopsies
   E. that the patient return in a year

10. The formula for DES is seen in

    A. Figure 15–2, *A*
    B. Figure 15–2, *B*
    C. Figure 15–2, *C*
    D. Figure 15–2, *D*
    E. Figure 15–2, *E*

11. Clear cell adenocarcinomas of the vagina and cervix associated with DES exposure are most likely to be diagnosed in patients in which of the age groups?

    A. younger than 9 years
    B. 9 to 14 years
    C. 15 to 21 years
    D. 22 to 28 years
    E. older than 29 years

FIGURE 15–1 (From DiSaia PJ, Creasman WT: *Clinical Gynecologic Oncology*, 4th ed. St Louis, Mosby, 1993.)

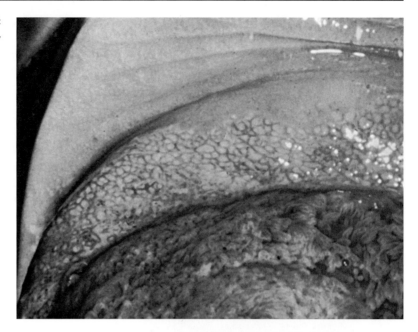

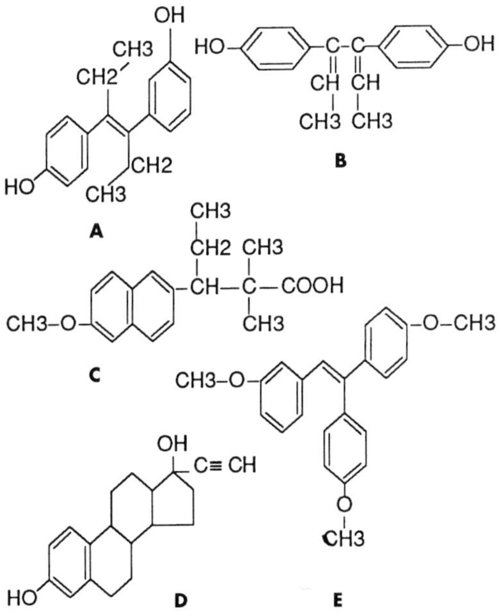

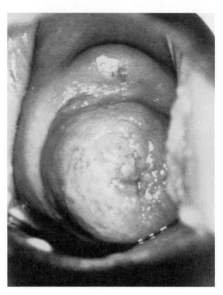

FIGURE 15–2

FIGURE 15–3 (From Robboy SJ, Scully RE, Herbst AL: Pathology of vaginal and cervical abnormalities associated with prenatal exposure to diethylstilbestrol [des]. J Reprod Med 15 : 13–18, 1975.)

12. A 25-year-old gravida 0 with exposure to DES has a Pap smear and biopsy diagnosis of cervical intraepithelial neoplasia II (CIN II) of the cervix. The biopsies were obtained under colposcopic direction. Colposcopy was satisfactory. The appearance of the cervix is depicted in Figure 15–3. Acceptable care of this patient at this juncture is

   A. laser vaporization
   B. cryotherapy
   C. trachelectomy
   D. repeat Pap smear in 6 months
   E. repeat colposcopy in 6 months

13. Of the following, the most likely abnormality to be found in a male because of in utero DES exposure is

   A. infertility
   B. carcinoma of the prostate
   C. epididymal cysts
   D. carcinoma of the testis
   E. hyperplasia of the testis

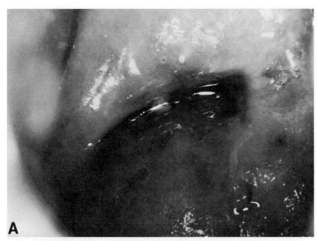

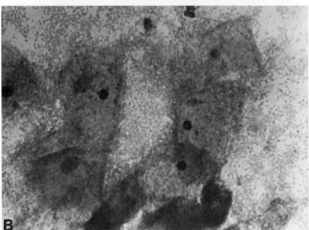

FIGURE 15–4

14. A 25-year-old gravida 0 is referred to a rural health clinic with a complaint of heavy vaginal discharge. The history includes known in utero exposure to DES. Results of previous Pap smears and colposcopy have been negative. On examination, the cervix appears as pictured in Figure 15-4, *A*. A sample of the vaginal discharge is placed on a slide and allowed to dry. The sample is then stained, as shown in Figure 15-4, *B*. The next best step in the treatment of this patient is

A. laser vaporization
B. cryotherapy
C. a biopsy of the cervix at the 7 o'clock position
D. antibiotic therapy
E. excisional biopsy (LEEP)

DIRECTIONS:

for Questions 15–18: For each numbered item, select the one heading most closely associated with it. Each lettered heading may be used once, more than once, or not at all.

A patient has known intrauterine exposure to DES. For each of the conditions listed in Questions 15–18, there is

(A) a great increase in incidence (>25%)
(B) a moderate increase in incidence (>5% but <25%)
(C) a slight increase in incidence (<5%)
(D) a suspected increase in incidence based on clinical studies, but this has not been proved
(E) no data to support an increase in incidence

15. Altered immune response

16. Breast carcinoma

17. Adenosis

18. Ectopic pregnancy

DIRECTIONS:

for each numbered item 19–21, indicate whether it is associated with:

(A) steroidal estrogen only
(B) stilbene-type estrogen only
(C) both steroidal estrogen and stilbene-type estrogen
(D) neither steroidal estrogen nor stilbene-type estrogen

19. Constriction rings near the entrance of the fallopian tube

20. Cervical collar

21. Neural tube defect

DIRECTIONS:

for each numbered item 22–24, indicate whether it is associated with:

(A) DES exposure at 25 weeks
(B) DES exposure at 10 weeks
(C) both (A) and (B)
(D) neither (A) nor (B)

22. Duplication of a ureter

23. Smaller than normal endometrial cavity

24. T-shaped uterus

DIRECTIONS:

for Questions 25–29: Select the one best answer or completion.

25. The probability of a patient exposed in utero to DES having a structural abnormality of the cervix or vagina is increased by a history of

    A. menarche at age 15
    B. pregnancy
    C. DES exposure after week 22 of gestation
    D. DES exposure of less than 2 weeks' duration

26. A 27-year-old gravida 0 who has had follow-up for a cervicovaginal ridge associated with in utero exposure to DES is planning to become pregnant. The most likely outcome of this patient's attempt to have children is

    A. an ectopic pregnancy
    B. infertility
    C. stillbirth
    D. premature delivery
    E. normal pregnancy

27. A 23-year-old gravida 0 who gives a history of in utero exposure to DES requests contraceptive advice. The choice of contraceptive methods is most directly influenced by

    A. gestational age of first exposure
    B. duration of exposure
    C. dosage of DES used
    D. gestational age when therapy stopped
    E. normal contraceptive considerations

28. The approximate number of vaginal cancers reported in DES-exposed women is

    A. 50
    B. 200
    C. 350
    D. 500
    E. 750

29. Which of the following patterns of menarche, menstrual duration, and menstrual flow is most likely to be true of women with in utero exposure to DES?

	Menarche	Menstrual duration	Menstrual flow
A.	Early	Short	Light
B.	Normal	Average	Heavy
C.	Normal	Short	Light
D.	Normal	Prolonged	Heavy
E.	Delayed	Irregular	Light

ANSWERS

1. **B,** Pages 401, 407. It appears that the clear cell adenocarcinomas arise from the tuboendometrial cell.

2. **E,** Page 408. A solid core of squamous cell epithelium that arises from the vaginal plate replaces müllerian-derived columnar epithelium. The vaginal plate grows cephalad from the urogenital sinus, and the solid core of squamous cell epithelium ultimately canalizes to form the permanent lining of the vagina. In mice, when squamous cell transformation of columnar epithelium is arrested by estrogen treatment, persistence of müllerian-type columnar epithelium results in the upper vagina and cervix. In utero exposure to DES in humans may have a similar effect—that is, a DES-induced persistence of glandular epithelium in the vagina leading to adenosis.

3. **B,** Page 403. Tissues having a normal diploid (2N) distribution are euploid and normal. Polyploidy refers to the nuclear DNA measurement being increased by multiples of the diploid amount. Aneuploidy occurs when the DNA content reveals a wide distribution of intermediate modal values that differ from the diploid or polyploid ranges, and often a wide range of intermediate values are encountered. Metaplasia usually contains diploid values and occasionally some polyploid values. Tissues showing an aneuploid distribution usually consist of moderate or severe dysplasia (CIN II or CIN III, respectively) or frank malignancy.

4. **E,** Page 402. The intervals for follow-up examinations depend on the findings and the completeness of the initial examination. Yearly intervals are adequate for most persons.

5. **E,** Page 403. Adenosis, ectropion, and cervicovaginal ridges heal spontaneously in many (but not all) DES-exposed females. The risk of cancer in the DES-exposed female is less than 1 cancer per 1000 exposed women.

6. **D,** Page 399. Insofar as clear cell adenocarcinomas developed in the DES-exposed women through their 20s and early 30s, the cancers will continue to be diagnosed for a number of years, since limited DES usage in pregnancy is known to have continued until 1971.

7. **E,** Page 405. Cerclage is not indicated as an interval procedure. In fact, it should be considered during pregnancy only in patients who have undergone midtrimester losses. Indications for cerclage are no different than if the woman had not been exposed to DES. Although there may be an increased risk for an unfavorable outcome in DES-exposed females with an abnormal hysterosalpingogram, the results of the examination have not been correlated with any individual or specific adverse pregnancy outcome. Routine hysterographic evaluation of DES-exposed females is therefore not warranted. Ablation of the adenosis could destroy a large portion of the reproductive tract. Unless the condition is associated with dysplasia or malignancy, ablation is not indicated. In view of the higher rates of ectopic pregnancy among those exposed to DES, some structural or functional alteration of the fallopian tubes appears likely. This is generally not recognized by laparoscopic examination. This patient requires only routine preconception counseling and evaluations such as the determination of rubella immunity.

8. **E,** Page 407. The risk of clear cell adenocarcinoma of the vagina and cervix is increased in DES-exposed women, but these tumors occur in less than 1 per 1000 exposed women.

9. **E,** Pages 402–403. This woman's age places her at low risk for DES-associated changes. Figure 15–1 depicts a heavy mosaic pattern (histologically proven metaplasia) in a hood surrounding the cervix of a DES-exposed offspring. Squamous cell metaplasia may give rise to an atypical-appearing transformation with areas of "mosaicism" and "punctuation," findings that often suggest the presence of intraepithelial neoplasia in the unexposed female. However, in the DES-exposed offspring, such changes often indicate the presence of active immature squamous cell metaplasia rather than a dysplastic process. Colposcopy does allow for the careful evaluation of the transformation zone in the DES-exposed woman; it provides a guide for biopsy sites in persons whose Pap smears indicate atypia of the squamous cells. In this case, with known negative Pap smears for 5 years, it would be reasonable to do nothing and see the patient again in 1 year.

10. **A,** Page 400; Figure 15–1 in Stenchever. Both *A,* DES, and *B,* dienestrol, are members of the stilbene group and differ only in the location of double bonds. Methallenestril (Vallestril), *C,* is a naphthalene. *D* is chlorotrianisene (TACE), and *E* is ethinyl estradiol.

11. **C,** Page 407; Figure 15–8 in Stenchever. Clear cell adenocarcinomas are extraordinarily rare before age 14. Then there is a rapid rise in the age-incidence curve that plateaus at about age 19, followed by a drop to lower levels through the 20s.

12. **A,** Page 403. Figure 15–3 depicts a vaginal hood. Local destruction of the entire area of intraepithelial neoplasia is important. In the cervix, laser treatment can be used, and occasionally local surgical therapy in the form of conization is

indicated. Although cryotherapy has been used extensively and successfully to treat intraepithelial neoplasia of the cervix in the unexposed woman, it has been reported to be followed by cervical stenosis in many DES-exposed women. For that reason, this type of therapy should be avoided if possible. Trachelectomy (cervicectomy) is unwarranted in a young woman without any children. It represents undertreatment for a malignant process and overtreatment for a benign one.

13. **C,** Page 408. Cryptorchidism, hypoplasia of the testis, epididymal cysts, and abnormalities in semen analyses (though not infertility) have been described in DES-exposed males. The testicular and semen changes have not been verified by some studies. An increased incidence of cancer has not yet been reported. If cryptorchidism is verified, however, an increased incidence of carcinoma could be expected because cryptorchidism is a risk factor for testicular cancer.

14. **D,** Pages 401, 671–672. Figure 15–4 depicts a normal cervix. The smear contains clue cells indicating the presence of bacterial vaginosis. Thus, the patient should be treated. There is no area to ablate with laser or cryotherapy. Vaginal adenosis occurs in about one third, not one half, of DES-exposed females.

15–18. 15, **D;** 16, **D;** 17, **A;** 18, **B;** Pages 403–406; Table 15–2 in Stenchever. On the basis of experimental animal studies, there has been concern that DES-exposed offspring may have an altered immune state and may be subject to an increased frequency of autoimmune disease. Although not establishing a definitive clinical association, these data do raise concern about a possibility of altered immune function in DES-exposed females. The answer to Question 16 is tricky. Because of the high doses of estrogen taken during pregnancy by DES-exposed mothers, there have been concerns of an increased risk of estrogen-sensitive tumors in this group. The question, however, addressed the woman exposed in utero, not the woman actually *ingesting* DES. Recent studies suggest that there may be a mild increase in the risk of breast cancer for those who ingested the drug but that the increased risk is small enough that no change in clinical screening is warranted. Adenosis has been reported to occur in 30% to 90% of DES-exposed subjects. However, data from case-control studies, which are not influenced by the potential bias of self-selection or physician referral, suggest that the overall prevalence is closer to 30% to 40%. Unfavorable pregnancy outcomes, including premature live birth, ectopic pregnancy, and nonviable birth, have been reported more commonly among DES-exposed females. The most

reliable source of data to evaluate these outcome comes from case-control studies that have calculated the outcome of first pregnancies. Of DES-exposed women, 7% experienced ectopic pregnancy.

19–21. 19, **B;** 20, **B;** 21, **D;** Pages 401–403. A constriction ring near the entrance of the fallopian tube and a cervical collar have been associated with DES exposure. Ingestion of steroidal estrogens during pregnancy has not been reported to be associated with such changes. Neither DES exposure nor steroidal estrogen use has been reported to increase the incidence of neural tube defect.

22–24. 22, **D;** 23, **B;** 24, **B;** Pages 401–403. DES exposure does not appear to cause anatomic abnormalities of the urinary tract. Various types of abnormalities of the shape and size of the endometrial cavity have been identified by hysterosalpingograms performed on DES-exposed women. These associations appear in part to be related to the increased risk of uterine changes in persons whose mothers began DES treatment in early pregnancy.

25. **A,** Pages 401–402. (Jeffries JA, Robboy SJ, O'Brien PC, et al: Structural anomalies of the cervix and vagina in women enrolled in the Diethylstilbestrol Adenosis [DESAD] Project. Am J Obstet Gynecol 148 : 59, 1984.) Factors that appear to increase the frequency of structural changes of the cervix and vagina include nulliparity and late menarche. The dosage of DES and the time DES use was started during pregnancy are important interrelated factors. A larger dosage of the drug or initiation of treatment early in pregnancy (ie, before the 18th week) leads to a greater risk of adenosis.

26. **E,** Page 405. Unfavorable pregnancy outcomes, including premature live birth, ectopic pregnancy, and nonviable birth, have been reported more commonly among DES-exposed females. Although reproductive performance in DES progeny has been associated with an increased proportion of unfavorable outcomes, more than 80% of DES-exposed women who desire pregnancy have delivered at least one live-born infant. Primary infertility is more common in DES-exposed females, and tubal factors appear to be a contributory cause.

27. **E,** Page 403. No data indicate that any contraceptive method, including contraceptive steroids, is contraindicated in the DES-exposed female. There has been concern regarding the potential increased risk of endocrine-related tumors. In spite of these concerns, no current evidence indicates increased risk of such malignancies associated with the use of estrogen-containing compounds. Also, there has been concern about prescribing an IUD because of the abnormal

contours of the endometrial cavity shown on hysterosalpingography. It has not yet been demonstrated, however, that the IUD increases the risk in the DES-exposed female.

28. **E,** Page 4. Only about 715 cases of cancer have been identified in the thousands of women regularly examined because of exposure to DES.

29. **C,** Pages 404–405; Figure 15–6 in Stenchever. Studies indicate that women exposed to DES are more likely to have shorter duration and diminished amounts of menstrual flow than other women. There is no difference in the age of menarche when DES-exposed patients are compared with controls.

Spontaneous and Recurrent Abortion

DIRECTIONS:

for Questions 1–17: Select the one best answer or completion.

1. A 23-year-old gravida 4, para 1, ab 3, registered for prenatal care. The patient's first pregnancy, 5 years ago, went to term. She delivered a 3800-g male. This was followed by spontaneous abortions at 18, 16, and 14 weeks. The patient is again pregnant and, according to her last menstrual period, is 14 weeks pregnant. An ultrasound examination was requested and is depicted in Figure 16–1. The next step in management should be

   A. dilatation and curettage (D&C)
   B. amniocentesis for karyotype
   C. a progestational agent
   D. cerclage
   E. bed rest

2. The evidence for an immunologic cause of repetitive abortions is based on

   A. randomized controlled trials
   B. observational data
   C. retrospective studies
   D. epidemiologic data
   E. conjecture

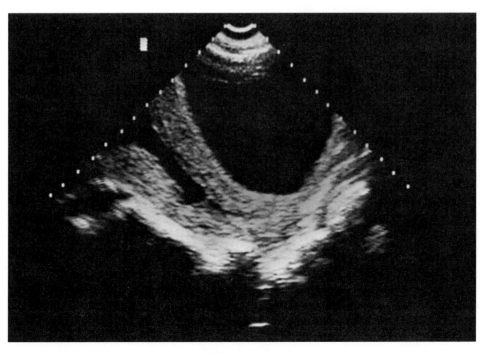

FIGURE 16–1

3. A gravida 3, para 0, ab 3, has just undergone hysterosalpingography, the result of which is shown in Figure 16–2. While discussing this finding, the patient tells you that she had in utero diethylstilbestrol (DES) exposure. This new information suggest that your management should be modified to include

   A. Strassman metroplasty
   B. Jones metroplasty
   C. Tompkins metroplasty
   D. cervical cerclage
   E. no modification indicated

4. A 31-year-old gravida 2, para 1, is 9 weeks pregnant by dates. She reports having bled for 2 days last week. An ultrasound image is obtained and is depicted in Figure 16–3. The most appropriate diagnosis is

   A. missed abortion
   B. threatened abortion
   C. incomplete abortion
   D. complete abortion
   E. blighted ovum

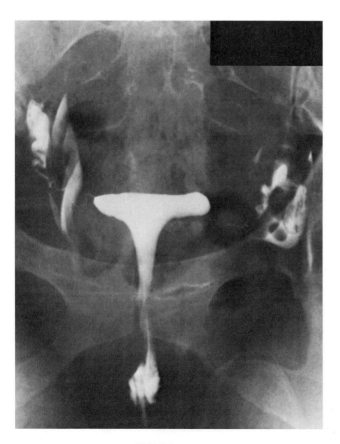

FIGURE 16–2

5. The most common cause of fetal loss is errors in

   A. maternal gametogenesis
   B. paternal gametogenesis
   C. fertilization
   D. zygote division
   E. implantation

6. A 25-year-old unsensitized Rh-negative gravida 4, para 1, ab 2, whose last menstrual period was 10 weeks ago, has just passed some products of conception. This woman states that she has always had regular periods. Current studies indicate that the best management of this patient is

   A. oxytocin
   B. curettage
   C. misoprostol
   D. serial determinations of β-human chorionic gonadotrophin (β-hCG)
   E. observation only

7. An 18-year-old woman and her 20-year-old husband want an explanation for the fact that they have no live-born children. She has a history of two spontaneous abortions at 8 and 10 weeks. The last abortus was submitted for karyotyping and was 45X. The survival rate of 45X conceptions is about 1 in

   A. 300
   B. 200
   C. 100
   D. 50
   E. 2

8. Compared with persons who have aborted once, women who have repetitive abortions and have had no living children are most likely to have

   A. a balanced translocation
   B. 45X abortuses
   C. a uterine or cervical problem
   D. abortuses with trisomy
   E. lupus anticoagulant

9. On examination, an 18-year-old gravida 1, para 0, is noted to have blood coming through her closed cervix. Her last menstrual period was 8 weeks ago, and her uterus is 6 weeks in size. A β-hCG titer is positive. To her knowledge, this woman has not passed any tissue. This constitutes a(n)

   A. incomplete abortion
   B. inevitable abortion
   C. threatened abortion
   D. septic abortion
   E. missed abortion

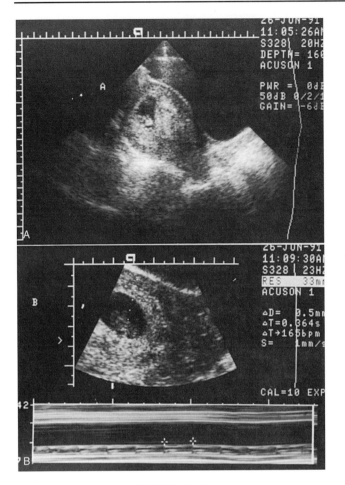

FIGURE 16–3

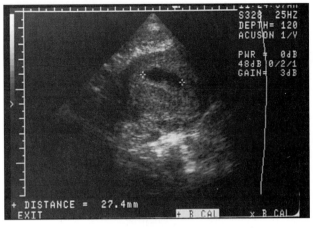

FIGURE 16–4

10. A 30-year-old moved to the United States from India 5 years ago. She has never had a live-born infant, and she has been trying to become pregnant for 8 years. The woman thinks that she aborted on at least two occasions 6 years ago, when she was 4 to 6 weeks late for her period. She showed her physician the material she passed, and he assured her that she had aborted, but there was no histologic proof. For the last 5 years, the woman's periods have been very scant and infrequent. She denies pelvic pain or dysmenorrhea. She does have premenstrual tension, but it is not severe enough to require medication. Her physical examination is completely normal. Her pelvic examination is also normal. The uterus is normal in size, anterior in position, and smooth. The ovaries are easily palpated. There is no pain. The procedure most likely to establish the diagnosis is

A. hysterosalpingogram
B. D&C
C. hysteroscopy
D. laparoscopy
E. laparotomy

11. Patients with systemic lupus erythematosus who have circulating lupus anticoagulant have an increased likelihood of aborting. It has been postulated that this immunoglobulin is responsible for the abortion by

A. promoting the activation of prothrombin
B. decreasing platelet adhesiveness
C. causing complete fetal heart block
D. decreasing prostacyclin formation
E. interfering with the maternal blocking factor

12. A 26-year-old gravida 2, para 1, is 14 weeks pregnant by dates. On pelvic examination, the uterus felt smaller than you would have anticipated. A representative ultrasound image is depicted in Figure 16–4. The most appropriate next step in this patient's treatment is

A. determination of her serum fibrinogen level
B. diagnostic laparoscopy
C. a quantitative serum β-hCG level
D. uterine evacuation
E. culdocentesis

13. The management of a patient with a threatened septic abortion who is not in shock should include

A. single-agent antibiotics
B. an intraarterial line
C. corticosteroids
D. digitalis
E. uterine evacuation

14. A 33-year-old gravida 4, para 0, ab 4, is now 8 weeks pregnant. Ultrasound imaging shows a gestational sac containing a fetus of appropriate size. Cardiac activity is recorded at 140 beats/min. Although the patient has bled for 3 days, a source is not visible on this scan. A serum β-hCG level is at the mean for 8 weeks. The patient states that she is currently staining 6 to 7 pads a day. She does not have cramps. Your management would include

A. thyroid replacement therapy
B. iron replacement therapy
C. absolute bed rest
D. progesterone suppositories
E. aspirin

15. You are counseling a young couple with a history of repetitive abortions. The couple asks about a karyotype on each of them. The most likely finding would be

A. a maternal balanced translocation
B. paternal polyploidy
C. an X chromosome mosaicism of the father
D. a robertsonian translocation
E. no abnormality for either partner

16. The most frequent chromosomal trisomy found in abortuses is

A. 13, 15
B. 16
C. 18
D. 21
E. 22

17. The patient is a 35-year-old gravida 4, para 0, who is interested in attempting another pregnancy. Of the following, which test is most likely to determine the cause of this patient's recurrent pregnancy loss?

A. serum thyroid-stimulating hormone (TSH) level
B. midluteal phase serum progesterone level
C. test for lupus anticoagulant activity
D. hysterosalpingogram
E. culture for *Chlamydia trachomatis*

DIRECTIONS:

for Questions 18–22: For each numbered item, select the one heading most closely associated with it. Each lettered heading may be used once, more than once, or not at all.

18–20. Incidence of embryonic loss

A. 1%–2%
B. 15%–20%
C. 40%
D. 70%
E. 80%

18. Clinically recognized abortions

19. Total human pregnancy loss

20. Percentage of abortions occurring in the first trimester

21–22. In answering Questions 21 and 22, consider Figure 16–5.

A. Figure 16–5, *A*
B. Figure 16–5, *B*
C. Figure 16–5, *C*
D. Figure 16–5, *D*

21. Greatest incidence of spontaneous abortion

22. Metroplasty by the Strassman technique

DIRECTIONS:

For each of the following questions, one of the responses is correct. Select the one best answer or completion.

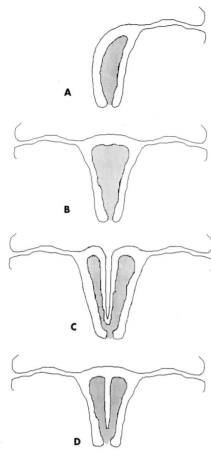

FIGURE 16–5

23. **A woman who smokes two packs per day is at risk for which of the following?**

A. increased likelihood of abortion of a chromosomally normal fetus
B. increased likelihood of trisomy 18
C. increased likelihood of triploidy
D. increased likelihood of monosomy
E. no increase in the risk of abortion

24. **A woman who has undergone a gastrointestinal series and intravenous pyelography at about the time of implantation asks about the most likely impact this x-ray exposure will have on her pregnancy. You should counsel her that she is at**

A. increased risk for abortion of a chromosomally normal fetus
B. increased risk for trisomy 18
C. increased risk for triploidy
D. increased risk for monosomy
E. no increased risk for abortion

25. **A woman who imbibes an alcoholic beverage an average of three times a week should be counseled that she is at**

A. increased risk for abortion of a chromosomally normal fetus
B. increased risk for trisomy 18
C. increased risk for triploidy
D. increased risk for monosomy
E. no increased risk for abortion

26. **Antiphospholipid antibodies have been found in the circulation of women with**

A. recurrent abortions
B. systemic lupus erythematosus only
C. a history of thrombocytopenia
D. a false-negative test result for syphilis
E. chronic users of prostaglandin synthetase inhibitors

27. **A 23-year-old is 5 weeks late for her menstrual period. She started spotting 8 days ago. You obtained a serum β-hCG level 7 days ago that was 3770 mIU/mL and a second β-hCG level yesterday that was 4500 mIU/mL. The most likely diagnosis is a(n)**

A. ectopic pregnancy
B. threatened abortion
C. missed abortion
D. complete abortion
E. normal pregnancy

28. **In counseling a woman about the possibility of a spontaneous abortion in a subsequent pregnancy, the factor in her history that would give the poorest prognosis would be**

A. a history of three previous abortions
B. a maternal age of 35 years
C. a neonatal death
D. a paternal age of 55 years
E. conception within 3 months of her previous pregnancy loss

29. **Embryonic death is established if no cardiac activity is identified by ultrasonography when the embryo is**

A. 2 mm long
B. 4 mm long
C. 6 mm in circumference
D. >10 mm in smallest diameter

ANSWERS

1. **D,** Page 420. The ultrasound image depicted in Figure 16–1 is a longitudinal view through the pelvis. A well-filled bladder and the lower uterine segment and cervix are visible. Since there is fluid in the cervical canal itself, the diagnosis of an incompetent cervix is strongly suggested. The best treatment of cervical incompetence is placement of a concentric nonabsorbable silk or Mersilene suture at the level of the internal os (cerclage), using the technique described by either Shirodkar or McDonald. This ultrasound image does not show the fetus. For a D&C to be indicated, either the history or the ultrasound image should have suggested an embryonic pregnancy, an inevitable or incomplete abortion, or intrauterine fetal death. Nothing in the history suggests a threatened abortion. Besides, although some physicians recommend that patients with threatened abortion restrict their physical activities or be confined to bed rest, there is no evidence that these measures or any active medical therapy improves the prognosis of the threatened abortion. Treatment with progestins was previously advocated, but there is no evidence that such therapy improves the prognosis.

2. **D,** Pages 424–425. An immunologic cause of repetitive abortions is not well established. There are conflicting studies. Some suggest greater sharing of more than one human leukocyte antigen (HLA) at the A, B, and DR locus. An immunologic cause would be supported by a decreased, rather than an increased, maternal blocking factor. This factor, the circulating immunoglobulin G (IgG) antibody, coats the foreign fetal antigens and prevents the fetus from being rejected. Progesterone provides some protection of the fetus from an immunologic effect. This neither supports nor refutes the immunologic cause.

3. **E,** Page 420. No therapy has been shown to be beneficial in lowering the abortion rate in women exposed to DES who have abnormalities of the uterine cavity (see Figure 16–2) and recurrent abortion.

4. **B,** Pages 429–430. This sonogram depicts a 7-week viable pregnancy, as evidenced by the normal fetal heart rate seen in Figure 16–3, *B,* making the diagnosis threatened abortion. It had been quoted that there is a 50% chance of aborting if a patient bleeds before 20 weeks. The recent literature suggests that the risk of abortion is greater among women who bleed for 3 or more days (24%) than in those who bleed only 1 or 2 days (7%). Sonographic studies reveal that in groups of women with threatened abortion and a live fetus, about 85% of these fetuses subsequently are delivered and survive. There is no evidence that women with gestational bleeding who do not abort have an increased incidence of complications of pregnancy, but they may have a slightly increased incidence of fetal anomalies and preterm birth.

5. **A,** Pages 416. Of all fetal losses, 26% are due to errors of maternal gametogenesis; 5% to errors of paternal gametogenesis; 4% to errors of fertilization; and 4% to errors of zygote division.

6. **C,** Page 430. A complete abortion usually occurs before 6 weeks of gestation or after 14 weeks of gestation. In this question, it is fair to assume that the abortion is incomplete. A patient with an inevitable or incomplete abortion may receive intravenous oxytocin, though the small number of oxytocin receptors present in uterine muscle at this stage of pregnancy usually results in poor contractions that are insufficient to reliably empty the uterus. In the past, it was routine to treat these patients with sharp or suction curettage on an outpatient basis. Recent data suggest that it is equally effective to use oral misoprostol, which avoids the possibility of operative complications such as perforation or intrauterine adhesion formation. The evacuation should be complete to minimize the chance of a septic abortion. Since there is always a significant loss of blood, the patient should receive iron supplementation. If the patient is Rh-negative and the father is Rh-positive (or if the Rh is unknown), the woman should receive 50 µg of anti-D γ-globulin.

7. **A,** Page 417. The survival rate of 45X conceptions is about 1 in 300. This is the most common single chromosomal abnormality found in abortus material. The most common type of chromosomal abnormality is an autosomal trisomy. There is evidence that monosomy 45X is associated with a younger maternal age than other aneuploid or euploid abortions. Karyotypes of abortuses of women who have had more than one abortion tend to be similar to the karyotype of the first if the first abortus was either normal or an autosomal trisomy. Chromosomal abnormalities in the parents are an infrequent cause of abortions; in fact, more than 95% of couples who have two or more spontaneous abortions are chromosomally normal.

8. **C,** Pages 419–420, 432, 434. Women with recurrent abortions have a tendency to abort later in gestation, with two thirds of such abortions occurring beyond 12 weeks of gestation. The abortuses of women who have three or more abortions are more likely to be chromosomally

normal (80% to 90%) than those of women with a single spontaneous abortion. If the cause of repetitive abortion is found, it is likely to be associated with a uterine or cervical problem, such as a fusion anomaly, leiomyomata, intrauterine adhesions, or cervical incompetence. If a woman has had no live births and three abortions, she has an approximately 50% chance of having a full-term gestation in her next pregnancy; if she has had one live birth, this chance is increased to about 70%.

9. **C,** Page 430. An incomplete abortion is the passage of some, but not all, fetal or placental tissue through the cervix before 20 weeks of gestation. An *inevitable abortion* is uterine bleeding from a gestation of less than 20 weeks accompanied by cervical dilation but without expulsion of any placental or fetal tissue through the cervix. A *threatened abortion* is the presence of any uterine bleeding from a gestation of less than 20 weeks without any cervical dilation or effacement. A *septic abortion* is any type of abortion that is accompanied by uterine infection. A *missed abortion* is fetal death before 20 weeks of gestation without expulsion of any fetal or maternal tissue for at least 8 weeks thereafter.

10. **C,** Pages 420–421. This woman has a history that is compatible with intrauterine adhesions. The cause is not clear, but perhaps she contracted genital tuberculosis, which is still encountered in India. Adhesions in the uterine cavity can cause partial or complete obliteration of the endometrium, leading to menstrual abnormalities and amenorrhea as well as being a cause of abortion. The best means of diagnosis is hysteroscopy. The problem may be strongly suspected at the time of D&C and can be recognized by hysterosalpingogram. On occasion, adhesions are missed on the hysterosalpingogram. A laparotomy and laparoscopy would not be helpful.

11. **D,** Pages 425–427. It is thought that abortion occurs because of thrombosis in the placental blood supply. Abortions associated with lupus erythematosus often occur during the second trimester. The antibody interferes with formation of prostacyclin, leading to a relative excess of thromboxane, thus causing a thrombotic tendency. There is interference with the activation of prothrombin by the prothrombin activator complex. Decreased platelet adhesiveness is a feature of von Willebrand disease and is implicated in bleeding, not abortion. The fetus of a mother with systemic lupus erythematosus sometimes has a complete heart block. It is unlikely that this is the cause of the increased rate of spontaneous abortion in patients with systemic lupus erythematosus. It has been hypothesized that a maternal

blocking factor coats the foreign fetal antigens and prevents the fetus from being rejected. This concept is still theoretical, and no evidence has been presented to suggest that the lupus anticoagulant in any way interferes.

12. **D,** Pages 430. The ultrasound image suggests the diagnosis of a blighted ovum or a missed abortion. A large gestational sac can be seen, but a fetal pole cannot. There is no evidence of free fluid, making a culdocentesis or laparoscopy unnecessary because the diagnosis of a heterotopic pregnancy is extremely unlikely. A quantitative β-hCG titer is unnecessary. The incidence of hypofibrinogenemia is uncommon in gestations of less than 14 weeks or when the duration of fetal death is less than 6 weeks. The uterus may be evacuated by sharp or suction curettage, although recent studies indicate equal efficacy with greater safety with the use of oral misoprostol.

13. **E,** Page 431. Patients with a septic abortion should receive combination antibiotics, including an agent that is effective against anaerobic bacteria. Newer antibiotics such as imipenem may become an exception to this rule. The uterine cavity should be evacuated to provide drainage of the infected material. Evacuation may be accomplished surgically or medically. Use of an intraarterial line and digitalis may be considered if septic shock develops, but this approach is unnecessary in the case of a septic abortion without shock. Likewise, corticosteroids are not indicated in this patient, and their use in septic shock is controversial.

14. **B,** Page 431. Thyroid and progesterone have not been proved effective in preventing an abortion. In some cases, the presence of vaginal bleeding is the first sign of uterine evacuation of an already nonviable conceptus. The administration of a progestin may increase the probability of a missed abortion. Iron replacement is indicated in women who are bleeding, especially when there is a good chance that the blood loss will be significant. There is no evidence that bed rest is of value. If the woman aborts, the longer she stays in bed, the greater the emotional (and possibly even the financial) loss to the family. Both corticosteroids and aspirin, which inhibit platelet aggregation, have been suggested for patients who have had recurrent abortions, not for patients with a threatened abortion.

15. **D,** Page 417. A maternal and paternal karyotype is an accepted part of the workup of a couple with repetitive abortions. The yield is not large, however. More than 90% of couples in this category are chromosomally normal. Abnormalities occur in the female parent about twice as frequently as in the male. About one half of all

chromosomal abnormalities are balanced recipro-cal translocations, and one fourth are robertsonian translocations. If the karyotype is abnormal, mosaicism in one of the parents (usually X chromosome mosaicism of the mother) is a frequent finding. If a translocation is found in one parent, about 80% of the pregnancies will abort.

16. **B**, Page 417. In most surveys of chromosomal anomalies of abortuses, the relative frequency of the types of anomalies is similar. The most frequent type is autosomal trisomy, which accounts for about half the abnormal karyotypes. Trisomies of all autosomes except for autosome 1 have been reported after karyotyping of abortions, with trisomy 16 being the most frequent. About one third of all autosomal trisomies in abortuses are trisomy 16, with trisomy 13, 15, 21, and 22 the next most common.

17. **D**, Pages 414, 432, 434. The most common cause of recurrent pregnancy losses for patients with more than three losses is a uterine or cervical abnormality. Numerous infectious agents present in the cervix, uterine cavity, or seminal fluid have been postulated to be etiologic factors for abortion. *Chlamydia trachomatis* is a common sexually trans-mitted pathogen, but there is no evidence that it causes abortion in asymptomatic women. This test should be considered as a part of this patient's routine care based on the prevalence of *Chlamydia* in the local population or the presence of specific risk factors in the patient's history. The workup for a couple with a history of recurrent abortion should include a history and physical examination with pertinent questions regarding cervical incompetence. Even though the likelihood of detecting an abnormality is low, it should also incorporate a complete blood count, a serum TSH level, a midluteal phase serum progesterone measurement, and tests to detect lupus anticoagu-lant. A hysterogram should be obtained. If no abnormalities are found, karyotyping of the husband and the wife is indicated.

18–20. 18, **B**; 19, **D**; 20, **E**; Pages 414–415. About 15% to 20% of all known human pregnancies terminate in clinically recognized abortion. However, the incidence of total human embryonic loss is estimated to be much higher. The rate of human pregnancy loss is estimated to be as high as 70%. About 80% of abortions occur in the first trimester, with the incidence decreasing with increasing gestational age.

21–22. 21, **A**; 22, **C**; Pages 419–420. Figure 16–5, *A*, shows a unicornuate uterus; *B* shows a normal uterus; *C* shows a bicornuate uterus; and *D* shows a sep-tate uterus. The unicornuate uterus is associated with the greatest incidence of spontaneous abortion: about 50%. This figure is higher than the

25% to 30% reported with either a septate or a bicornuate uterus. A bicornuate uterus can be unified with the Strassman technique. Either a transfundal metroplasty, as described by Jones or Tompkins, or a transcervical hysteroscopic resection of the uterine septum is the method used to correct a septate uterus. Surgical correction should not be considered if the woman has never aborted, and it should not be performed until other causes of abortion have been ruled out.

23. **A**, Page 427. In one study, for women who smoked more than 14 cigarettes per day, the risk of having an abortion was 1.7 times greater than for women who did not smoke. There was no increased risk of an aneuploid abortion in smokers.

24. **E**, Pages 428–429. There is little likelihood that irradiation of less than 0.05 Gy (several times greater than the amount used in all diagnostic procedures listed) causes an abortion in a person, even if irradiation is administered during the time of implantation.

25. **A**, Page 428. The risk of abortion is three times normal with daily ingestion of alcohol; it is twice normal in women who drink at least 2 days a week. As with smokers, the risk of abortion is confined to chromosomally normal embryos.

26. **A**, Pages 425–426. Lupus anticoagulant and antiphospholipid antibodies have been found in women with systemic lupus erythematosus as well as in those with other connective tissue diseases. These substances have been found in women with a history of recurrent thrombotic episodes and in women with no other disease process. About 50% of women with lupus antico-agulant have a false-positive serologic test result for syphilis. Lupus anticoagulant is found in a subset of women with recurrent abortions.

27. **C**, Page 433. A β-hCG level of 3770 mIU/mL is not compatible with a normal pregnancy of 8 to 9 weeks. In normal gestations, the level of hCG doubles about every 2 days, and the rate of increase in a particular patient can be compared with the expected normal rate of increase. By definition, this cannot be called a normal preg-nancy because the patient is bleeding. The finding that the β-hCG is not rising as expected strongly suggests that this pregnancy will be lost. While this pattern of inappropriate β-hCG occurs in ectopic pregnancies, the most likely cause is a failing pregnancy or missed abortion.

28. **A**, Pages 432–434. When talking to a woman who is contemplating pregnancy, it is important to know the facts about previous pregnancies. The risk of a pregnancy terminating in a spon-taneous abortion increases with increasing mater-nal and paternal age, but the change is small compared with other risk factors. For women with

no live births and a reproductive history of three pregnancies that terminated in abortion, the chance of having an abortion in a subsequent pregnancy is about 50%. For women with at least one live birth and three spontaneous abortions, there is only a 30% chance that the next pregnancy will terminate in abortion. Since the mid-1970s, the incidence of a spontaneous abortion in a woman with diabetes, when the condition is controlled either by diet or by insulin, is the same as in the general population. If conception occurs within 3 months after a live birth, the incidence of abortion is slightly increased compared with the relatively stable rate if conception occurs more than 3 months after a live birth.

29. **B,** Page 430. Embryonic death is established when no cardiac activity is demonstrated by ultrasonography of an embryo greater than 4 mm in length.

CHAPTER
17

Ectopic Pregnancy

for Questions 1–14: Select the one best answer or completion.

1. An 18-year-old woman is seen in the emergency department. She is 5 weeks late for her period. She is sexually active and has used foam irregularly for contraception. At the time you see her, her blood pressure is 90/60 and her pulse is 110. She is receiving Ringer's lactate. The intern has performed a pelvic ultrasound examination, which shows free fluid in the abdominal cavity. A pregnancy test is negative. You would

   A. admit and observe
   B. obtain computed tomography of the abdomen and pelvis
   C. perform culdocentesis
   D. obtain a radioimmunoassay for β-human chorionic gonadotropin (β-hCG)
   E. perform laparotomy

2. The overall subsequent conception rate for women who have had an ectopic pregnancy is

   A. 30%
   B. 40%
   C. 50%
   D. 60%

3. Of women who have had an ectopic pregnancy, the number who have a subsequent live birth is about

   A. one quarter
   B. one third
   C. one half
   D. two thirds
   E. three quarters

4. In patients with a ruptured tubal pregnancy, nonclotting blood is almost always found in the peritoneal cavity. The reason that this blood does not clot is that the blood

   A. has not been outside of the body
   B. has been mixed with peritoneal fluid
   C. has previously clotted
   D. is diluted to a hematocrit of less than 15%
   E. is of fetal origin

5. Women with ectopic pregnancies should receive Rh(D) immunoglobulin if they are

   A. Rh negative, antibody negative
   B. Rh negative, antibody positive
   C. Rh positive, antibody negative
   D. Rh positive, antibody positive
   E. Du positive, antibody negative

6. In cases in which a salpingectomy is the treatment of choice for a ruptured tubal pregnancy,

   A. the ipsilateral ovary should also be removed
   B. the contralateral ovary should also be removed
   C. both ovaries should be removed
   D. both ovaries should be preserved if possible

7. With currently available equipment for abdominal ultrasonography, a "fetal pole" or embryonic sac in the oviduct can be visualized in approximately what percentage of patients with tubal pregnancies?

   A. 75%
   B. 65%
   C. 50%
   D. 35%
   E. 25%

8. According to current epidemiologic data, the single largest factor contributing to the number of women with ectopic pregnancy is

   A. an increase in the fertility rate
   B. an increase in the number of adolescents becoming pregnant
   C. gamete intrafallopian transfer (GIFT)
   D. an increase in the incidence of salpingitis
   E. a decrease in the use of barrier contraception

9. Although the overall death rate/case rate ratio of ectopic pregnancy has decreased sevenfold since 1970, the annual percentage of all maternal deaths in the United States resulting from ectopic pregnancy has nearly doubled. The main reason for this is a(n)

   A. increase in pregnancy rates among unmarried women
   B. death rate/case rate ratio in black women that has increased threefold
   C. decrease in maternal mortality associated with term pregnancy
   D. decrease in the rate of complications from legal abortion

10. The greatest risk of a subsequent ectopic pregnancy follows

    A. one induced abortion
    B. two induced abortions
    C. prior postpartum endometritis
    D. previous pelvic surgery
    E. a previous ectopic pregnancy

11. β-hCG levels in patients with a tubal ectopic pregnancy follow a pattern of change that is characterized by being

    A. identical to an intrauterine gestation
    B. more gradual than an intrauterine gestation
    C. generally flat
    D. marked by periodic rises and falls
    E. highly variable

12. The most consistent symptom of ectopic pregnancy is

    A. amenorrhea
    B. vaginal bleeding
    C. subjective symptoms of pregnancy
    D. abdominal pain
    E. passage of tissue

13. The main advantage of not removing the oviduct at the time of surgery for an unruptured tubal pregnancy is a(n)

    A. increase in the subsequent live birth rate
    B. decreased repeat ectopic pregnancy rate
    C. reduction in overall maternal mortality
    D. decreased incidence of future anovulatory bleeding

14. The chemotherapeutic agent used for the medical treatment of an ectopic pregnancy is

    A. doxorubicin
    B. mifepristone (RU486)
    C. cyclophosphamide
    D. methotrexate
    E. chlorambucil

DIRECTIONS:

for Questions 15–20: For each numbered item, select the one heading most closely associated with it. Each lettered heading in Figure 17–1 (*A–E*) may be used once, more than once, or not at all.

15. Associated with the highest morbidity

16. Most common location of ectopic gestations

17. Location of less than 1% of ectopic gestations

18. Most common location for implantation in women with an intrauterine device (IUD)

19. Most common location for implantation in a conception after an ectopic pregnancy

20. Associated with a "tubal abortion"

FIGURE 17–1 Sites of implantation.

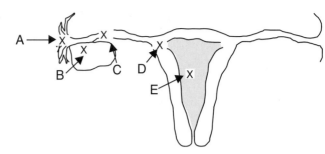

DIRECTIONS:

for Questions 21–29: Select the one best answer or completion.

21. Which of the following hormones is responsible for both the decidual change and the Arias-Stella reaction in ectopic pregnancies?

    A. β-hCG
    B. progesterone
    C. estradiol
    D. estrone

22. What level of serum progesterone is associated with an almost universally bad outcome for a gestation when the β-hCG level is 3,000 mIU/mL?

    A. 10 ng/mL
    B. 20 ng/mL
    C. 30 ng/mL
    D. 40 ng/mL
    E. 50 ng/mL

23. An assay for β-hCG is obtained and reported to be 800 mIU/mL. A second test is performed 72 hours later. This time the value is 1200 mIU/mL. A sonogram is obtained and no abnormalities are reported, but no gestation can be identified. The most likely diagnosis is

    A. an ectopic pregnancy
    B. complete abortion
    C. an early intrauterine pregnancy
    D. a missed abortion

24. Factors that contribute to or cause death from ectopic pregnancy in more than three quarters of cases include

    A. physician delay
    B. blood loss
    C. anesthetic complications
    D. misdiagnosis
    E. infection

25. You are an expert witness. The plaintiff, a 35-year-old woman, claims that she no longer can become pregnant as a result of the defendant's mismanagement. The plaintiff has been under the defendant's care for several years, during which time he hospitalized her for acute pelvic inflammatory disease and the surgical removal of the organ depicted in Figure 17–2. On the witness stand, you might emphasize that the most likely diagnosis associated with this history and pathologic specimen is

    A. chronic endometritis
    B. Arias-Stella reaction
    C. cervical pregnancy
    D. intrauterine gestation
    E. endometrial carcinoma

26. The most common contributing factor in ectopic implantation is

    A. aneuploidy
    B. family history of this condition
    C. previous sterilization
    D. pelvic infection
    E. intrauterine contraceptive devices

27. Which of the following patients would be at greatest risk for ectopic pregnancy if a pregnancy should occur?

    A. a gravida 3, para 3, sterilized by laparoscopically placed clips at age 35
    B. a gravida 1, para 1, sterilized by laparoscopically directed bipolar cautery at age 38
    C. a gravida 4, para 4, sterilized by postpartum tubal ligation (Pomeroy) at age 38
    D. a gravida 2, para 1, sterilized by laparoscopically directed bipolar cautery at age 22
    E. a gravida 4, para 3, whose husband was sterilized by vasectomy at age 25

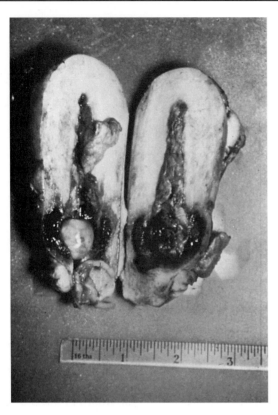

FIGURE 17–2

28. **The use of laparoscopy to establish the diagnosis of ectopic pregnancy carries a**

   A. 15% false-negative rate
   B. 5% false-negative rate
   C. <1% false-negative rate
   D. 5% false-positive rate
   E. <1% false-positive rate

29. **Which of the following is a relative contraindication to the use of methotrexate for medical management of a suspected ectopic pregnancy?**

   A. an adnexal gestational mass 3 cm in diameter
   B. lower abdominal crampy pain
   C. 50 mL of blood in the peritoneal cavity (estimated by ultrasonography)
   D. a serum β-hCG level of 1500 mIU/mL
   E. fetal cardiac activity

ANSWERS

1. **E,** Page 462. This patient appears to be in shock and should receive immediate attention. A radioimmunoassay would delay definitive treatment. A radioimmunoassay may be more sensitive, but regardless of the results, the diagnosis is a hemoperitoneum with hypovolemia. In this case, the most likely diagnosis is a ruptured corpus luteum. On occasion, an arteriole in the ovary is bleeding and requires suturing. The role of colocentesis in the diagnosis and management of ectopic pregnancy is changing. When results are positive, this procedure can help to establish the presence of blood or pus in the peritoneal cavity, but the ready availability of ultrasonography in most institutions and its less invasive nature make ultrasonography preferable.

2. **D,** Pages 470–472. The overall subsequent conception rate for women with an ectopic pregnancy is about 60% to 80%. Also see the comment for Answer 3.

3. **B,** Pages 470–472. A little less than half of pregnancies subsequent to an ectopic pregnancy terminate in another ectopic gestation or spontaneous abortion. Since the conception rate for women in this group is 60% to 80%, only about one third

have a subsequent live birth. However, these general figures are modified by several factors, particularly age, parity, evidence of contralateral tubal disease, and whether the tube containing the ectopic pregnancy was ruptured.

4. **C,** Page 457. Blood is almost always found in the peritoneal cavity in patients with ruptured ectopic pregnancies of any location except cervical implantation. As we begin to make the diagnosis before rupture, the number of patients with blood in the peritoneal cavity is likely to fall. The blood is from the mother. It is able to clot and does so in the same way that peripheral blood does. After clotting, this blood undergoes lysis to yield the nonclotting blood found. In patients with rapid catastrophic blood loss, the blood found may clot on occasion because it has not had time to undergo lysis. The blood found in the peritoneal cavity generally has a hematocrit of only slightly less than that of peripheral blood.

5. **A,** Page 470. Although the risk of Rh sensitization of an Rh-negative mother by an ectopic pregnancy is low, all Rh-negative patients who are not already sensitized should receive Rh(D) immunoglobulin. A person who is classified as RhDu-positive rarely

develops antibodies when challenged by Rho(D) antigen.

6. **D,** Page 464. Although data concerning the removal of the ipsilateral ovary conflict, most authors agree that as little as possible should be done to or around the ovary to preserve future fertility options.

7. **E,** Pages 460–461. In 1987, with abdominal scanning techniques, the visualization of an ectopic gestation occurred in only about 25% or less of patients. Transvaginal scanning techniques eventually may raise this rate to 50% or better. Imaging is improving at such a rapid rate that its efficacy in the future is difficult to predict. Visualization of an intrauterine gestational sac containing a fetal pole is possible at 5 to 7 weeks of gestational age (menstrual dates).

8. **D,** Pages 446, 157. The Centers for Disease Control and Prevention reported a marked increase in ectopic pregnancy in the United States between 1970 and 1989. During this time, there was a fivefold increase in the annual number of women hospitalized for ectopic pregnancies (from 17,800 to 88,400); there was a tripling of the rate reported per 1000 pregnancies. In the United States, these numbers have since declined. The increased incidence of ectopic pregnancies during this earlier period is thought to have been mainly the result of an increased incidence of salpingitis, which is a major risk factor for ectopic pregnancy. The improvement in diagnostic techniques may also contribute to this reported increase.

9. **B,** Page 444. About 40 to 50 deaths from ectopic pregnancy occur annually. Even though the percentage of maternal deaths rose from 8% in 1970 to 14% in 1980, the percentage of ectopic pregnancies that result in death has decreased (Fig. 17–2 in Stenchever). The overall death rate/case rate ratio of ectopic pregnancy has decreased sevenfold in all women with ectopic pregnancy and is similar in all age groups, but it is about three times higher in African-American women. Because the incidence of ectopic pregnancy is also higher in African Americans in the United States, a pregnant African-American woman is about five times more likely to die of ectopic pregnancy than a Caucasian woman. Ectopic pregnancy is the most common single cause of all maternal deaths among African-American women, causing about one fifth of such deaths.

10. **E,** Page 450; Table 17–1 in Stenchever. Although some studies have suggested that a prior induced abortion increases the risk of ectopic pregnancy, it has been shown that when techniques are used to control the effects of other risk factors, the history of one prior induced abortion does not significantly increase the risk of an ectopic pregnancy. Another study suggests that two or more prior induced abortions do not increase the risk of an ectopic pregnancy. Previous pelvic surgery and previous pelvic infection pose an extra risk, but not the same as a prior ectopic pregnancy, which confers a relative risk of 7.7.

11. **E,** Pages 457–458. Because of limited space or inadequate nourishment, the trophoblastic tissue of most ectopic pregnancies does not grow as rapidly as that of pregnancies located within the uterine cavity, resulting in an unpredictable rise in β-hCG. In general, β-hCG is lower in ectopic pregnancies compared with normal intrauterine pregnancies. The rate of increase in β-hCG is much slower in ectopic pregnancies compared with the normal doubling time of 48 to 72 hours. This difference is not in itself diagnostic of an ectopic pregnancy and cannot be used to establish the diagnosis. Serum values often plateau or fall before surgical intervention occurs. These values also fall after a tubal abortion or the demise of the pregnancy. Despite these observations, no changes in serum level can be used to predict either rupture of the tube or the eventual outcome of the ectopic pregnancy.

12. **D,** Page 456; Table 17–2 in Stenchever. The most common symptoms associated with an ectopic pregnancy are abdominal pain, absence of menstrual bleeding, and irregular bleeding. Pain is nearly a universal symptom but is not type-specific. Before rupture, the pain may be only a vague soreness or a colicky type of pain. The location of pain may be generalized, unilateral, or bilateral. Shoulder pain occurs in about one fourth of patients with an ectopic pregnancy as a result of diaphragmatic irritation from a hemoperitoneum.

13. **A,** Page 464. With increasing frequency, conservative management (not removing the oviduct) of an unruptured ectopic pregnancy is the preferred surgical choice for a woman who desires future fertility. When conservative surgery is correctly performed, the repeat ectopic pregnancy rate is not increased compared with salpingectomy. Furthermore, the subsequent live-birth rate is increased. Current operations appear to have an unappreciable effect on overall maternal mortality, and there is little information about the effects of these operations on regular cyclic bleeding. The best results of conservative operation occur after salpingotomy or salpingostomy, the latter being used more frequently in the United States.

14. **D,** Page 467. After initial reports of the successful treatment of ectopic pregnancies with methotrexate in 1982, a number of studies have critically analyzed this treatment alternative. These protocols prescribed methotrexate over a 5-day course of treatment in doses ranging from 60 to 300 mg

intramuscularly. Although mifepristone shows promise for similar purposes, its use in the United States is currently limited. The other chemotherapeutic agents are not efficacious in treating trophoblastic disorders. The disadvantages of methotrexate treatment include the need for subsequent laparotomy for bleeding and the unacceptable toxic side effects of the drug.

15–20. 15, **D**; 16, **C**; 17, **B**; 18, **E**; 19, **E**; 20, **A**; Pages 450–453; Figure 17–8 in Stenchever. Although most ectopic gestations implant in the middle to distal portion of the tube, the area of implantation associated with the greatest morbidity and mortality is the interstitial portion because of the catastrophic consequences of a rupture in that area. Implantations at or near the fimbrial end of the tube may abort without causing tubal rupture. Less than 1% of ectopic pregnancies are found implanted in the ovary. About 2% of all ectopic pregnancies are interstitial. Most pregnancies that follow an ectopic pregnancy or that occur while an IUD is in position are intrauterine.

21. **B**, Pages 458–460. The progesterone produced by the corpus luteum is responsible for both the decidual and the Arias-Stella reaction.

22. **A**, Page 460. When the hCG level is above 3000 mIU/mL, a serum progesterone level of less than 12 ng/mL has been associated with a 97% pregnancy loss rate. This observation allows the clinician to anticipate a bad prognosis for these patients, but the level of serum progesterone does not differentiate between an ectopic implantation and an intrauterine gestation that is failing.

23. **D**, Pages 458–459. The β-hCG level has increased 40% in 72 hours. This indicates an abnormal pregnancy—a blighted ovum, an ectopic implantation, or a missed abortion, the most common of which is missed abortion. In a normal pregnancy, the β-hCG level should be at least 66% higher than the initial value in 48 hours. Therefore, it is highly unlikely that this is a normal pregnancy. The possibility of an ectopic pregnancy must always be considered in patients like this and if risk factors are present, additional testing may be warranted.

24. **B**, Pages 445–446. More than 85% of deaths from ectopic pregnancy result from blood loss. Physician delays or misdiagnosis contributes to maternal death in roughly half of cases. Anesthetic complications and infection account for less than 2% of all ectopic pregnancy deaths.

25. **C**, Page 452. This is a hysterectomy specimen from a cervical pregnancy. Most cervical pregnancies occur after sharp uterine curettage. More than half of patients with a cervical pregnancy require hysterectomy for treatment. Even if a hysterectomy is not performed, the prognosis for future fertility is poor.

26. **D**, Pages 446–447. The most common contributing factor in ectopic pregnancies is previous pelvic infection. Although the rate of ectopic gestations is higher in patients who have undergone tubal sterilization or who use IUDs, these patients account for only a fraction of the ectopic pregnancies that occur each year. There is no evidence that either family history or aneuploidy contributes significantly to the risk of an ectopic pregnancy.

27. **D**, Page 449. The highest risk of ectopic pregnancy after sterilization failure is following bipolar cautery. The risk is estimated to be in the range of 1% to 2%, but this risk rises almost threefold if the procedure is performed when the patient is younger than 28 years. The risk of failure is not influenced by the patient's parity, and there is no evidence that previous vasectomy alters the risk of ectopic gestation.

28. **D**, Page 457. The use of laparoscopy to establish the diagnosis of ectopic pregnancy carries a 5% false-positive rate; that is, in roughly 5% of patients with an intrauterine gestation, an ectopic pregnancy is incorrectly diagnosed.

29. **E**, Pages 467–469. For successful medical treatment of an ectopic pregnancy, the adnexal mass must be less than 4 cm in diameter, the patient must be asymptomatic or minimally symptomatic, and there must be no evidence of active bleeding. The success rate is higher if there is less than 100 mL of blood in the cul-de-sac and there is no sonographic evidence of fetal heart activity. Serum β-hCG levels should be below 1500 mIU/mL, and serum progesterone levels should be below 10 ng/mL. Studies suggest that when fetal cardiac activity is present, success rates fall to approximately 85%, making the presence of fetal cardiac activity a relative, but not absolute, contraindication to methotrexate therapy.

Benign Gynecologic Lesions

for Questions 1–23: Select the one best answer or completion.

1. A 28-year-old gravida 1, para 0, at 24 weeks of gestation with a known history of leiomyomata has severe uterine pain. The fetal status is normal. On palpation, a 6-cm tender area is noted and is thought to be located on the uterus. The examination is otherwise unremarkable. The most likely diagnosis is

   A. a ruptured uterus
   B. a placental abruption
   C. hyaline degeneration of a myoma
   D. carneous degeneration of a myoma
   E. premature labor

2. Which of the following is best treated by wide excision?

   A. contact dermatitis
   B. psoriasis
   C. lichen planus
   D. hidradenitis suppurativa
   E. seborrheic dermatitis

3. A 32-year-old patient has a 6-month history of dyspareunia, dysuria, and dribbling of urine. A palpable tender mass is apparent in the anterior vagina. The most likely diagnosis is

   A. a Skene gland cyst
   B. chronic cystitis
   C. a vaginal inclusion cyst
   D. a Gartner duct cyst
   E. a urethral diverticulum

4. During a routine gynecologic examination of an asymptomatic, sexually active 28-year-old, a 3-cm sausage-shaped cystic mass is found protruding from the anterolateral wall of the upper vagina. The treatment of choice is

   A. expectant management
   B. oral antibiotics
   C. laparoscopy and cystoscopy
   D. marsupialization of the cyst
   E. excision of the cyst

5. A 25-year-old gravida 1, para 1, who is 6 weeks postpartum and breast-feeding, comes to the emergency department with heavy vaginal bleeding since having intercourse 2 hours ago. This was the first time in several months she had attempted coitus. Although the examination is difficult, a 1-cm transverse laceration of the posterior fornix is identified. The proper management is

   A. vaginal estrogen cream
   B. vaginal packing
   C. suturing the laceration
   D. hospitalization for observation
   E. discharge to be followed up in the office in the AM

6. A 37-year-old patient complains of inter-menstrual and postcoital spotting. The findings on speculum examination are illustrated in Figure 18–1. Appropriate therapy for this patient's condition is

   A. hysterectomy
   B. fractional dilatation and curettage (D&C)
   C. removal of the mass in the office
   D. laser conization
   E. vaginal estrogen cream

7. An asymptomatic 25-year-old gravida 5, para 5, who has had a tubal ligation has a 20-week irregular pelvic mass, which you suspect is uterine myomata. The next step in evaluation should be

   A. magnetic resonance imaging (MRI)
   B. ultrasound imaging
   C. computed tomography (CT)
   D. hysteroscopy
   E. no additional testing is required

8. A 47-year-old asymptomatic patient is found to have an 8-week-size irregular myomatous uterus. Appropriate management should be

   A. reevaluation in 6 to 12 months
   B. administration of GnRH analogues
   C. fractional D&C
   D. myomectomy
   E. hysterectomy

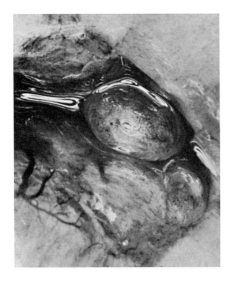

FIGURE 18–1   (From Kolstad P, Stafl A, eds: Atlas of Colposcopy, 2nd ed. Baltimore, University Park Press, 1977, p 66.)

9. A 23-year-old graduate student is found to have an asymptomatic 4-cm ovarian cyst. Her menstrual periods are regular. She is not sexually active and does not use oral contraceptives. The cyst is freely mobile and nontender to palpation. The treatment of choice is

   A. reexamination in 6 weeks
   B. oral contraceptives
   C. needle aspiration guided by ultrasonography
   D. laparoscopy
   E. laparotomy

10. A 28-year-old gravida 0 whose last normal menstrual period was 6 weeks ago has a 1-week history of left lower quadrant pain. She uses a diaphragm for contraception. Her previous menstrual history was normal. She denies any history of pelvic inflammatory disease. Abdominal examination results are normal. On pelvic examination, a tender 3-cm left adnexal mass is noted. The hematocrit is 38%, the white blood cell count is 6000, and the serum pregnancy test yields negative results. The most likely diagnosis is

    A. ectopic pregnancy
    B. tuboovarian abscess
    C. salpingitis
    D. endometriosis
    E. corpus luteum cyst

11. After the delivery of twins at term by cesarean section and closure of the uterine incision, bilateral ovarian masses similar to those in Figure 18–2 are found. Your next step would be to

    A. perform a total abdominal hysterectomy with bilateral salpingo-oophorectomy
    B. perform a bilateral oophorectomy
    C. perform a bilateral wedge resection
    D. aspirate the cysts
    E. close the abdomen

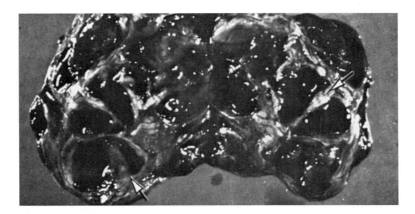

FIGURE 18–2   (From Blaustein A: In Blaustein A, ed: Pathology of the Female Genital Tract. New York, Springer-Verlag, 1977, p 397.)

12. The most common complication of a cystic teratoma is

    A. infection
    B. torsion
    C. rupture
    D. hemorrhage
    E. malignant degeneration

13. A 25-year-old woman taking birth control pills whose last normal menstrual period was 1 week ago complains of a sudden onset of severe left lower quadrant pain, which awoke her from sleeping. She had several milder episodes over the last week for which she did not seek medical care. She is nauseated and has vomited three times. On physical examination, her temperature is 100°F. There is tenderness in the left lower abdominal quadrant, and an exquisitely tender 5-cm left adnexal mass is found. A β-human chorionic gonadotropin (β-hCG) titer is negative. The most appropriate action is to

    A. administer parenteral broad-spectrum antibiotics
    B. perform intravenous pyelography
    C. perform a barium enema
    D. perform laparoscopy or laparotomy
    E. perform culdocentesis

14. A 25-year-old gravida 1, para 1, complains of pain during intercourse. This has been a problem for 3 months and is noted primarily on entry. Physical examination is normal except for several punctate ulcers in the vestibule, which are primarily located around the Bartholin glands. These ulcers are exquisitely tender when touched with a cotton-tipped applicator stick. The complaint is most likely due to

    A. contact dermatitis
    B. vulvar vestibulitis
    C. psoriasis
    D. hidradenitis suppurativa
    E. syringoma

15. During pregnancy, most myomata

    A. grow
    B. shrink
    C. enlarge and undergo degeneration
    D. shrink and undergo degeneration
    E. remain the same size and do not undergo degeneration

16. The most common type of degeneration to occur within a myoma is

    A. calcific
    B. red
    C. hyaline
    D. myxomatous
    E. sarcomatous

17. Medical treatment of myomata is best accomplished with

    A. danazol
    B. medroxyprogesterone (Depo-Provera)
    C. GnRH analogues
    D. estrogens
    E. testosterone

18. A 35-year-old gravida 0 is undergoing surgery for a solid left ovarian mass. The frozen section of the ovary is pictured in Figure 18–3. The pelvis is otherwise normal. According to this histologic picture, the patient should undergo

    A. total abdominal hysterectomy with bilateral salpingo-oophorectomy
    B. total abdominal hysterectomy with left salpingo-oophorectomy
    C. bilateral salpingo-oophorectomy
    D. left salpingo-oophorectomy
    E. left oophorectomy

19. Optimal therapy for the lesion pictured in Figure 18–4 is

    A. vulvectomy
    B. excisional biopsy
    C. irradiation
    D. 5-fluorouracil
    E. methotrexate

20. The most common large cyst of the vulva is a(n)

    A. epidermal inclusion cyst
    B. Bartholin duct cyst
    C. Gartner duct cyst
    D. nabothian cyst
    E. sebaceous cyst

21. A 72-year-old patient asks about several 1-mm dark-blue lesions on the vulva that have appeared since her last annual visit. The most likely diagnosis is a(n)

    A. pyogenic granuloma
    B. cherry angioma
    C. angiokeratoma
    D. strawberry hemangioma
    E. nevus

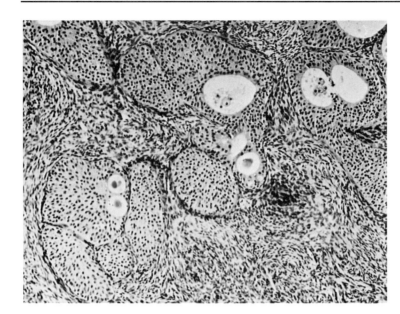

FIGURE 18–3

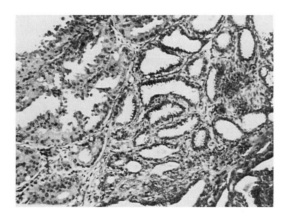

FIGURE 18–4

22. A 55-year-old patient has the lesion shown in Figure 18–5. She complains of mild dysuria. The initial therapy for this condition is

   A. topical estrogen
   B. operative excision
   C. laser ablation
   D. fulguration
   E. cryosurgery

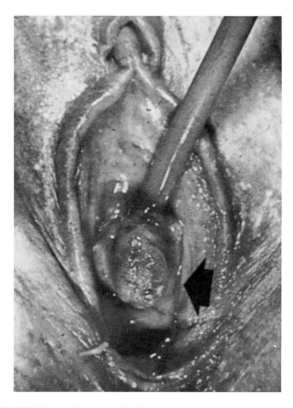

FIGURE 18–5   (From Marshall FC, Uson AC, Melicow MM: Surg Gynecol Obstet 110:724, 1960.)

23. The chromosomal makeup of benign cystic teratomas is most often

   A. 46,XX
   B. 46,XY
   C. 45,X
   D. 47,XXX
   E. 47,XXY

DIRECTIONS:

for Questions 24–29: For each numbered item, select the one heading most closely associated with it. Each lettered heading may be used once, more than once, or not at all.

24–26. **Match the description with the most closely associated vulvar lesion.**

A. fibroma
B. lipoma
C. hidradenoma
D. granular cell myoblastoma
E. Bowen disease

24. Most commonly benign solid vulvar tumor

25. Arises from neural sheath cells

26. Histologically similar to adenocarcinoma

27–29. **Match the association with the ovarian neoplasm.**

A. cystic teratoma
B. fibroma
C. serous cystadenoma
D. dysgerminoma
E. endometrioma

27. Tubercle of Rokitansky

28. Meigs syndrome

29. Brenner tumor

DIRECTIONS:

for Questions 30–39: Select the one best answer or completion.

30. Which of the following is the appropriate management for hematometra?

A. hysterectomy
B. hysteroscopy
C. cold-knife conization
D. relief of the obstruction

31. Which of the following ultrasound descriptions would be most compatible with a dermoid?

A. multiple dense echogenic areas within the adnexa
B. cyst filled with bands of mixed echoes
C. multiple simple cysts in the ovary
D. a sausage-shaped cystic dilation lateral to the uterus
E. free fluid in the posterior cul-de-sac

32. Which of the following is most likely to undergo torsion?

A. leiomyoma of oviduct
B. paratubal cyst
C. cystic teratoma
D. submucous leiomyoma

33. Which of the following is of mesonephric duct origin?

A. leiomyoma of oviduct
B. paratubal cyst
C. cystic teratoma
D. fibroma

34. Conservative management would be appropriate for which of the following patients with an adnexal mass?

A. a patient with a solid tumor
B. a prepubertal patient with a 2-cm solid mass
C. a reproductive-age patient with a cystic mass greater than 8 cm
D. a 55-year-old with a 3-cm unilateral cystic mass

35. A hysterectomy should be performed if a myomatous uterus

A. is the size of a 10-week gestation
B. appears to be enlarging and the patient is menopausal
C. on ultrasound evaluation is found to contain echogenic areas
D. contains more than eight individual myomas

36. Which of the following suggest that a pigmented lesion is malignant?

A. a regular border
B. symmetrical shape
C. variation of color
D. diameter < 3 mm

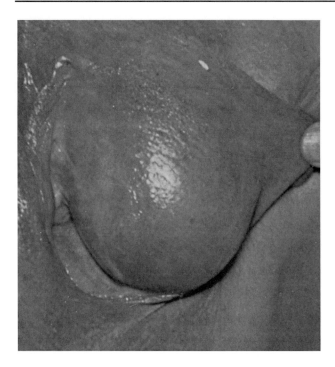

FIGURE 18–6   (From Friedrich EG, ed: Vulvar Disease, 2nd ed. Philadelphia, WB Saunders, 1983, p 233.)

37. A 65-year-old patient is undergoing office endometrial sampling because of vaginal spotting. With difficulty, a 1-mm dilator is passed into the endometrial cavity, resulting in discharge of pus from the cervical os. This patient should

   A. be given intravenous broad-spectrum antibiotics
   B. undergo pelvic ultrasonography
   C. undergo fractional D&C at a later date
   D. undergo hysterectomy

38. A 28-year-old patient is concerned about a growth on her labia. The significant finding on pelvic examination is shown in Figure 18–6. The most likely diagnosis is

   A. fibroma
   B. lipoma
   C. Bartholin duct cyst
   D. hidradenitis suppurativa

39. The appropriate management of a recurrent granular cell myoblastoma is

   A. radiation therapy
   B. 5-fluorouracil chemotherapy
   C. radical vulvectomy
   D. wide local excision

ANSWERS

1. **D,** Pages 501–502. The blood supply to myomas is less than that to a similar-sized area of normal myometrium. Therefore, as a myoma grows, it outgrows its blood supply, resulting in degeneration. The most acute form of degeneration is red, or carneous, degeneration typified by the rapidly growing myoma during the midtrimester of pregnancy. The sudden muscular infarction causes pain and localized peritonitis. Treatment should be medical because surgical intervention in a pregnant patient results in profuse blood loss. Placental abruption at 24 weeks is unusual, and the uterus would be expected to be diffusely tender.

2. **D,** Pages 488–489. Hidradenitis suppurativa is a chronic refractory infection of the skin and subcutaneous tissue. It may progress from subcutaneous nodules to draining abscesses and sinuses. The treatment of choice is early aggressive wide excision. Dermatologic conditions such as contact dermatitis, psoriasis, lichen planus, and seborrheic dermatitis can all be treated with a topical steroid.

3. **E,** Pages 489–490. The most common symptoms associated with a urethral diverticulum are urinary urgency, frequency, and dysuria. Dyspareunia and dribbling after micturition have also been reported by the 80% of patients with a urethral diverticulum who are symptomatic. The diagnosis may be confirmed by several techniques, including urethrography, cytourethroscopy, and positive-pressure urethrography with a Davis catheter.

4. **A,** Page 479. Gartner duct cysts are dysontogenetic cysts of mesonephric origin, usually found in the upper half of the vagina. They occur in approximately 1 of 200 women and are usually asymptomatic. Unless symptoms such as vaginal pain, dyspareunia, difficulty with urination, or a large palpable mass occur, these cysts may be followed up conservatively.

5. **C,** Pages 491–492. Coitus is the most common cause of trauma to the lower genital tract of adult women. Predisposing factors include virginity, pregnancy, postpartum state, postmenopausal vaginal epithelium, prolonged abstinence, hysterectomy, and inebriation. The most prominent symptom of a coital vaginal laceration is profuse or prolonged vaginal bleeding. Many women in whom a laceration develops experience sharp

pain during intercourse, and about 25% note persistent abdominal pain. The most troublesome, but extremely rare, complication of a vaginal laceration is vaginal evisceration. Management includes suturing the laceration with the patient under adequate anesthesia. Patients such as the one described have vaginas that show little estrogen effect and are thereby at greater risk for trauma.

6. **C,** Page 492. A patient with intermenstrual and postcoital spotting has symptoms suggestive of a cervical polyp. The differential diagnosis for the lesion in Figure 18–1 includes an endocervical or endometrial polyp, a prolapsed myoma, a squamous papilloma, products of conception, sarcoma, and a cervical malignancy. In most instances, an endocervical polyp can be removed by twisting it off its base with a surgical clamp. This can usually be done in the office. If the intermenstrual and postcoital spotting continue after removal of the polyp, endometrial sampling is indicated to identify an endometrial lesion whose symptoms mimicked those of a polyp.

7. **E,** Pages 502–503. This question raises several issues. First, what is most cost-effective? The diagnosis of uterine myomas is usually confirmed by palpation of an enlarged, firm, irregular uterus during pelvic examination. In experienced hands, further verification is unnecessary—it is a clinical diagnosis. In difficult cases, concentric calcifications on abdominal radiography or characteristic findings on ultrasonography, CT, and MRI may aid diagnosis. Ultrasound imaging remains the most cost-effective single imaging technique. Submucous myomas may be observed during hysteroscopy. They also appear as filling defects on the hysterosalpingogram. The second issue is the availability of expert assistance if an ovarian malignancy is encountered at laparotomy. In communities without an oncologist, ultrasonography should be employed if the diagnosis is in doubt. The third issue is that medical therapy is also an option for this patient if myomas are confirmed. At this patient's age, and given the size of the myomata, medical therapy provides only a short-term response. If the patient does not desire surgery, frequent follow-up is mandatory.

8. **A,** Pages 503–504. Most women with uterine myomas do not require surgery. This is particularly true for asymptomatic perimenopausal patients since the condition tends to improve with declining levels of circulating estrogen. Reexamination allows determination of the rate of growth. Symptomatic patients must be evaluated appropriately, with therapy ultimately depending on severity and persistence of symptoms, age, parity, and reproductive plans. D&C

would be warranted in cases of abnormal bleeding. Myomectomy, both transabdominal and hysteroscopic, is reserved for symptomatic women who have not completed childbearing. A few small series of cases using danazol, GnRH analogues, or medroxyprogesterone have reported reduction in tumor size. Myomas tend to return after the medication is discontinued.

9. **A,** Page 507. The initial management of a suspected functional ovarian cyst is observation. Since most follicular cysts are reabsorbed spontaneously or silently rupture in 4 to 8 weeks, reevaluation in 6 weeks is acceptable. A 6-week, rather than a 4-week, interval is preferable so that the patient can be examined at a different point in her cycle. Oral contraceptives remove any influence by pituitary gonadotrophins and may be prescribed for a short-term trial. Recent data demonstrate that oral contraceptives do not bring about the disappearance of functional ovarian cysts better than observation alone. Surgical intervention is not warranted in the asymptomatic patient initially.

10. **E,** Pages 456–457, 1087. *Halban syndrome* describes a persistently functioning corpus luteum cyst that clinically mimics an ectopic pregnancy. This triad includes a delay in normal menses with subsequent spotting, unilateral pelvic pain, and a small tender adnexal mass. With the advent of rapid, sensitive pregnancy tests that measure β–hCG, the distinction between ectopic pregnancy and persistent corpus luteum cyst is made more easily because the pregnancy test result is almost always positive in the presence of an ectopic pregnancy.

11. **E,** Pages 510–511. Pregnancies producing large placentas, such as those associated with twins, diabetes, and Rh sensitization, are more likely to be associated with theca-lutein cysts. The ovaries should be handled delicately to avoid cyst rupture and hemorrhage. No further surgery is warranted because the cysts will regress as the gonadotrophin stimulation disappears.

12. **B,** Page 479. The most frequent complication of a cystic teratoma is torsion, which occurs in approximately 11% of patients. The overall incidence of rupture is less than 5%, occurring more commonly in pregnancy and the puerperium with resultant leakage and incitement of a chemical peritonitis. Infection, hemorrhage, and malignant degeneration are all unusual complications, occurring in less than 1% of patients.

13. **D,** Pages 519–520. The differential diagnosis includes an ectopic pregnancy, pelvic inflammatory disease (PID), and ovarian torsion. A pregnancy test yields negative results, and the last menstrual period was 1 week ago. This makes the

diagnosis of an ectopic pregnancy unlikely. This patient is obviously sick and has a low-grade fever. PID is unlikely. Most patients with adnexal torsion, like the one described, are ill enough to warrant operative intervention. When the diagnosis is in doubt, laparoscopy may be needed to rule out conditions such as abscess or a ruptured corpus luteum. In selected cases of partial torsion, it is acceptable to untwist the pedicle, perform cystectomy, and then stabilize the ovary. This does carry the risk of releasing venous thrombi. In cases of vascular compromise, unilateral salpingo-oophorectomy is the operation of choice.

14. **B,** Page 487. Vulvar vestibulitis appears as vulvar burning and pain at the introitus. Typical signs include focal ulceration and inflammation of the vestibular mucosa with punctate 3- to 10-mm lesions, particularly between the two Bartholin glands. The condition spontaneously remits in one third of patients and is usually treated conservatively, initially with anesthetics. Only if vestibulitis is refractory should laser surgery or surgical excision be contemplated. Contact dermatitis is due to either true allergies or a contact irritant. Psoriasis usually affects intertriginous areas and is manifested by red-yellow papules. Hydradenitis suppurativa is a chronic infection of the skin and subcutaneous tissue that typically progresses to draining abscesses and sinuses. Syringoma is a rare benign tumor of the exocrine sweat glands. It starts as small subcutaneous papules and may coalesce to form cords of tissue.

15. **E,** Page 502. Serial ultrasound examinations have shown that 80% of myomata do not change size during pregnancy. If the myoma does change size, there is usually no associated pain. The most acute form of degeneration is red, or carneous, infarction, which occurs in approximately 5% to 10% of pregnant women with myomas.

16. **C,** Page 502. Ultimately, most myomata outgrow their blood supply, resulting in some type of cellular degeneration. The most common form of degeneration of a myoma is hyaline degeneration. On a cellular level, the smooth muscle cells are replaced by fibrous connective tissue. Degenerative change occurs in 65% of cases. The other extreme is malignant degeneration, which is known to occur in 0.3% to 0.7% of cases.

17. **C,** Page 503. Myomata can be medically treated by decreasing the circulating level of estrogens. GnRH analogues successfully reduce the size of myomata in as many as 80% to 100% of patients. In some patients, the size decreases by as much as 90%. Maximum reduction occurs within 8 months. Unfortunately, after the therapy is discontinued, most myomata return to their pretreatment size within 6 months. Thus, GnRH agonists have been used most successfully preoperatively to reduce the size of the myomata—to reduce blood loss at the time of operation. Since myomata tend to get smaller after patients are climacteric, the perimenopausal use of a GnRH agonist obviates the need for a hysterectomy in selected patients.

18. **E,** Pages 515–519; Figure 18–43 in Stenchever. (From Czernobilsky. In Blaustein A, ed: Pathology of the Female Genital Tract. New York, Springer-Verlag, 1977, p 490.) The ovarian tumor in Figure 18–43 is a Brenner tumor, a smooth, solid ovarian tumor that is usually asymptomatic. Typically, they occur in women 40 to 60 years old, with 90% of these neoplasms discovered as an incidental finding during a gynecologic procedure. Histologically, the Brenner tumor is identified by solid masses or nests of epithelial cells with a surrounding fibrous stroma. The appropriate management of a Brenner tumor is simple excision.

19. **B,** Pages 484–485; Figure 18–7 in Stenchever. (From Kaufman RH: Cystic tumors. In Gardner HL, Kaufman RH, eds: Benign Diseases of the Vulva and Vagina, 2nd ed. Boston, GK Hall, 1981, p 101.) Although possibly mistaken for an adenocarcinoma, the lesion pictured in Figure 18–7 is a hidradenoma, a small benign vulvar tumor that originates in the apocrine sweat glands in the inner surface of the labia majora. The therapy for hidradenomas is excisional biopsy. No medical therapy is indicated, and vulvectomy is a type of surgical excision that is far too great in scope.

20. **B,** Page 482. The most common large cyst of the vulva is a cystic dilation of an obstructed Bartholin duct. Treatment is not necessary unless it becomes infected or symptomatic. Sebaceous and inclusion cysts are the most common small vulvar cysts. Sebaceous cysts are typically multiple, freely mobile, and found in the anterior half of the labia majora. Inclusion cysts may develop after traumatic injury. Gartner duct cysts are found in the vagina, and nabothian cysts are found in the cervix.

21. **B,** Page 483. Senile or cherry angiomas are commonly found small lesions arising on the labia majora of postmenopausal women. They are typically less than 3 mm in diameter, multiple in number, and dark blue or red-brown. Pyogenic granulomas are an overgrowth of inflamed granulation tissue and are usually approximately 1 cm in diameter. They may be clinically mistaken for nevi, vulvar condylomas, or cancer. Angiokeratomas are purple and twice the size of cherry angiomas. They typically occur in patients between ages 30 and 50. They tend to grow rapidly and may bleed during strenuous

exercise. Strawberry or cavernous hemangiomas are congenital defects usually found in young children.

22. **A,** Pages 481–482; Figure 18–1 in Stenchever. A urethral caruncle is a fleshy outgrowth from the edge of the urethra. It is most commonly found in postmenopausal women and may respond to topical or oral estrogen. If the caruncle does not regress or is symptomatic, therapeutic modalities include operative excision, laser ablation, fulguration, or cryosurgery.

23. **A,** Pages 511–512. Benign cystic teratomas contain elements from all three germ cell layers, ectodermal tissue being predominant. Malignant transformation of a benign cystic teratoma occurs in no more than 1% to 2% of cases, usually in patients over 40. The malignant component is usually a squamous carcinoma. Benign teratomas are bilateral 10% to 15% of the time. The chromosomal makeup is 46,XX. A series of experiments using chromosome banding techniques and electrophoretic variance found that the chromosomes of dermoids are different from the chromosomes of the host. It has been postulated that dermoids begin by parthenogenesis from secondary oocytes. An alternative hypothesis is that the dermoid results from the fusion of the second polar body with the oocyte.

24–26. 24, **A;** 25, **D;** 26, **C;** Pages 483–485. Fibromas are the most common solid tumor of the vulva; lipomas are the other common benign tumor of mesenchymal origin. Both are slow-growing, have a low-grade malignant potential, and are typically excised to establish the diagnosis. Granular cell myoblastomas arise from neural sheath (Schwann) cells and are sometimes called *schwannomas*. These rare, slow-growing, solid tumors are painless and benign but infiltrate surrounding tissue. If the initial excision is not wide enough, these tumors tend to recur. A hidradenoma may be mistaken histologically for adenocarcinoma because of its hyperplastic adenomatous pattern. There is, however, a lack of mitotic figures and nuclear pleomorphism. The tumor arises from apocrine sweat glands and may be solid or cystic. It typically occurs in Caucasian women between the ages of 30 and 70. The treatment of choice is excisional biopsy.

27–29. 27, **A;** 28, **B;** 29, **C;** Pages 479, 511–514, 516. Most of the solid elements in a cystic teratoma are contained in a nipple of the cyst wall called the *protuberance* or *tubercle of Rokitansky*. Meigs syndrome is the association of an ovarian fibroma with ascites and hydrothorax. Both the ascites and hydrothorax resolve when the tumor is removed. Although classically described with an ovarian fibroma, these clinical features are also found with

other ovarian tumors. Thirty percent of Brenner tumors are associated with a serous or mucinous cystadenoma of the ipsilateral ovary.

30. **D,** Page 479. Management of hematometra depends on operative relief of the lower tract obstruction. Appropriate biopsy specimens of the endocervical canal and endometrium should be obtained to rule out malignancy when the cause of hematometra is not obvious. If the uterus is significantly enlarged or if there is any suspicion that the retained fluid is infected, drainage should be accomplished first. Biopsy should be postponed for approximately 1 month to diminish the chances of infection or uterine perforation. Hematometra following operations or cryocautery usually resolves with cervical dilation. Hematometra following a first-trimester abortion is treated by repeat suction aspiration of the products of conception that are blocking the internal os.

31. **B,** Pages 513–514. The diagnosis of a dermoid cyst is often established when a semisolid mass is palpated anterior to the broad ligament. Approximately 50% of dermoid cysts have pelvic calcifications on x-ray examination. Often, an ovarian teratoma is an incidental finding during radiologic investigation of the genitourinary or gastrointestinal tract. Many, but not all, dermoids have a characteristic ultrasound picture. These characteristics include a dense echogenic area within a larger cystic area, a cyst filled with bands of mixed echoes, and an echoic dense cyst. Laing and coworkers found that only one of three dermoids has this "typical picture." In their series of 45 patients with 51 biopsy-proven dermoid cysts, 24% of the dermoid cysts were predominantly solid, 20% were almost entirely cystic, and 24% were not visible.

32. **C,** Pages 519–520. The most common structure to undergo torsion is a cystic teratoma. Both tubal myomas and paratubal cysts may undergo acute torsion, resulting in acute lower abdominal and pelvic pain. Most cases of paratubal cyst torsion are associated with pregnancy or the puerperium.

33. **B,** Pages 504–505. Tubal myomas arise from smooth muscle cells, as do the commonly coexistent uterine myomas. Paratubal cysts may be of mesonephric, paramesonephric, or mesothelial origin. Both tubal myomas and paratubal cysts may mimic an ovarian tumor. The former simulates a solid tumor, whereas the latter is often indistinguishable from a cystic ovarian mass.

34. **D,** Page 172. Growing evidence supports the conservative treatment of postmenopausal women with small simple adnexal cysts. Any solid adnexal mass that is discovered before puberty or after menopause requires surgical intervention. It should be noted that approximately 50% of

ovarian cysts in prepubertal girls are follicle cysts. Similarly, a solid adnexal mass of any size or a cystic mass larger than 8 cm warrants surgery. A 5- to 8-cm cystic mass that persists several months despite either oral contraceptive suppression or normal menstruation should also be evaluated surgically. Increasingly, simple cysts in young women are managed through laparoscopy.

35. **B,** Page 503. In addition to symptomatic myomas, there are situations in which asymptomatic uterine myomas may be removed. Myomas larger than the size of a 12- to 14-week gestation are expected to produce symptoms eventually and may obscure the palpation of the adnexa. The growth of myomata after menopause is the classic finding in cases of leiomyosarcoma. Myomas that expand into the broad ligament may compress the ureter, resulting in hydroureter and possibly even renal compromise. Calcium deposits within a myoma are indicative of benign degeneration and are not an indication for hysterectomy.

36. **C,** Pages 482–483. Although vulvar nevi are usually asymptomatic, it should be recalled that approximately 30% of malignant melanomas arise from a preexisting nevus. Since a disproportionate number of malignant melanomas (5% to 10%) arise in the vulvar area, all vulvar nevi should be excised and examined histologically. Characteristic clinical features of an early malignant melanoma may be remembered by thinking of "ABCD," as described by Friedman: *a*symmetry, *b*order irregularity, *c*olor variegation, and a *d*iameter greater than 6 mm.

37. **C,** Page 495. Cervical stenosis that results in a pyometra in a postmenopausal patient may be caused by a previous operation, radiation, infection, neoplasia, or atrophic changes. A pyometra in a postmenopausal patient usually does not require antibiotics since the primary goal of therapy is achieved with transcervical drainage. Ultrasonography has no diagnostic or therapeutic value at this time. After the acute infection has subsided, however, fractional D&C should be performed to rule out carcinoma of the endometrium.

38. **C,** Page 482. The lesion visualized in Figure 18–6 is most likely a Bartholin duct cyst since a Bartholin duct cyst is the most common large cyst found within the vulva. A fibroma is less likely but is the most common benign solid tumor of the vulva. A lipoma, another common benign solid tumor of the vulva, is softer and usually larger than a fibroma. Hidradenitis suppurativa causes a more diffuse inflammatory reaction and is often found with weeping areas in various stages of infection and healing. For a symptomatic patient, surgical management is indicated. Fibromas and lipomas are surgically excised, while a Bartholin duct cyst can be excised or marsupialized.

39. **D,** Page 485. A granular cell myoblastoma is typically painless. Treatment involves wide excision to remove the filamentous projections into the surrounding tissue. If the initial excisional biopsy is not adequate and aggressive enough, these benign tumors tend to recur. Recurrence takes place in approximately one in five of these vulvar tumors. The appropriate therapy is a second operation with excision of wider margins since these tumors are not radiosensitive.

Endometriosis and Adenomyosis

Select the one best answer or completion.

1. **Of the following side effects of gonadotrophin-releasing hormone (GnRH) agonist therapy, the *least* common is**

    A. hot flashes
    B. hot flushes
    C. insomnia
    D. reduced bone mineral content
    E. vaginal dryness

2. **In a 25-year-old with pelvic pain, endometriosis is best confirmed by**

    A. the initial history
    B. a repeat pelvic examination on the first day of menstrual flow
    C. laparoscopic visualization and biopsy
    D. speculum visualization
    E. hysterosalpingogram

3. **The most common site for endometriosis is the**

    A. rectosigmoid
    B. ovary
    C. appendix
    D. uterosacral ligament
    E. fallopian tube

4. **A 22-year-old gravida 0 undergoes laparoscopy for progressive dysmenorrhea and chronic pelvic pain. She is found to have minimal endometriosis. She is not sexually active, uses no contraception, but does plan to marry in 6 months. She and her fiancé look forward to having children someday. Optimal therapy for this woman would be**

    A. conception
    B. oral contraceptives
    C. danazol therapy
    D. GnRH agonist
    E. laparotomy and resection of the endometriosis

5. **At laparoscopy performed for progressive dysmenorrhea and dyspareunia, a 42-year-old gravida 3, para 3, is found to have endometriosis with extensive ovarian involvement. The recommended therapy should be**

    A. danazol
    B. oral contraceptives
    C. laparotomy and resection of endometriotic lesions
    D. total abdominal hysterectomy
    E. total abdominal hysterectomy, bilateral salpingo-oophorectomy

6. **The chemical structure of danazol is depicted in**

    A. Figure 19–1, *A*
    B. Figure 19–1, *B*
    C. Figure 19–1, *C*
    D. Figure 19–1, *D*
    E. Figure 19–1, *E*

7. **Of the five photomicrographs shown in the figures listed below, the one diagnostic of endometriosis is**

    A. Figure 19–2
    B. Figure 19–3
    C. Figure 19–4
    D. Figure 19–5
    E. Figure 19–6

8. **Of the five photomicrographs shown in the figures listed below, the one diagnostic of adenomyosis is**

    A. Figure 19–2
    B. Figure 19–3
    C. Figure 19–4
    D. Figure 19–5
    E. Figure 19–6

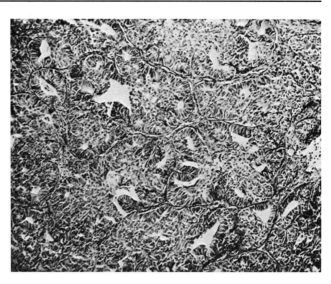

FIGURE 19–1

FIGURE 19–4 (From Kurman RJ, Norris HJ: In Blaustein A, ed: Pathology of the Female Genital Tract, 2nd ed. New York, Springer-Verlag, 1982.)

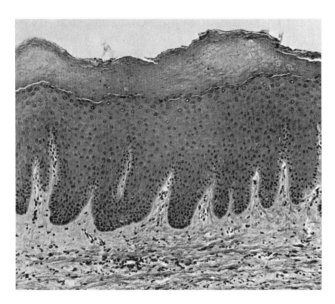

FIGURE 19–2 (From Friedrich EG, Wilkinson EJ: The vulva. In Blaustein A, ed: Pathology of the Female Genital Tract, 2nd ed. New York, Springer-Verlag, 1982.)

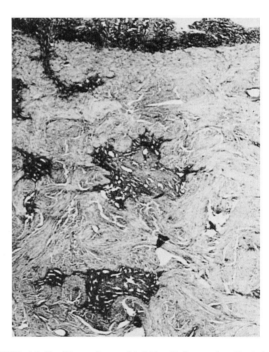

FIGURE 19–5 (From Janovski NA, Dubranszky V: Atlas of Gynecologic and Obstetric Diagnostic Histopathology. New York, McGraw-Hill, 1967, p. 217.)

9. A 42-year-old gravida 4, para 4, has bothersome dysmenorrhea and menorrhagia. On pelvic examination the uterus is globular, tender, boggy, and approximately twice normal size. The most likely diagnosis is

   A. endometriosis
   B. adenomyosis
   C. leiomyoma uteri
   D. leiomyosarcoma
   E. endometrial carcinoma

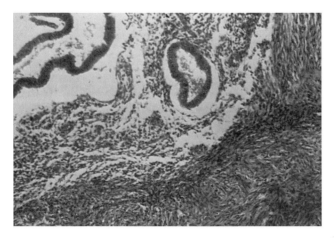

FIGURE 19–3 (From Stenchever MA, Droegemueller W, Herbst AL, Mishell DR: Comprehensive Gynecology, 4th ed. St Louis, Mosby, 2001.)

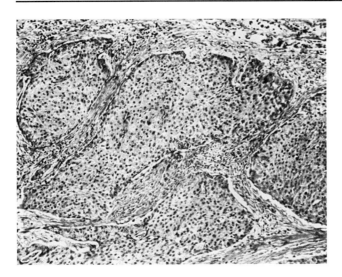

FIGURE 19–6 (From Clement PB, Scully RE: Carcinoma of the cervix: histologic types. Semin Oncol 9:251, 1982.)

10. In a patient with endometriosis who has undergone 6 months of treatment with a GnRH agonist, ovarian function will generally return within

A. 1–2 weeks
B. 3–5 weeks
C. 6–12 weeks
D. 14–20 weeks
E. 24–30 weeks

11. Of the following, the *least* common symptom associated with endometriosis involving the gastrointestinal tract is

A. abdominal cramping
B. lower abdominal pain
C. pain with defecation
D. constipation
E. intermittent rectal bleeding

12. A 30-year-old has completed her child-bearing. She has mild endometriosis, which was confirmed by laparoscopy 1 year ago. Since that procedure, the patient's dyspareunia and dysmenorrhea have gotten worse. The most reasonable operative procedure at this point is a

A. dilatation and curettage (D&C)
B. uterine suspension
C. total abdominal hysterectomy
D. presacral neurectomy
E. resection of the uterosacral ligaments

13. A 29-year-old patient has documented mild endometriosis and chooses high-dose continuous progestin therapy over the alternative medical treatments offered. She should be informed that her chance of having abnormal bleeding with progestin therapy is approximately

A. 5%
B. 10%
C. 20%
D. 40%
E. 60%

14. Effects of GnRH therapy for endometriosis include all the following *except*

A. decreased follicle-stimulating hormone (FSH)
B. decreased luteinizing hormone (LH)
C. amenorrhea
D. decreased high-density lipoprotein

15. Danazol treatment of endometriosis is associated with an increase in

A. FSH
B. LH
C. low-density lipoprotein
D. high-density lipoprotein

16. Which treatment for endometriosis appears to alter immunologic function?

A. danazol
B. GnRH
C. oral contraceptives
D. Depo-Provera

17. What is the postulated level of estradiol that protects against bone loss while not interfering with the suppressive effects of GnRH agonist?

A. 10 pg/mL
B. 20 pg/mL
C. 30 pg/mL
D. 40 pg/mL

18. The choice of medical therapy for any given patient depends on

A. cost of treatment
B. drug side effects
C. patient compliance
D. all the above

19. If GnRH therapy is begun in the follicular phase, amenorrhea is induced in

A. <1 week
B. 2–3 weeks
C. 4–5 weeks
D. 6–8 weeks

20. **If GnRH therapy is begun in the luteal phase, amenorrhea is induced in**

    A. <1 week
    B. 2–3 weeks
    C. 4–5 weeks
    D. 6–8 weeks

21. **Which of the following is a nasal spray?**

    A. leuprolide acetate (Lupron)
    B. nafarelin acetate (Synarel)
    C. goserelin acetate (Zoladex)
    D. all the above

22. **The most common surgical approach to endometriosis is**

    A. hysteroscopy
    B. laparoscopy
    C. laparotomy
    D. transvaginal

23. **Endometriosis is associated with all the following *except***

    A. anovulation
    B. pain
    C. first-trimester abortion
    D. dyspareunia

24. **Clinical descriptors of young women at a higher than normal risk for endometriosis include all the following *except***

    A. 13-year-old girl with imperforate hymen
    B. 22-year-old woman with regular menses lasting 8 days
    C. 20-year-old woman with irregular menses lasting 3 days
    D. all the above

25. **In an effort to explain the etiologic basis of endometriosis, it has been postulated that**

    A. endometriosis is due to implantation of endometrial cells shed as a result of retrograde menstruation
    B. cells of the müllerian duct, derived from coelomic epithelium, undergo metaplasia to form endometrial tissue
    C. endometrial tissue can be transplanted via both the lymphatic and the vascular system
    D. all the above

26. **Laparoscopy for pelvic pain reveals several lesions. Those that should undergo biopsy to confirm a diagnosis of endometriosis include a**

    A. 0.5-cm blood-filled cyst
    B. powder burn area
    C. clear vesicle
    D. all the above

27. **The classic signs of endometriosis include all the following *except***

    A. a uterosacral ligament nodularity
    B. a fixed retroverted uterus
    C. bilateral symmetrical adnexal enlargement
    D. tenderness on examination

28. **Systematic documentation of the extent of endometriosis includes**

    A. physical findings
    B. location of adhesions
    C. appearance of endometriosis
    D. all the above

29. **Indications for treatment with danazol include**

    A. hereditary angioneurotic edema
    B. benign cystic mastitis
    C. endometriosis
    D. all the above

30. **The therapeutic effect of danazol is due to its binding to**

    A. progesterone receptors
    B. androgen receptors
    C. sex hormone–binding globulin
    D. all the above

31. **A 26-year-old woman has started taking danazol for the treatment of moderate endometriosis. She should be instructed to**

    A. take 200 mg 4 times a day
    B. use mechanical contraceptives during the first month
    C. start treatment on the first day of the menstrual cycle
    D. all the above

32. **A 29-year-old gravida 0 presents with a chief complaint of progressive dysmenorrhea for 2 years. She has had dyspareunia for 12 months, the duration of her marriage. She has never used contraception. Her underlying problem is probably due to**

    A. adenomyosis
    B. chronic pelvic inflammatory disease
    C. endometriosis
    D. leiomyoma

33. **Surgery is mandatory in the treatment of endometriosis for cases in which there is**

    A. ureteral obstruction
    B. compromise of large bowel function
    C. an 8-cm ovarian endometrioma
    D. all the above

34. **The glands and stroma of adenomyosis are**

    A. derived from aberrant glands of the basalis layer of the endometrium
    B. comparable in estrogen and progesterone receptors with the glands and stroma of the endometrium
    C. primarily confined to that part of the myometrium nearest the endometrium
    D. more responsive to hormone stimulation than the glands and stroma of the endometrium

35. **Steroid hormone therapy after definitive surgical treatment for endometriosis should be used to manage**

    A. menopausal symptoms
    B. residual macroscopic endometriosis
    C. suspected microscopic endometriosis
    D. all the above

36. **GnRH agonist therapy for endometriosis is effective when**

    A. there is severe adhesive disease
    B. there is only one endometrioma that is <4 cm in diameter
    C. all lesions are < 1 cm in diameter
    D. all the above

37. **The side effects of GnRH agonists can be made more tolerable with the addition of**

    A. danazol
    B. low-dose estrogen
    C. triphasic oral contraceptives
    D. monophasic oral contraceptives

38. **In patients with moderate to severe endometriosis, in what percentage of cases is the cervix deviated/laterally displaced?**

    A. 15%
    B. 33%
    C. 75%
    D. 90%

39. **How long does it take to recover the bone density lost with 6 months therapy with GnRH agonist**

    A. 1–3 months
    B. 6–9 months
    C. 12–24 months
    D. 36–48 months

ANSWERS

1. **D,** Page 547. Side effects of GnRH agonist therapy are primarily those of estrogen deficiency—that is, hot flashes, hot flushes, vaginal dryness, and insomnia. There are conflicting data about bone mineral content. Any decrease in bone density is, partially or completely, reversible.

2. **C,** Pages 537–542. In most cases, the diagnosis of endometriosis is confirmed by direct laparoscopic visualization and biopsy. Often, it is discovered during an infertility workup. Some persons think that pelvic examination on the first day of the cycle allows evaluation at the time of maximal swelling and tenderness. As with the history, the pelvic examination does not confirm the diagnosis. Because vaginal implants are rare, confirmation via speculum examination is unlikely. Abnormalities found on hysterosalpingogram are not specific for the diagnosis of endometriosis. Endometriosis does not have a specific pattern on either ultrasonography or MRI. The specificity and sensitivity of MRI for endometriosis are approximately 60%. Assays for CA-125 have a low specificity because they are also increased in other conditions, such as pelvic inflammatory disease and epithelial ovarian tumors. The CA-125 level, however, is elevated in a majority of patients with

endometriosis and does tend to increase with advancing stages.

3. **B,** Page 535. The ovaries are the most common site for endometriosis in two of three patients.

4. **B,** Pages 542–552. For a symptomatic young patient with minimal endometriosis, medical suppression is a logical first step in therapy. Laparoscopic laser ablation is a surgical modality often used at the time of diagnosis and could have been performed in this patient. Danazol and GnRH agonist are appropriate drugs for patients whose symptoms persist or whose disease progresses despite administration of oral contraceptives. Laparotomy with resection of endometriotic lesions and hysterectomy with bilateral salpingo-oophorectomy are procedures reserved for more advanced or debilitating endometriosis. Recommending conception must be individualized to the patient's personal needs and circumstances. Such a recommendation carries with it an inherent paradox since infertility is common in patients with endometriosis.

5. **E,** Page 552. In a 42-year-old multigravida, the most logical recommended approach to ovarian endometriosis is hysterectomy with bilateral salpingo-oophorectomy. The extirpative procedure

removes not only macroscopic disease but also the potential stimulus for future endometriosis (ie, the ovaries). Although this is optimal treatment, the patient must share in the decision regarding oophorectomy. Any medical regimen would be considered less acceptable because of the patient's age and the extent of disease. It should also be noted that with pelviscopic surgical techniques, even moderately advanced endometriosis often can be managed at the initial laparoscopic procedure by using laser vaporization.

6. **A,** Page 544. Danazol is an attenuated, orally active androgen. Chemically, it is a synthetic steroid, the isoxazole derivative of ethisterone (17'-ethinyltestosterone). Choice B is testosterone, C is progesterone, D is estradiol, and E is estrone.

7. **B,** Page 536. The three cardinal histologic features of endometriosis are ectopic endometrial glands, ectopic endometrial stroma, and hemorrhage into adjacent tissue. In addition, previous hemorrhage can be discovered by identifying large macrophages filled with hemosiderin near the periphery of the lesion. It has been estimated that no specific pathologic diagnosis can be made in about one third of typical endometriosis cases. Figure 19–2 is hyperplastic dystrophy of the vulva. Figure 19–4 is adenocarcinoma of the endometrium. Figure 19–5 is adenomyosis. Figure 19–6 is squamous cell carcinoma of the cervix.

8. **D,** Page 555. The standard criterion for diagnosis of adenomyosis is the finding of endometrial glands and stroma more than one low-power field (2.5 mm) from the basalis. The glands are typically inactive or proliferative. Cystic hyperplasia occurs occasionally, but secretory patterns are rare. The myometrium reacts to the ectopic endometrium by undergoing both hypertrophy and hyperplasia, thus producing the globular enlargement of the uterus.

9. **B,** Page 556. Patients with adenomyosis are usually asymptomatic. Symptomatic adenomyosis usually appears in women between 35 and 50 years of age; affected women often are parous. The classic symptoms are menorrhagia, dysmenorrhea, and occasionally dyspareunia. The tender, boggy, and enlarged uterus described in this patient is typical. The degree of tenderness and the consistency of the uterus may vary, depending on the time in the patient's menstrual cycle that she is examined.

10. **C,** Page 548. After 6 months of GnRH agonist therapy, ovarian function returns to normal within 6 to 12 weeks. The greatest advantage of a GnRH agonist over danazol appears to be the production of medical castration without androgenic side effects.

11. **E,** Page 552. Gastrointestinal involvement occurs in 5% of cases of endometriosis. Involvement of the small bowel is rare. Most cases of gastrointestinal endometriosis are asymptomatic. If they are symptomatic, however, rectal bleeding is less likely than cramping, lower abdominal pain, pain on defecation, or constipation.

12. **C,** Pages 551–552. No well-controlled studies have documented the benefit of D&C or uterine suspension in endometriosis. Occasionally, presacral neurectomy or uterosacral resection is performed for midline pain. In women who have completed childbearing and are in their late 20s or early 30s, hysterectomy with ovarian preservation can be optimal. In 5% to 10% of women, the disease is subsequently progressive and a second operation, a bilateral oophorectomy, is necessary.

13. **D,** Page 550. The most persistent side effect of progestin therapy for endometriosis is bleeding or spotting. It is reported that approximately 40% of patients who take high-dose progestin therapy for endometriosis experience abnormal bleeding. This can be alleviated somewhat by adding small doses of oral estrogen.

14–16. 14, **D;** 15, **C;** 16, **A;** Pages 554–560. Both GnRH and danazol decrease the levels of FSH and LH. Recent studies have demonstrated that danazol may also modulate immunologic functions by way of affecting macrophages or T lymphocytes. Both drugs induce amenorrhea and have been found to be effective in the treatment of endometriosis, with several double-blind trials demonstrating comparable efficacy. Danazol decreases high-density lipoprotein levels and elevates low-density lipoprotein levels, thereby having a potential effect on atherosclerotic disease. GnRH agonists have no effect on sex hormone–binding globulin, so the androgenic side effects seen with danazol are not observed. This is due to an increase in free serum testosterone that results with decreased sex hormone–binding globulin.

17. **C,** Page 548. Currently, many clinicians "add back" very low doses of estrogen, low doses of progestins, or both in combination with long-term GnRH agonist therapy. The daily add-back therapy is begun after 2 to 3 months of agonist therapy. It is postulated that the addition of low-dose estrogen or progestins will make the side effects less bothersome and diminish or overcome the demineralization of bone. Barbieri has suggested that there is a therapeutic window that he estimates is a circulating level of approximately 30 pg/mL of estradiol. He postulates that this level of estradiol is enough to protect the body from substantial bone loss and is not high enough to interfere with the inhibition of endometriosis.

18. **D,** Page 544. To date, no hormonal therapy has been able to produce long-lasting cures with ablation of all foci of endometriosis after discontinuation of hormonal management. The choice of medical therapy for the individual patient depends on the clinician's evaluation of adverse effects, side effects, cost of therapy, and expected patient compliance. The recurrence rate following medical therapy is 5% to 15% in the first year; it increases to 40% to 50% in 5 years. Obviously, the chance of recurrence is directly related to the extent of initial disease.

19–20. 19, **D;** 20, **C;** Pages 546–548. A patient's response to agonist therapy depends on when therapy is initiated. If during the follicular phase, estradiol levels rise for approximately 3 weeks, after which they rapidly decline, there is no LH surge, and amenorrhea is induced within 6 to 8 weeks. If, on the other hand, after it has been determined that the patient is not pregnant, agonist therapy is begun during the luteal phase, LH levels are elevated for 1 week, and estradiol levels are suppressed to those of a castrated female within 2 weeks. Amenorrhea is induced within 4 to 5 weeks.

21. **B,** Page 546. Multiple GnRH agonists have been developed. These agonists may be administered by the intravenous, intramuscular, subcutaneous, intravaginal, or intranasal route. The oral route is not practical because the hormone is inactivated by enzymes in the gastrointestinal tract. Representative agonists are leuprolide acetate (Lupron, injectable), nafarelin acetate (Synarel, intranasal), and goserelin acetate (Zoladex, subcutaneous implant). The usual dose of leuprolide acetate is 3.75 mg intramuscularly once per month or 11.25 mg depot injection every 3 months. Nafarelin acetate nasal spray is given in a dose of 1 spray (200 g) in one nostril in the morning and 1 spray (200 g) in the other nostril in the evening. Goserelin acetate is given in a dosage of 3.6 mg every 28 days in a biodegradable subcutaneous implant.

22. **B,** Pages 550–552. Laparoscopy is employed frequently for both diagnostic and therapeutic reasons. The major advantage of treating endometriosis with laparoscopy, using either the laser or electrocautery, is that the patient may be treated at the time of diagnosis. Depending on the operative technique chosen, endometriosis is coagulated, vaporized, resected, or subjected to a combination thereof. The vast majority of surgical treatment for endometriosis occurs via laparoscopy rather than laparotomy because of a shorter recovery period and reduction in the extent of subsequent adhesions. Hysteroscopy allows visualization of the endometrium only and is therefore not appropriate for visualization of endometriosis.

Hysteroscopy may be used in conjunction with laparoscopy if an intrauterine pathologic condition is suspected. A transvaginal view is limited and is of no clinical benefit for suspected endometriosis.

23. **C,** Pages 537–538. Approximately 15% of women with endometriosis also have coincidental anovulation. Pain is a well-known symptom, but there is no correlation between pain severity or frequency and the stage of endometriosis. Although first-trimester abortion has been reported to be associated with endometriosis, more recent data call this into question.

24. **C,** Page 532. The theory of retrograde menstruation as a cause of endometriosis is supported by clinical observations that women with a menstrual flow longer than 7 days have a two times greater prevalence of endometriosis. Endometriosis is also found frequently in women with outflow obstruction of the genital tract.

25. **D,** Page 532. Most authorities think that several factors are probably involved in causing endometriosis. These include retrograde menstruation, metaplasia of coelomic epithelium, and transport of endometrial cells via blood or lymphatics. A genetic predisposition has also been identified. Abnormalities of both humoral and cell-mediated components of the immune system also have been implicated. In addition, iatrogenic dissemination of endometriosis has been reported.

26. **D,** Page 539. Endometriotic lesions have a myriad of appearances. The gross appearance of the lesion depends on the site, the activity and chronicity of the endometriosis, and the day of the menstrual cycle. The predominant color depends on the blood supply, the amount of hemorrhage, and the degree of fibrosis. New lesions are small, usually blood-filled cysts of less than 1 cm in diameter. Clinically, they are often described as "raspberry spots" or "powder burns." Initially, they are raised above the surrounding tissue. With time, they become larger and assume a light- or dark-brown color associated with intense scarring. These may appear as blood-filled or chocolate cysts. They are usually puckered or retracted from the surrounding tissue. The pattern of ovarian endometriosis varies. Individual areas vary from 1 mm to 14 cm, with associated adhesions that may be filmy or dense. Larger cysts are usually densely adherent to the pelvic sidewall or the broad ligament.

27. **C,** Page 539. The most constant pelvic findings associated with endometriosis are a fixed retroverted uterus with scarring and tenderness posterior to the uterus. Characteristic nodularity of the uterosacral ligaments and the cul-de-sac of Douglas may be palpated on the rectovaginal

examination. The ovaries may be enlarged and tender and often are fixed. The adnexal enlargement is rarely symmetrical.

28. **D,** Page 540. A committee of the American Society of Reproductive Medicine developed a detailed form to help the clinician document the most important features of endometriosis and pelvic pain (see Figure 19–10 in Stenchever). The key elements of this form are a complete description of the patient's symptoms, documenting physical findings of tenderness, commenting on the presence of adhesive disease by location and points of attachment, illustrating the operative appearance of peritoneal endometriosis, and documenting posttreatment symptoms and physical findings at regular intervals using additional dated forms.

29. **D,** Pages 544–546. Danazol has been an important medication in the treatment of endometriosis since its FDA approval in the mid-1970s. It is also useful in cases of menorrhagia, benign cystic mastitis, and hereditary angioneurotic edema.

30. **D,** Pages 544–546. Danazol binds to androgen and progesterone receptors and also to sex hormone–binding globulin. It directly inhibits several steroidogenic enzymes in both the ovary and the adrenal gland.

31. **D,** Pages 544–546. The standard prescribed dosage of danazol is 400 to 800 mg/day for approximately 6 months. The half-life of this oral drug is between 4 and 5 hours. Therefore, for the 800-mg dosage regimen, it is best to recommend 1 tablet 4 times/day rather than 2 tablets in the morning and 2 tablets at night. Prescribing danazol, 200 mg every 6 hours, results in mean serum estradiol concentrations that are 40% lower than with the alternative regimen, 400 mg 2 times/day. Traditionally, the drug is started on the fifth day after the onset of menses. The length of therapy of oral danazol should be individualized, depending partly on the stage of endometriosis. Women should use mechanical contraceptives for the first month because danazol has produced female pseudohermaphroditism in a developing fetus. If it is certain that the patient is not pregnant, danazol is begun on the first day of the menstrual bleeding. By starting the hormone earlier in the cycle, the patient experiences less breakthrough bleeding during the first 4 to 6 weeks.

32. **C,** Pages 531–532. The patient described is most likely to have endometriosis. There is no history of prior infection to warrant a diagnosis of chronic PID, but this condition must still be included in the differential diagnosis. Adenomyosis is most likely in a multiparous patient. There is no clinical suspicion or evidence of leiomyoma. If this condition is suspected, ultrasound could help make this diagnosis.

33. **D,** Pages 550–552. Although the choice between medical and surgical management for endometriosis depends on many considerations, certain findings warrant surgical management. Ureteral obstruction can ultimately lead to renal failure. Large bowel involvement by endometriosis must be managed surgically to avoid extensive compromise of bowel function. A large endometrioma poses the risk of an acute accident such as torsion, rupture, and hemorrhage. Furthermore, it should be remembered that an ovarian malignancy and an endometrioma can present the same clinical picture.

34. **A,** Page 554. Adenomyosis and endometriosis are different clinical entities. The glands in adenomyosis, derived from the basalis layer, are not as responsive to hormones as are those in the endometrium. This may, in part, be due to the relative lack of estrogen and progesterone receptors in the glands and stroma of adenomyosis. In most instances, adenomyosis is diffusely distributed throughout the myometrium.

35. **D,** Page 552. Postoperative hormones can be given for a variety of indications. If all the endometriosis has not been removed, administration of medroxyprogesterone is recommended for 1 year. To treat menopausal symptoms, cyclic estrogen and progestin can be used. Postoperative danazol or oral contraceptives may help eradicate microscopic endometriosis.

36. **C,** Pages 546–548. GnRH agonist therapy improves symptoms in up to 90% of patients, depending on the extent of the disease. The greatest effects occur in patients whose endometriotic lesions are <1 cm in diameter. On the other hand, endometriomas and severe adhesive disease do not respond to hormonal therapy.

37. **B,** Page 548. "Add-back" hormone therapy is now commonly used in combination with chronic use of GnRH agonist regimens. The daily add-back is begun simultaneously with the initial dose of agonist. This is meant to reduce or eliminate vasomotor symptoms and vaginal atrophy and to overcome bone demineralization. Both estrogen and progestin can be used in this way. Oral contraceptives, either monophasic or triphasic, do supply adequate amounts of estrogen and progestin but have greater pharmacologic impact than is required for symptomatic relief.

38. **A,** Page 539. Lateral displacement or deviation of the cervix is visualized or palpated by digital examination of the vagina and cervix in approximately 15% of women with moderate or severe endometriosis.

39. **C,** Page 547. Side effects associated with GnRH agonists are those associated with estrogen deprivation and are similar to menopause. A 2% to 7% decrease in bone mineral content of trabecular bone in the lumbar spine has been reported. This decrease does not occur in the compact bone of the distal radius. The decrease in bone density completely recovers in 12 to 24 months after therapy is discontinued.

Anatomic Defects of the Abdominal Wall and Pelvic Floor

DIRECTIONS:

for Questions 1–9: Select the one best answer or completion.

1. A 72-year-old para 3 has a history of a recently noticed "bulge" protruding through the vaginal introitus. Fifteen months before this visit a vaginal hysterectomy was performed on this patient for uterine descensus. This "bulge" is most likely a(n)

   A. cystocele
   B. rectocele
   C. enterocele
   D. prolapsed ovary
   E. sigmoid diverticulum

2. In performing a lower abdominal midline incision, the major anatomic landmark encountered in the abdominal wall that involves a change in the fascial investiture of the rectus muscle is

   A. Hesselbach's triangle
   B. linea semilunaris
   C. linea nigra
   D. linea alba
   E. umbilicus

3. A 52-year-old para 4 complains of a bulging vaginal mass, constipation, and incomplete stool evacuation. The anatomic defect most likely to contribute to these is

   A. a cystourethrocele
   B. uterine prolapse
   C. poor anal sphincter tone
   D. a rectocele
   E. an enterocele

4. An 82-year-old woman with total vaginal vault prolapse is referred to you with a 2-month history of noticing a "bulge" between her labia. She is being treated for congestive heart failure. She underwent total abdominal hysterectomy and bilateral oophorectomy 25 years earlier and has been sexually inactive for more than 15 years. The best choice of a surgical procedure to correct this problem is a(n)

   A. abdominal suspension from the rectus fascia
   B. abdominal sacral colpopexy
   C. abdominal enterocele reduction
   D. vaginal colpocleisis
   E. vaginal sacrosphinous ligament suspension

5. A defect in pelvic anatomy that can be correctly called a true hernia is a(n)

   A. cystocele
   B. enterocele
   C. rectocele
   D. urethrocele
   E. ureterocele

6. The goal of an anterior colporrhaphy performed to correct stress urinary incontinence in a patient who has a cystourethrocele is to

   A. foreshorten the pubovesical fascia
   B. lengthen the urethra
   C. make the bladder smaller
   D. correct the urethrovesical angle
   E. replace the bladder neck behind the pubic symphysis

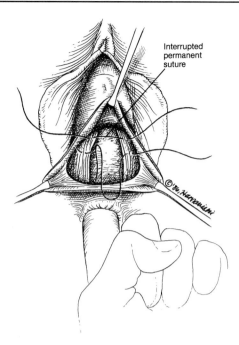

FIGURE 20–1   (From Mishell DR Jr, Stenchever MA, Droegemueller W, Herbst AL: Comprehensive Gynecology, 3rd ed., St. Louis, Mosby, 1997.)

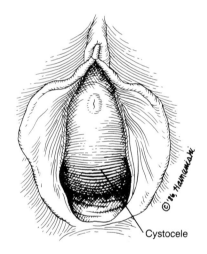

FIGURE 20–2

7. The structure, pictured in Figure 20–1, that provides the most support in the repair of a rectocele is the

A. levator ani muscle group
B. perirectal connective tissue
C. proximal fibers of the superficial transverse muscle of perineum
D. trimmed posterior vaginal mucosa
E. anal sphincter

8. At the time of preoperative evaluation of a patient on whom you anticipate performing a postpartum tubal sterilization, you notice a 5-cm umbilical hernia. You would now

A. proceed with the operation as planned and repair the hernia on completion of the sterilization
B. proceed with the tubal sterilization and plan repair of the hernia at a later date
C. schedule a sterilization procedure at a time when a general surgeon can assist with a herniorrhaphy
D. proceed with the sterilization only and make a lower midline vertical incision
E. proceed with the operation using the laparoscope

9. A 48-year-old patient with the anatomic findings illustrated in Figure 20–2 has symptoms of pelvic pressure, urethral irritation, and constant stress urinary incontinence with mild Valsalva maneuver. If the appropriate urologic workup documents stress urinary incontinence, the procedure most likely to obtain good results is a(n)

A. Marshall-Marchetti-Krantz procedure
B. vaginal hysterectomy with anterior colporrhaphy
C. anterior wall colporrhaphy
D. Burch procedure
E. Pereyra operation

DIRECTIONS:

for Questions 10–19: For each numbered item, select the one heading most closely associated with it. Each lettered heading may be used once, more than once, or not at all.

10–13. Choose the most appropriate surgical procedure for the patients described below.

(A) vaginal hysterectomy and anteroposterior colporrhaphy
(B) Manchester-Fothergill and anterior colporrhaphy
(C) LeFort (modified)
(D) Watkins interposition
(E) Goodall-Power

10. An 85-year-old widowed woman with congestive heart failure and total procidentia

11. A 45-year-old with an elongated cervix, a well-supported uterus, and a cystourethrocele who has stress urinary incontinence. This patient has a long history of pelvic inflammatory disease.

12. A 78-year-old sexually inactive woman with a second-degree cystocele and rectocele

13. A 45-year-old woman with a second-degree cystourethrocele who has stress urinary incontinence

14–16. Operative procedures involving use of the abdominal approach for the management of descensus of the vaginal vault posthysterectomy have included fixation of the vaginal vault to various structures.

(A) anterior abdominal wall
(B) lumbar spine
(C) sacral promontory
(D) sacrospinous ligament
(E) none of the above

14. Which of the above increases the risk of enterocele?

15. Which of the above can be done via the vaginal route?

16. Which of the above does *not* require repair of an existent enterocele to repair a vaginal vault prolapse successfully?

17–19. Match the anatomic finding with the appropriate statement.

(A) cystocele
(B) enterocele
(C) rectocele
(D) urethrocele

17. Is considered a true hernia.

18. Contributes to urinary incontinence.

19. Contributes to urinary retention.

DIRECTIONS:

for Questions 20–39: Select the one best answer or completion.

20. The following anatomic descriptions are true for the inguinal canal *except*

A. This aperture results from the embryonic descent of the testes from their original retroperitoneal site to the scrotum.
B. Herniated peritoneum into this space may occur in both sexes.
C. In a woman, the round ligament courses through this aperture.
D. It runs from the internal ring vertically to the external ring at Hesselbach's triangle.

21. The following are factors that increase the occurrence of incisional hernias *except*

A. chronic cough
B. fascial necrosis from sutures being too tight
C. poor nutrition
D. recent pregnancy
E. wound infection

22. Nonoperative management of hernias of the ventral wall and groin is often feasible in women. Strategies that work include all the following *except*

A. corset for small incisional hernia
B. nothing during pregnancy for an uncomplicated umbilical hernia
C. truss for inguinal hernia
D. waiting until age 3 or 4 years to repair congenital umbilical hernia

23. During the performance of a vaginal hysterectomy, a postoperative enterocele is prevented by appropriate surgical disposition of all the following *except*

A. broad ligaments and round ligaments
B. cardinal ligaments
C. cul-de-sac peritoneum
D. uterosacral ligaments

24. Although the appropriate surgical correction of vaginal vault (stump) prolapse includes a recognition of many factors, the *least* important is

A. desire for sexual activity
B. enterocele
C. normal axis of the vagina in a standing position
D. perineal body anatomy
E. urethrocele

25. A cystourethrocele is more likely to develop if a woman has

A. an anthropoid pelvis
B. an episiotomy at the time of vaginal delivery
C. had two or more cesarean sections for abnormal fetal lie
D. prominent ischial spines
E. a wide pubic arch

26. **The characteristics of an umbilical hernia include the fact that**

    A. during repair, remnants of the umbilical cord are often found
    B. the herniation is at the point where the vertical linea semilunaris joins the lateral border of the rectus muscle
    C. this fascial defect in its more severe form appears as a gastroschisis
    D. this fascial defect usually closes during the first 3 years of life

27. **The following are true regarding abdominal hernias in adults** *except*

    A. They are congenital in origin.
    B. They contain visceral organ structures (eg, bowel).
    C. They contain a reflection of peritoneum (sac).
    D. They represent a fascial defect.

28. **After a hysterectomy, surgical culdoplasty may be performed by all the following** *except*

    A. fixing the uterosacral ligaments to the cul-de-sac peritoneum
    B. obliterating the cul-de-sac by concentric purse-string sutures in the endopelvic fascia
    C. shortening the cul-de-sac by suturing the uterosacral ligaments in the midline and to the edge of the proximal vaginal incision
    D. suturing the round ligaments and the ovarian ligaments to the edge of the proximal vaginal incision

29. **Refer to Figure 20–3. For vaginal sacrospinous ligament fixation, proper placement of sutures is indicated by**

    A. label *1*
    B. label *2*
    C. label *3*
    D. none of the above

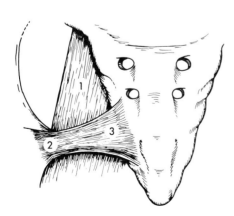

FIGURE 20–3

30. **Among women reporting urinary incontinence, what is the percentage who also have fecal incontinence?**

    A. 3%
    B. 15%
    C. 30%
    D. 60%

31. **What structure provides the voluntary squeeze pressure that prevents fecal incontinence despite increasing rectal or abdominal pressure?**

    A. internal anal sphincter
    B. external anal sphincter
    C. puborectalis
    D. pubococcygeus

32. **What important reflex is missing in patients with Hirschprung disease?**

    A. rectoanal inhibitory reflex
    B. gastrocolic reflex
    C. patellar reflex
    D. Babinski reflex

33. **Fecal incontinence is most commonly due to**

    A. pelvic floor denervation
    B. diet
    C. aging
    D. obstetric injury
    E. surgical misadventure

34. **Chronic constipation can be caused by which of the following drugs?**

    A. narcotics
    B. antidepressants
    C. anticholinergics
    D. all of the above

35. **The dovetail sign or loss of anterior perineal folds indicates a defect in**

    A. internal anal sphincter
    B. external anal sphincter
    C. bulbocavernosus muscle
    D. superficial transverse perineal muscle

36. **In a woman complaining of fecal incontinence in whom the results of physical examination are normal including normal rectal tone, which of the following tests is initially indicated?**

    A. anal manometry
    B. pudendal nerve latency
    C. anal ultrasound imaging
    D. thyroid-stimulating hormone level

37. **The integrity, thickness, and length of both the internal and the external sphincters can be determined by**
    A. transanal ultrasonography
    B. colonoscopy
    C. anal manometry
    D. electromyography

38. **Surgical management of fecal incontinence includes all of the following** *except*
    A. anal sphincteroplasty
    B. repair of rectal prolapse
    C. posterior levatorplasty
    D. implantation of artificial sphincters

39. **The most common cause of rectovaginal fistula is**
    A. obstetric trauma
    B. inflammatory process
    C. neoplasm
    D. foreign body

ANSWERS

1. **C**, Page 576. Enteroceles frequently occur after hysterectomy and generally are due to weakened support of the pouch of Douglas. Lack of attention to the surgical repair of the supporting structures at the time of original operation may contribute to the formation of a postoperative enterocele, especially one that appears this soon after the antecedent hysterectomy. A small preexisting herniation of peritoneum may have been overlooked during the vaginal hysterectomy. Lack of obliteration of this hernia sac and improper attention to the plication of uterosacral or cardinal ligaments may contribute to the development of an enterocele shortly after operation. In this situation, there is often a degree of total vault prolapse perceived by the patient as a "bulge" passing through the vaginal introitus. Although a cystocele and a rectocele may be associated with an enterocele, they are usually secondary rather than primary offenders. Prolapsed adnexal structures are rare and usually are not involved in cases of vaginal vault prolapse. Likewise, prolapse of the sigmoid colon or parts of the sigmoid colon does not appear in this fashion.

2. **B**, Page 566; Figure 20–1 in Stenchever. The investing fascia of the external oblique, internal oblique, and transversus abdominis muscles completely encases the rectus abdominis muscles cephalad to the linea semilunaris. Caudally from the semilunar line, the muscle is completely posterior to the aponeurosis of the fascia of these muscles and lies directly on the peritoneum. In making a midline incision, this change is apparent after the rectus muscle is mobilized laterally and just before entry into the peritoneal cavity. In the repair of this incision, it is important to remember that this area of relative weakness contributes to a higher-than-normal incidence of postoperative abdominal incisional hernias. Hesselbach's triangle defines that anatomic area in which a defect in the fascia transversalis may result in a femoral type of groin hernia. The linea alba is the midline fusion of the rectal fascia and is not used as a superficial anatomic landmark. The linea nigra is a vertical discoloration of the skin occurring between the umbilicus and the top of the pubic symphysis.

3. **D**, Page 574. In a patient with these complaints, referable primarily to lower bowel dysfunction, the most likely contributing anatomic defect is a rectocele. The other anatomic defects may be associated with the presence of a rectocele but do not contribute to these symptoms. Patients may often need to "splint" the posterior vaginal wall to ameliorate those symptoms associated with difficulty in bowel movements. Chronic constipation in these patients, with retention of firm stool in the lower colon, can be associated with degrees of discomfort during sexual intercourse. Poor anal sphincter tone may be secondary to an incompletely healed perineal laceration incurred during childbirth. Symptoms related to this defect, such as incontinence of stool or flatus, did not manifest in this patient and, when present, are not necessarily associated with other disorders of pelvic support. Operative management of a rectocele is generally carried out at the time of other vaginal surgery. Likewise, perineal body reconstruction (perineorrhaphy) is also indicated in patients with a marked defect in perineal support. However, this does not routinely imply reconstruction of the anal sphincter.

4. **D**, Page 583. Although there are a variety of procedures to manage vaginal vault (stump) prolapse, selection of the appropriate procedure is guided by a number of factors. These include the

age of the patient, sexual activity, the specific anatomic defects involved, and the general health of the patient. In this geriatric patient who is sexually inactive and has congestive heart failure, an extensive abdominal operation involving either suspension of the vaginal wall to the rectus fascia or any of a variety of sacral suspensions using inert gauze material is not needed. Because this patient is sexually inactive, a more extensive procedure such as vaginal sacrospinous ligament suspension is not necessary. The logical choice for this situation is some form of vaginal closure or colpocleisis. This could be a vaginectomy or vaginal colpocleisis modified after the LeFort procedure. In performing this procedure, it is important to identify an enterocele if it is present so that the appropriate dissection, ligation, and excision of redundant peritoneum can be accomplished to prevent an enterocele from forming posterior to the colpocleisis.

5. **B,** Page 576. An enterocele is a true hernia of the peritoneal cavity emanating from the pouch of Douglas between the uterosacral ligaments and into the rectovaginal septum. The enterocele may be noticed as a separate bulge above the rectocele, and at times it may be large enough to prolapse through the vagina. A hernia by definition must contain a serosal sac, and it may also contain bowel or omentum. The other defects noted in the other choices are not true hernias in that they do not contain herniated peritoneum through a fascial defect. They are prolapsed distal bowel (rectocele), bladder (cystocele), or urethra (urethrocele). A urethrocele is usually a detachment of the urethra rather than a ballooning out of this structure. It is the most unusual of those listed and represents sacculation of the distal ureter into the bladder as a result of stenosis of the ureteral meatus.

6. **E,** Pages 571–572. The overall goal of anterior colporrhaphy to correct urinary incontinence is to replace the bladder neck behind the symphysis pubis in order to increase the amount of pressure transmitted to the proximal urethra during Valsalva maneuvers. The anatomic abnormality associated with urinary incontinence is discussed in Chapter 21 of Stenchever. The other corrections noted in this question may all occur in the process of performing an adequate anterior colporrhaphy; that is, the pubovesical fascia may be drawn more closely toward the midline by appropriately placed Kelly plication sutures. Depending on the degree of urethrocele, the urethra may be somewhat lengthened, although this is not thought to lend appreciably to urinary continence. Bladder capacity may be reduced by a cystocele repair, which results in the urge to void sooner

than when there is marked laxity in the vaginal wall. Finally, the urethrovesical angle may be increased in the process of anterior colporrhaphy because of appropriate elevation of the bladder neck behind the symphysis. However, the angle in and of itself is probably not important in correcting incontinence.

7. **A,** Page 575. In performing a posterior colporrhaphy, the major contribution to the restoration of the pelvic floor anatomy is made by reducing the aperture of the levator hiatus. Although the levator plate is made up of a number of muscles, restoration of the anatomy of the pubococcygeus and puborectalis is probably most important. Plication of the lower margins of the bulbocavernosus and transverse perinei muscles also strengthens the support of the urogenital diaphragm. During dissection in the operating room, separation and identification of these muscles are difficult. The superficial transverse perinei do not lend appreciably to pelvic muscle support, nor does the relatively attenuated perirectal connective tissue. The trimmed vaginal mucosa likewise does not strengthen the posterior vaginal wall. The anal sphincter is usually not involved in this repair procedure. Knowledge of the anatomy of the levator plate is important in planning the appropriate operation for patients with marked posterior vaginal wall defects.

8. **A,** Page 569. In this unexpected situation, the presence of a small umbilical hernia need not deter the surgeon from performing the original operation. A Pomeroy tubal sterilization can be carried out with appropriate repair of the umbilical hernia after completion of the sterilization. Care should be taken to completely dissect the peritoneal sac away from the point of intraperitoneal entry. Likewise, care should be taken to find the lateral extent of the fascial defect and to repair this by direct approximation from superior to inferior using nonabsorbable sutures; the fascia is closed in a "vest over pants" manner. There is no point in delaying the repair of this hernia to a later date if it can be repaired at the time of this operation. A gynecologist should have the competence to perform an umbilical herniorrhaphy without assistance from a general surgeon. There is no need to change the incision, nor is there any need to use the laparoscope. Knowledge of this anatomic defect at the time of operation should alert the surgeon to the possibility of adherent bowel just under the peritoneal sac or the presence of a Meckel's diverticulum just beneath the peritoneal surface. Another consideration in this question has to do with the issue of informed consent. Appropriate informed consent must be obtained for all surgical procedures. With the

potential alteration of the umbilicus, the surgeon should be aware that surgical alteration of this structure may carry with it the risk of patient dissatisfaction.

9. **B,** Pages 571–572. Although a number of options exist for surgical correction of stress urinary incontinence, certain principles can be used to guide surgical decisions. The point of this question is to consider a general approach based on specific anatomic findings. Accordingly, this patient, with marked anterior wall relaxation (cystourethrocele) and related pelvic pressure and irritation, should undergo a vaginal procedure. This will best treat the anatomic defect (cystourethrocele) while offering a high degree of success in curing the incontinence. Most surgeons would agree that in a patient of this age, concomitant vaginal hysterectomy is also indicated. Although it could be argued that a combined operation might be better, it should be appreciated that the performance of a retropubic operation, such as in a Marshall-Marchetti-Krantz or a Burch procedure, is not indicated as the sole operation. Likewise, the Pereyra operation performed without correction of the cystourethrocele will not correct the vaginal wall defect.

10–13. 10, **C;** 11, **B;** 12, **C;** 13, **A;** Pages 571–585. This series of questions deals with the choice of surgical treatment for symptomatic pelvic relaxation under different circumstances. It must be realized that there is no consensus among surgeons about the appropriate surgical treatment in every case; however, the situations described here do delineate the types of operations to be considered in certain instances. In general, eponyms should be avoided, but certain surgical procedures are named for the surgeon or surgeons who first described and popularized them. It is realized that some of these operations are rarely indicated. This series of operations underscores the need for the consultant to know a wide range of surgical options and thus assist the occasional individual patient. The LeFort operation is usually considered the procedure of choice in geriatric patients with total prolapse. This is in contrast with the Goodall-Power modification, which is used with lesser degrees of prolapse in the geriatric age group. This operation involves removing smaller triangular portions of the anterior and posterior vaginal wall mucosa instead of the traditional rectangular portions removed in the LeFort operation. Thus, when sutured together after reduction of the uterus, effective colpocleisis has been accomplished. Both operations obliterate the vagina and should be reserved for sexually inactive women. Both usually are done in conjunction with a perineorrhaphy as an additional measure to ensure a better long-term result. The Manchester-Fothergill operation is rarely indicated today. It is reserved for the occasional patient who has appreciable stress urinary incontinence, an elongated cervix, and excellent uterine support either by previous operation or by intercurrent inflammatory or adhesion disease. An adequate anterior colporrhaphy and plication of the vesical neck can be accomplished with this operation, which involves amputating the elongated cervix and using the cardinal ligaments to improve support. The Watkins interposition or transposition operation was used extensively for uterine prolapse in patients with a large cystocele. The operation consists of amputating the elongated cervix and suturing the fundus of the uterus beneath the large cystocele. The fundus therefore was used as an obturator to fill the defect in the anterior segment of the pelvic diaphragm. This operation is rarely used today in lieu of more popular forms of vaginal plastic procedures and because of the possibility of endometrial cancer developing in a relatively inaccessible uterus. Most instances of symptomatic vaginal relaxation associated with uterine prolapse can be surgically treated by vaginal hysterectomy and anterior and posterior colporrhaphy. This maintains a degree of vaginal depth and caliber suitable for sexual function while correcting anatomic defects that may be associated with urinary incontinence or problems with bowel evacuation. The gynecologic surgeon should realize that although vaginal hysterectomy with colporrhaphy usually can be performed, another operation is available when indicated by special circumstances to ensure the overall health of the patient.

14–16. 14, **A;** 15, **D;** 16, **E;** Pages 583–585. A variety of vaginal or abdominal procedures are available to correct vaginal stump prolapse. Within each category, specialized surgical nuances may be applied to individual cases. In choosing an abdominal colpopexy of some variety, attention should be paid to the restoration of the anatomy so that after the procedure the anatomy will be as nearly normal as possible. With either a vaginal or an abdominal colpopexy, an enterocele must be identified if one is present. In vaginal reconstructive surgery, recognition of a dissecting enterocele sac should prompt its removal. In the abdominal operation the deep cul-de-sac or beginning enterocele should be closed before the vaginal vault is attached to a fixed structure. If the surgical approach does not consider an existing enterocele, sac dissection may take place despite adequate support of the vaginal vault. If fixation to the anterior abdominal wall is chosen, the diameter of the pouch of Douglas is increased. This frequently adds to the risk of subsequent enterocele development if steps are not taken to obliterate the cul-de-sac. Both abdominal and vaginal procedures may preserve sexual function. This is especially important to consider when an associated vaginal repair is performed. Adequate caliber and depth can be maintained with careful attention to anatomic principles. The sacrospinous ligaments may be used for additional vaginal vault support in selected vaginal cases. This operation is technically more difficult and potentially riskier than routine vaginal colporrhaphy, but occasionally it should be chosen as a means of ensuring vaginal vault support.

17-19. **17, B; 18, D; 19, A; Pages 571–577.** A rectocele, a cystocele, and a urethrocele are not considered true hernias because these conditions do not include the protrusion of a peritoneal reflection or sac through a true fascial defect. Only the enterocele meets the definition of a true hernia. Attenuation or rupture of the pubovesical cervical fascia for any reason may allow the descent of the urethra (urethrocele), bladder neck, or bladder (cystocele) into the vaginal canal. Often a cystocele is present, and in this situation the patient is generally continent of urine. When a urethrocele is also present, the woman usually suffers from stress urinary incontinence because the urethra has rotated posteriorly. The urethra and bladder neck now lie in a position where intraabdominal pressure is not transmitted to the periurethral tissues. In other words, there is little compensatory pressure around the bladder neck and proximal urethra during times of Valsalva maneuver. In this situation, relatively more pressure is exerted on the bladder and relatively less pressure is placed on the urethra, thereby creating urinary incontinence. Even in the presence of a cystocele, with maintenance of normal intraurethral pressures, patients generally remain continent of urine. Women whose only defect is a cystocele with good urethral support may have difficulty with urinary retention because of marked caudal rotation of the bladder, effectively "kinking" the urethra. Such women may need to reposition the cystocele vaginally before they can void. This observation is useful when considering surgical techniques to correct anatomically related stress urinary incontinence.

20. **D, Page 567; Figure 20–2 in Stenchever.** Because of embryonic descent of the testis from its original retroperitoneal site to the scrotum, the internal inguinal ring is formed at the level of the transversalis fascia. The inguinal canal runs from the internal inguinal ring obliquely in a medial and caudal direction, emerging through the external inguinal ring, opening in the external oblique aponeurosis just above the pubic tubercle, and continuing into the scrotum. In the female, the round ligament courses similarly and ends just short of the labium majus. (The femoral canal represents a potential space under the inguinal ligament medial to the femoral vessels and lateral to the lacunar ligament. With a femoral hernia, the defect is in the transversalis fascia at Hesselbach's triangle.) Because there is no embryonic movement of the testicle in women, their inguinal canal is less likely to be associated with herniated peritoneum. Femoral hernias are more common in women than in men. Either potential space (canal) may be involved with a hernia that includes a portion of the bowel.

21. **D, Page 567.** Incisional hernias generally occur because of poor healing of the fascia. This may be due to intrinsic fascial problems associated with poor nutrition, infection of the incision, or fascial necrosis resulting from either infection or strangulation of the tissue by a closure that was too tight. An absorbable suture, especially in the setting of a wound infection, may lose its tensile strength before healing is complete. Repetitive stress and strain on the incision may interfere with healing. This can be caused by chronic cough or emesis postoperatively or by abdominal distention from marked ileus, ascites, or ongoing pregnancy. Postpartum operations do not involve increased risk simply because they are postpartum.

22. **C, Page 567.** Nonoperative management of hernias is often feasible. Congenital umbilical hernias often undergo spontaneous closure within the first 3 or 4 years of life. Small uncomplicated incisional hernias can be managed through application of abdominal wall pressure such as a corset. This tends to prevent incarceration. Unincarcerated groin hernias that are small may not need repair unless there is an increase in intraabdominal pressure (eg, associated with pregnancy, chronic cough, or frequent Valsalva maneuvers such as in repetitive lifting or straining). In pregnancy the risk of incarceration is actually lessened because of the uterus pushing the bowel and the omentum away from the true pelvis and the anterior abdominal wall. Since the surgical repair may be compromised by the increasing uterine size, hernia repairs are often delayed until the postpartum period unless incarceration or strangulation occurs. Trusses and other supports are generally difficult to fit and are of little value in women.

23. **A, Pages 576–577.** Enteroceles may occur after abdominal or vaginal hysterectomy and generally are due to a weakened support system around the cul-de-sac or pouch of Douglas. Inasmuch as an enterocele may form by herniation of the cul-de-sac past the uterosacral ligaments into the

rectovaginal septum, appropriate surgical disposition of the uterosacral ligaments, cardinal ligaments, and peritoneum overlying the cul-de-sac is imperative. Generally, if redundant peritoneum is beginning to herniate into the rectovaginal septum, this space should be closed after removal of the uterus to prevent further extension. Similarly, the uterosacral and cardinal ligaments should be plicated in the midline or into the vaginal cuff. The broad and round ligaments do not provide any functional support of the uterus or surrounding structures. They do not offer any benefit if incorporated into the vaginal closure for support. Each of these procedures has a number of variations, but all are considered types of culdoplasty.

24. **E,** Pages 583–585. There is some controversy with respect to the choice of procedure to correct a vaginal vault (stump) prolapse. Nevertheless, certain principles and facts are important. The first is that the normal position of the vagina in the standing position is against the rectum and no more than 30 degrees from the horizontal. This is important for the occasional patient in whom abdominal colpopexy is anticipated. The second principle is that pelvic relaxation is part of the problem and dictates that an existing cystocele, rectocele, or enterocele be repaired as part of this procedure to ensure long-term success. Defects are likely to recur when appropriate recognition and repair have not taken place during the initial surgery for vaginal prolapse. The third principle acknowledges that the perineal body is almost always severely weakened in women with total vaginal vault prolapse and therefore must be reconstructed. Although the recognition of a urethrocele is important relative to postoperative urinary continence, the lack of repair does not promote failure of the vaginal vault suspension. The patient's desire to be sexually active has significant impact on the choice of repair and maintenance of the caliber of the vaginal vault. It is clear that a LeFort procedure would not be appropriate in a sexually active person.

25. **E,** Page 571. The factors associated with the development of a cystourethrocele are numerous and difficult to state in specific terms, but some general associations can be noted. These include parity and a wide pelvic arch typical of the gynecoid type of pelvis. Although a cystourethrocele may develop in nulliparous women, this is unusual. In such cases, the patient often has concomitant neurologic or metabolic disease contributing to loss of pelvic support, or she may be overweight or have chronic obstructive pulmonary disease. The presence of a wide pubic arch in a gynecoid type of pelvis allows the full force of the fetal head to compress against this area during descent in the second stage of labor. Narrower arches, such as those associated with the android or anthropoid pelvis, seem to protect this region during descent of the fetal head. This may account in part for the observation that a cystourethrocele is much less common in African-American women, in whom an android or an anthropoid pelvis is more common. Prominent ischial spines are more consistent with the latter two types of pelves than with the gynecoid type. Operative obstetric interventions in and of themselves should not cause an increase in cystourethroceles. Cesarean sections undertaken to advance labor should not increase the risk of pelvic relaxation over the background risk associated with 9 months of pregnancy and the increased abdominal pressure. Although it has been suggested that episiotomies offer protection from pelvic support damage, this issue is highly controversial. In all probability, an episiotomy is done too late to protect from anterior wall damage during childbirth. Episiotomies do not play a role in the development of a cystourethrocele.

26. **D,** Pages 567–568. An umbilical hernia is an example of a congenital malformation. Before 10 weeks of gestation, the abdominal contents are partially herniated through the umbilicus into the extraembryonic coelomic cavity. Shortly thereafter, the visceral contents return to the abdominal cavity and the defect in the abdominal wall closes during subsequent fetal growth. Generally, at birth this space contains only the umbilical cord. After the cutting of the umbilical cord, the area heals so that the skin in the area of the umbilicus fuses over the closed fascial layer. Small umbilical hernias at birth usually close in the first 3 years of life. In rare cases, with a less complete closure of the abdominal wall, an omphalocele forms, which is a hernia sac in the umbilicus covered only by peritoneum and including bowel and sometimes other abdominal contents. This is in contrast with gastroschisis, which is a failure of fusion to the right of the midline. There are two unusual ventral hernias. One is an epigastric hernia, which occurs in a defect of the linea alba above the umbilicus. The other is the rare spigelian hernia, which occurs at a point where the vertical linea semilunaris joins the lateral border of the rectus muscle. In the repair of an umbilical hernia, usually all that is encountered is an empty hernia sac protruding through the small fascial defect.

27. **A,** Pages 556–558. By definition, the characteristics of an abdominal hernia include a reflection of peritoneum through a fascial defect. When intraperitoneal organ structures are part of the

hernia, they are called *sliding hernias*. Although most hernias occur at anatomic weak spots, they generally are not considered congenital anomalies. The only exception is an omphalocele. When surgical repair of abdominal hernias is being considered, it is important to remember that there is almost always a peritoneal reflection to dissect and close, in addition to closing the original fascial defect.

28. **D,** Pages 576–577. If a significant redundancy exists in the cul-de-sac peritoneum after vaginal hysterectomy, it is important to obliterate this space to prevent a future enterocele. If uterosacral ligaments can be identified, they should be used in the repair. This can be accomplished by fixing the uterosacral ligaments to the peritoneum of the sac and the vaginal vault. The peritoneum of the sac and the uterosacral ligaments and vagina of the opposite side are similarly used, with closure of this potential space with multiple sutures if necessary. This effectively shortens the cul-de-sac and supports the attendant enterocele neck. Suturing the round ligaments and the ovarian ligaments will not prevent development of either an enterocele or vaginal prolapse. Suturing the ovaries can be a cause of dyspareunia.

29. **C,** Pages 583–585. In performing a sacrospinous ligament fixation, the proper placement of the supporting suture is critical. Usually, only one suture is used; it is placed approximately two finger-breadths (3 cm) medial to the ischial spine. This can be done with either a suture ligature carrier or an aneurysm needle. It is important not to place the suture around or adjacent to the ischial spine because of danger to the underlying pudendal vessels and nerve. The sacrotuberous ligament will not offer proper support because an aneurysm needle or suture ligature carrier will not surround this structure.

30. **C,** Page 585. The exact prevalence of fecal incontinence is unknown because of social embarrassment and psychological impact. Estimates range from 2% to 11% of community-dwelling women older than 64 years. Over 30% of women reporting urinary incontinence also report fecal incontinence. This is called *dual incontinence*.

31. **B,** Page 586. As long as the pressure in the anal canal is maintained at a higher level than the rectal pressure, continence is maintained. Anal canal pressure depends on both internal and external anal sphincters. It is the external anal sphincter that provides the voluntary squeeze pressure that prevents incontinence in the face of increasing rectal or abdominal pressure.

32. **A,** Page 587. When stool or gas is sensed in the rectum, the internal anal sphincter has a reflex relaxation that allows for colonic contents to be sampled by the anal canal in order to distinguish solid from liquid from gas. After this sampling occurs, the internal sphincter pushes the material back into the rectum. This is the rectoanal inhibitory reflex and is absent in patients with Hirschsprung disease.

33. **A,** Page 588. Fecal incontinence due to an abnormal pelvic floor may be due to congenital anorectal malformations, obstetric injury, aging, surgery, or pelvic nerve denervation. Historically, incontinence due to denervation has been designated as idiopathic and accounts for 80% of patients with fecal incontinence.

34. **D,** Page 589. Many medications can affect bowel function. Chronic constipation may be caused by anticholinergics, antidepressants, nonsteroidals, iron, narcotics, and pseudoephedrine. The constipation could contribute to overflow incontinence or pelvic floor neuropathy due to straining.

35. **B,** Page 589. On physical examination, the dovetail sign or loss of anterior perineal folds indicates a defect in the external anal sphincter or a chronic third-degree laceration.

36. **D,** Page 591. The algorithm in Figure 20–20 in Stenchever recommends evaluation based on history and rectal tone. Normal rectal tone directs the clinician away from anal incontinence and toward a metabolic or colonic cause. Metabolic tests such as thyroid-stimulating hormone and glucose measurements should be considered. Poor resting tone directs the clinician to a neuromuscular cause.

37. **A,** Page 592. Transanal ultrasonography has significantly enhanced the ability to delineate defects of both the internal and the external sphincters. The integrity, thickness, and length of both sphincters can be determined. The internal sphincter appears as a hypoechoic circle; the external sphincter appears as a hyperechoic circle.

38. **C,** Page 597. Surgical management of fecal incontinence includes repair of rectal prolapse, anal sphincteroplasty, anal sphincter neuromuscular flaps, and implantation of artificial sphincters. Postanal repair of posterior levatorplasty has not been shown to be effective in the treatment of fecal incontinence.

39. **A,** Pages 598–599. Obstetric injuries are, by far, the most common cause of rectovaginal fistulas. Most rectovaginal fistulas caused by obstetric injury occur in the lower third of the vagina and may be associated with an external anal sphincter defect. Fistulas due to malignancy, surgical trauma, or an inflammatory process may occur at any point in the vagina, including the apex.

Urogynecology

DIRECTIONS:

for Questions 1–16: Select the one best answer or completion.

1. A 24-year-old healthy-appearing woman complains of the recent onset of urgency with loss of urine. She has never had such symptoms before. The best single test to make a diagnosis in this case is

   A. residual urine
   B. cystometrics
   C. urinalysis
   D. Bonney test
   E. urethroscopy

2. The major action of urethral support operations is to

   A. decrease bladder activity
   B. increase urethral sphincter tone
   C. decrease the parasympathetic nerve supply to the urethra
   D. decrease the caliber of the urethral lumen
   E. increase the transmission of abdominal pressure to the urethra

3. The major risk for a patient who has undergone a Mersilene sling procedure for urethral suspension is

   A. intraoperative hemorrhage
   B. infection
   C. transection of the urethra by the Mersilene
   D. reabsorption of the Mersilene sling
   E. loss of bladder innervation

4. A 72-year-old woman with diabetes has been sent to you from a nursing home for evaluation because she is always incontinent. She has no complaints other than the wetness. The test most likely to demonstrate the cause is

   A. urinalysis
   B. urethroscopy
   C. determination of residual urine
   D. Bonney test
   E. transurethral injection of methylene blue

5. A woman complains that she is losing a large volume of urine shortly after coughing or jumping. She occasionally has a loss of urine while in bed at night if she happens to cough vigorously. She is unable to stop the urinary stream once it has begun. Given this history, the most likely diagnosis is

   A. genuine stress incontinence
   B. a urethrovaginal fistula
   C. detrusor dyssynergia
   D. a urinary tract infection
   E. an ectopic ureter

6. A 24-year-old woman complains of frequency, urgency, and dysuria of 2 days' duration. The most likely causative agent is

   A. *Enterobacter aerogenes*
   B. *Streptococcus faecalis*
   C. *Chlamydia trachomatis*
   D. *Klebsiella aerogenes*
   E. *Escherichia coli*

7. Four weeks after a Marshall-Marchetti-Krantz repair for stress incontinence, a patient complains of increased pain in the suprapubic area that is aggravated by walking. She is continent and afebrile and has a white blood cell count of 11,000. Her urinalysis is normal. On examination, she has tenderness over the mons pubis. The pelvic examination is unremarkable. The most likely diagnosis is

   A. a urinary tract infection
   B. a retropubic abscess
   C. osteitis pubis
   D. osteomyelitis
   E. a hematoma in the space of Retzius

8. A 44-year-old woman complains of copious (approximately one-half cup) urine loss that she is unable to stop once the flow begins. She states that the loss begins shortly after a cough or sneeze and that she frequently feels that she needs to void. If she does not void within a few minutes after this sensation, she will also lose urine. The most likely diagnosis is

   A. urge incontinence
   B. stress incontinence
   C. a urethrovaginal fistula
   D. a urethral diverticulum
   E. overflow incontinence

9. A premenopausal woman who has completed her family and has mild genuine stress incontinence requests treatment. Initial treatment would be

   A. estrogen
   B. Kegel exercises
   C. an alpha-adrenergic agent
   D. a Kelly plication
   E. a Marshall-Marchetti-Krantz procedure

10. A 50-year-old woman has a history of recurrent dysuria and frequency in addition to dyspareunia and dribbling after voiding. On examination, she has a tender nodule palpable through the anterior vaginal wall. The most likely diagnosis is a(n)

    A. ectopic ureter
    B. Bartholin duct abscess
    C. urethral diverticulum
    D. urethrocele
    E. Gartner duct cyst

11. A cystourethrocele is a herniation of

    A. the bladder
    B. the urethra
    C. both the urethra and the bladder
    D. the bladder and a detachment of the urethra
    E. the bladder and a diverticulum of the urethra

12. A patient with genuine stress incontinence is most apt to have

    A. a short urethra
    B. an abnormal-appearing bead-chain cystourethrogram
    C. loss of the pubourethral vesical angle
    D. a positive Q-tip test result
    E. lack of transmission of intraabdominal pressure to the urethra

13. Instructions for Kegel exercises include contraction of the pubococcygeal muscles and which of the following?

	Repetitions during one sitting	Repetitions during one day	Breathing	Position
A.	5	2–4	Panting	Sitting
B.	5	2–4	Deep breathing	Sitting
C.	5–10	>100	Doesn't matter	Doesn't matter
D.	5–10	6–8	Deep breathing	Supine
E.	5–10	6–8	Hold breath	Doesn't matter

14. A woman has genuine stress incontinence and signs and symptoms of anterior vaginal wall excoriation from a fourth-degree cystourethrocele. Her stress incontinence has improved minimally with adequately performed Kegel exercises. She wishes to remain fertile, but she wants surgery to relieve her symptoms. The appropriate recommendation is a(n)

    A. vaginal hysterectomy and anterior and posterior repair
    B. retropubic urethropexy such as a Marshall-Marchetti-Krantz procedure
    C. trial on an anticholinergic drug
    D. anterior colporrhaphy with a Kelly plication
    E. fascial sling procedure

15. A patient complains of leakage of urine. Which of the following facts, obtained while taking a history, will be most useful in developing a plan to relieve her symptoms?

    A. is 45 years old and stopped menstruating 9 months ago
    B. is not undergoing estrogen replacement therapy
    C. drinks 20 to 30 cups of coffee a day
    D. takes terbutaline for her asthma
    E. jogs 2 miles every morning

16. A patient whose history and assessment suggest detrusor dyssynergia is likely to benefit from

    A. digitalis
    B. edrophonium
    C. imipramine
    D. reserpine
    E. hydralazine

DIRECTIONS:

for Questions 17–20: For each numbered item, select the one heading most closely associated with it. Each lettered heading may be used once, more than once, or not at all.

17–20. Match the procedure with the technique.

(A) passing a needle with a suture from the rectus fascia through the space of Retzius to the paravaginal tissue
(B) suturing lateral paravaginal fascia together beneath the urethra to support the bladder neck
(C) suturing the paravaginal fascia to the symphysis pubis
(D) suturing the rectus fascia beneath the urethra
(E) suturing the paravaginal fascia to Cooper's ligament

17. Burch

18. Kelly

19. Marshall-Marchetti-Krantz

20. Pereyra

DIRECTIONS:

for Questions 21–28: Select the one best answer or completion.

21. Involuntary loss of urine associated with bladder pressure greater than urethral pressure in the absence of detrusor contractions is associated with which type of incontinence?

    A. urge
    B. genuine stress
    C. mixed
    D. overflow
    E. bypass

22. Involuntary loss of urine related to uninhibited detrusor contractions is associated with which type of incontinence?

    A. urge
    B. genuine stress
    C. mixed
    D. overflow
    E. bypass

23. Which of the following neural pathways or biochemical actions inhibits urination?

    A. loop I
    B. loop II
    C. parasympathetic system stimulation
    D. inhibition of alpha-adrenergic receptors

24. Genuine stress incontinence is diagnosed in a patient; it is recommended that she undergo retropubic urethropexy. Risk factors that should be discussed with her at this time include all the following *except*

    A. increased incontinence
    B. failure to achieve correction
    C. difficulty in urinating after the procedure
    D. infection of the graft material

25. Urinary continence is achieved by maintaining urethral pressures greater than intravesical pressures. Which of the following contributes most to the maintenance of intraurethral pressures?

    A. smooth and striated muscle in the urethral wall
    B. vascularity of the urethral epithelium
    C. the distal 1 cm of the urethra
    D. angle of the internal sphincter

26. The most probable cause of a urethral diverticulum is

    A. a congenital defect
    B. an infection
    C. nulliparity
    D. use of the "missionary position" during coitus
    E. use of "rear entry" during coitus

27. A 45-year-old woman complains of urinary urgency, frequency, and suprapubic pain that has lasted for several months. The patient is monogamous and denies history of sexually transmitted disease (STD). Urine cultures on three separate occasions have been negative, but the symptoms persist and are getting worse. She has stopped coffee, alcohol, and all fruit juices as these seem to increase the symptoms. Of the following, which treatment would be best for the most likely cause of this patient's symptoms?

A. psychiatric referral
B. ceftriaxone and tetracycline
C. pentosan polysulfate
D. trimethoprim normal rod sulfamethoxazole
E. oxybutynin

28. A history of traumatic forceps delivery is most likely in a patient with

A. neurogenic bladder
B. genuine stress incontinence
C. detrusor hyperactivity
D. urinary tract infection
E. interstitial cystitis

ANSWERS

1. **C,** Page 616. In an otherwise healthy woman who has experienced recent onset of urinary urgency and loss of urine, the differential diagnosis should include urethritis, trigonitis, and cystitis. If the clean-void urinalysis shows white blood cells and bacteria, cystitis is likely. If only white blood cells are found, urethritis with an organism such as *Chlamydia* is likely. In such a situation, treatment of the infection is the first priority; other tests (with the exception of urine culture to determine the type of organism) are not indicated unless symptoms persist later in the absence of an infection.

2. **E,** Page 621. The basic defect in genuine stress incontinence is lack of transmission of abdominal pressure to the urethra. The urethral support procedures all attempt to accomplish the same goal. This goal is to ensure adequate intraabdominal pressure transmission so that it, together with the sphincter muscles of the urethra and the epithelium of the urethra, combines to make the intraurethral pressure greater than the intravesical pressure, thereby ensuring continence.

3. **B,** Page 625. A foreign body left in place always creates a risk of infection. This is a major complication of a urethral sling, which uses synthetic materials. The Mersilene will not absorb, and it has been known to work its way into the urethra, with a resulting fistula. The patient is at no greater risk for hemorrhage or loss of bladder innervation than with any other suspension procedure.

4. **C,** Page 631. This patient is likely to have overflow incontinence secondary to a neurogenic bladder with incomplete emptying. Her age, history of diabetes, and constant wetting are significant clues to this etiologic complex. If this is the case,

large amounts of urine will remain in the bladder after voiding and may easily be detected by simple catheterization after an attempt to void. If the diagnosis of a neurogenic bladder is established, treatment of the underlying disease may be helpful to decrease incontinence, but usually it is not. Voiding frequently at specific times or using intermittent catheterization may be the best management. Catheterization does carry a risk of infection.

5. **C,** Page 630. Detrusor dyssynergia (also known as detrusor instability), detrusor irritability, or an unstable bladder is associated with uninhibited bladder contractions. These contractions are often triggered by an intraabdominal stress such as coughing. Therefore, the problem is easily confused with genuine stress incontinence. However, a careful history usually reveals that a few seconds elapse between the stress and the onset of the urine flow. The bladder hyperactivity should be demonstrated by a cystometrogram. Treatment with bladder retraining, which involves voiding at specific and progressively lengthening time intervals, and administration of anticholinergic or beta-adrenergic drugs is often helpful. A patient with a urethrovaginal fistula is likely to have a less predictable urinary stream during micturition and will complain of a watery vaginal discharge or that she loses urine on standing or at unpredictable times. A patient with a bladder infection is apt to have a hyperactive bladder that mimics detrusor dyssynergia. In addition, she usually experiences frequency, dysuria, and pyuria. The symptoms associated with an ectopic ureter include constant leaking of urine.

6. **E**, Page 616. *Escherichia coli* is the most frequently found bacterium in uncomplicated urinary tract infections. The causative bacteria are usually present in accumulations of more than 100,000 organisms per milliliter. The presence of as few as 100 organisms per milliliter may indicate an infection because of the dilution factor of bladder urine. At least 20% of all women have urinary tract infections at some time in their lives.

7. **C**, Page 626. It is possible that this patient, who has suprapubic pain 4 weeks after a Marshall-Marchetti-Krantz repair, could have a urinary tract infection, an abscess, or a hematoma. However, the lack of white blood cells in the urine, a normal white blood cell count, absence of fever, and no mass detected on examination make all these conditions unlikely. Osteitis pubis is rare, but with this presentation of pain over the symphysis without fever or mass, it is the most likely diagnosis. Osteomyelitis is another possibility, and clinical differentiation between osteomyelitis and osteitis pubis may be difficult. Diagnosing osteomyelitis requires changes in cortical bone shown on x-ray film, marrow biopsy demonstrating infection, and recovery of microorganisms. Osteomyelitis pubis may be the eventual end to the continuum of an inflammatory process involving the pubic bone. Osteitis pubis is an inflammation of the periosteum of the pubis, and it represents an early stage in this process.

8. **A**, Page 629. With a history of short delay after the cough, the copious uncontrollable urine loss, and the urgency that this patient often feels, urge incontinence is likely. Stress incontinence is usually described as loss of a small amount of urine. It occurs immediately after or during the cough or Valsalva maneuver. A urethrovaginal fistula causes an unpredictable urinary stream or loss of urine from the vagina. Typically, a patient with overflow incontinence complains of voiding small amounts of urine and still having the feeling that urine is present in the bladder. Such a patient almost constantly loses small amounts of urine without any control. A urethral diverticulum tends to leak after voiding. This patient should be evaluated for infection and detrusor contractility before any operation is performed.

9. **B**, Page 622. Because this woman is premenopausal, estrogen is probably not indicated, although it is helpful in treating postmenopausal women. Kegel pubococcygeal muscle exercises often yield good results if done correctly. Although the severity of the symptoms before therapy and the patient's age had no effect on outcome in one study evaluating the efficacy of Kegel exercises, the treatment was noted to be more effective when the symptoms were present for less than 1 year.

alpha-Adrenergic drugs are mildly effective in increasing urethral pressure, but they usually are not the best choice for the initial treatment of patients with mild symptoms of stress incontinence (although this approach might be tried in conjunction with Kegel exercises). Surgical treatment, whether by the vaginal or abdominal route, should be reserved until the effect of Kegel exercises can be evaluated.

10. **C**, Page 619. With a history of dysuria, urinary frequency, urinary dribbling, and dyspareunia, coupled with a palpable tender nodule, a urethral diverticulum is highly suspect. An ectopic ureter causes constant incontinence. The anatomic location is wrong for both Bartholin and Gartner duct pathologic conditions. A urethrocele is not detected as a tender nodule, whereas a urethral diverticulum often appears as a tender suburethral mass. Urethral diverticula are relatively uncommon, occurring in only 3% to 4% of all women during their lifetime. However, diverticula should be considered when these signs and symptoms occur.

11. **D**, Pages 566, 571–572, 621–622. *Urethrocele* is somewhat of a misnomer because the urethra commonly does not balloon out or herniate. The urethra instead becomes detached. Then both the urethra and the bladder rotate caudally out of the space beneath the symphysis pubis so that pressure from the intraabdominal cavity can no longer be transmitted to the urethra. Loss of this pressure transmission often results in genuine stress incontinence as the pressure transmission to the bladder continues, increasing the intravesical pressure above that of the intraurethral pressure.

12. **E**, Pages 621–622. Genuine stress incontinence is due mainly to a lack of transmission of intraabdominal pressure to the urethra. The length of the urethra or its angle, as measured by the Q-tip test, or the amount of funneling of the bladder neck, as determined by the bead-chain cystourethrogram, does not correlate well with the presence or absence of genuine stress incontinence. However, in all cases of genuine stress incontinence, the intravesical pressure exceeds the maximum urethral pressure in the absence of detrusor activity.

13. **C**, Page 622. Patients are frequently told to do Kegel exercises, but they are not told how often to perform them. If these exercises are not done frequently, they are ineffective. Kegel reported excellent results when the pelvic floor muscles were intermittently contracted and relaxed 5 times on waking, 5 times on rising, and 5 times every half hour throughout the day. Pelvic floor musculature must be adequate in order for the exercises to cause hypertrophy and yield a beneficial result. If the pelvic floor muscles have been attenuated or

are in any way obliterated, the exercise regimen is less helpful because muscles cannot be developed if they are not present. Five to 10 repetitions should be performed at any one time. These sets should be repeated several times a day. The critical point in this question is that Kegel exercises are isometric. Breathing deeply or panting does not help in doing Kegels.

14. **D,** Pages 572, 625. In this patient, who wishes to remain fertile, removal of the uterus is contraindicated. An anterior repair with a Kelly plication will support the bladder and urethra, thereby relieving her symptoms. There is no need for posterior repair if no symptoms of posterior relaxation are present. A retropubic urethropexy, such as a Marshall-Marchetti-Krantz procedure, will relieve the patient's stress incontinence but it will not replace the cystocele; therefore, the anterior vaginal wall will still be excoriated from extrusion. Modifications of the Marshall-Marchetti-Krantz procedure, such as the Burch procedure, also would be of little benefit in this case. Anticholinergics are of some value in the treatment of detrusor dyssynergia but not of genuine stress incontinence. A fascial sling procedure is usually reserved for patients with previous operative failures. It also would not correct the cystocele. An anterior colporrhaphy with a Kelly plication should correct this patient's problems.

15. **C,** Page 622. (American College of Obstetricians and Gynecologists: Technical Bulletin, No. 231, pp. 860–862.) It is important to take a complete history from patients complaining of leakage of urine. All answers are important. In this case, the fact that the patient is menopausal and not taking estrogen is probably not related to her incontinence. It is too soon for atrophy to have developed. The fact that the patient jogs 2 miles every day indicates that she is in good physical condition, but it does not tell us anything about her pelvic floor musculature. Terbutaline can cause urinary retention and should have a beneficial effect. Caffeine, on the other hand, can decrease the urethral closing pressure. This patient drinks an excessive amount of fluid. It would be important to know the specific gravity of her urine. Does she have diabetes insipidus? Does she have polyuria? It would be common to find that she is a nervous person and that frequent urination is a learned habit. Such a patient will benefit from bladder training if the rest of her history and physical examination results are normal. This patient should keep a diary and attempt to decrease the amount of fluid she drinks and the number of times she voids.

16. **C,** Pages 637–639. All are medications not usually associated with the urinary tract. Digitalis is a cholinergic agonist. It increases bladder wall tension. Edrophonium stimulates the parasympathetic nervous system, and the bladder contracts. Haloperidol is a neuroleptic agent. It blocks dopamine receptors and leads to internal sphincter relaxation. Imipramine is a tricyclic antidepressant with alpha-adrenergic enhancement characteristics that have been found to be beneficial in patients with detrusor dyssynergia. Both reserpine and hydralazine are antihypertensives. They block adrenergic activity.

17–20. 17, **E;** 18, **B;** 19, **C;** 20, **A;** Pages 625–627. In the Marshall-Marchetti-Krantz procedure, the paravaginal fascia is sutured to the symphysis pubis in the space of Retzius. The Burch procedure is a modification of the Marshall-Marchetti-Krantz procedure and requires suturing the paravaginal fascia to Cooper's ligament. The Kelly plication sutures lateral paravaginal fascia in the midline beneath the urethra. The Pereyra procedure involves passing a needle with a suture attached through the space of Retzius from the rectus fascia to the paravaginal fascia on either side of the urethra. Each procedure is designed to place the proximal third of the urethra in an area where the intraabdominal pressure can be transmitted to it, while maintaining support of the urethra in a way that will not allow it to move out of that pressure zone. This results in an increase in intraurethral pressure, which, together with the urethral sphincters and mucous membrane, creates an intraurethral pressure greater than the intravesical pressure, resulting in urinary continence.

21. **B,** Page 621. The various types of incontinence are defined according to the cause of the pressure gradient. Successful treatment is based on correcting the specific reason for the higher bladder pressure or the lower urethral pressure, or both. Therefore, it is important diagnostically to determine the reason for the pressure differential because the treatment differs depending on the underlying cause. Genuine stress incontinence is by definition the involuntary loss of urine associated with a bladder pressure greater than urethral pressure in the absence of detrusor contractions.

22. **A,** Pages 629–630. Motor urge incontinence is the desire to void along with the involuntary loss of urine associated with uninhibited detrusor contractions.

23. **A,** Pages 608–609; Figure 21–1. Loop I of the micturition feedback nervous system circuit runs from the cortex to the brain stem to inhibit urination by modifying sensory stimuli from loop II, thereby inhibiting the bladder. The parasympathetic system generally initiates voiding with detrusor muscle stimulation and relaxation of urethral sphincters. Activating the beta-adrenergic

CONTINENCE   MICTURITION

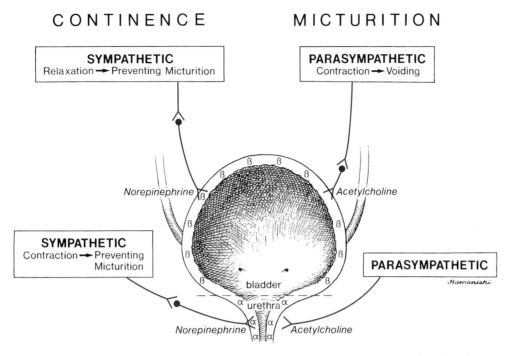

FIGURE 21–1 Innervation of bladder and urethra. Parasympathetic fibers arising in S_2 through S_4 have long preganglionic fibers and pelvic ganglia close to bladder and urethra. These fibers excrete acetylcholine. Sympathetic fibers, which have long postganglionic fibers, discharge norepinephrine to beta-receptors, primarily in the bladder, and to alpha-receptors, primarily in the urethra. (Redrawn and modified from Raz S: Urol Clin North Am 5:323, 1978.)

receptors of the sympathetic system inhibits the detrusor muscle through beta-receptors within the bladder, whereas activation of the alpha-adrenergic receptors causes urethral muscle constriction. Knowing these facts allows one to plan rational therapy for urge incontinence, which is due to uninhibited bladder muscle spasms.

24. **D,** Pages 625–627. Any surgical candidate should be informed of several basic surgical risks: infection, hemorrhage, damage to other structures, failure to achieve cure, and the risks associated with anesthesia. These general risks should all be documented on the patient's record. Specific procedures carry specific complications, and these should also be outlined. In the case of urethral suspension, failure to spontaneously void may be a major factor. The patient should recognize the possible need for long-term urinary catheterization. Eventually, nearly all patients with these repairs will void spontaneously. Some patients, particularly those who have minimal stress incontinence or have urge incontinence rather than stress incontinence, actually experience more incontinence postoperatively. Patients who have only genuine stress incontinence preoperatively sometimes experience detrusor instability after the operation and may require further medical therapy. Because graft material is not used in routine retropubic urethropexy, there is no graft material to become infected. The risk of soft tissue

infection should be no greater for these repairs than for any other carefully performed surgical procedure.

25. **B,** Page 610. The muscles, the vascularity, and the transmission of increased intraabdominal pressure are all important factors in maintaining a high urethral pressure with resultant continence, with the muscles being the most important factor listed. The vascularity of the submucosa and the overall mucosal thickness of the urethra increase in response to estrogen. This may be why estrogen helps in the treatment of incontinence in some estrogen-deficient women. The distal urethra is usually not important in maintaining continence because it is beyond the sphincter action of the striated muscle and beyond the area of intraabdominal pressure transmission. Similarly, the position or angle of the internal sphincter has little influence on the overall urethral pressure. Urethral pressure and the length of the urethra over which it acts determine continence.

26. **A,** Page 619. A urethral diverticulum may develop in several ways. These include a congenital defect, acute or chronic inflammation, and trauma. The congenital theory stems from the fact that cases have been reported in children and neonates. Infection of the periurethral glands with such organisms as *Gonococcus* or *Escherichia coli* can result in the formation of retention cysts, which when repeatedly infected may rupture into the

lumen of the urethra, giving rise to a diverticulum. Urethral trauma from multiple catheterizations or childbirth has been mentioned as an etiologic factor. There is little evidence that normal sexual practices have any influence on the development of urethral diverticula.

27. **C,** Page 618. This patient's symptoms suggest interstitial cystitis. The lack of positive urine cultures is common with this entity. Although this patient may be depressed because of her symptoms, psychiatric referral is not likely to help rectify her symptoms. A recent oral heparin analog, pentosan polysulfate (Elmiron), has provided relief for some patients. DNSO installation also may help. Ditropan is an anticholinergic that may relieve some frequency but does not help much with pain. It is best used for urge incontinence. Likewise, antibiotic treatment for STDs or urinary tract infection is unlikely to help.

28. **B,** Page 622. Women who delivered with forceps have been found to have a higher incidence of stress urinary incontinence than those who delivered spontaneously. There appears to be increased risk of anal incontinence as well.

Infections of the Lower Genital Tract

for Questions 1–31: Select the one best answer or completion.

1. **Bacteria that cause uncomplicated cystitis have become most resistant to which of the following antibiotics?**

   A. ampicillin
   B. cephalothin
   C. nitrofurantoin
   D. sulfamethoxazole
   E. eiprofloxacin

2. **A 19-year-old woman complains of headache, myalgia, dizziness, and low-grade fever with each menstrual period for the past 6 months. She feels well at other times and denies depression or dysmenorrhea. The woman takes birth control pills and uses tampons. Of the following, the most likely diagnosis is**

   A. Weil disease
   B. premenstrual syndrome
   C. Flu
   D. Lyme disease
   E. forme fruste of toxic shock syndrome

3. **A 22-year-old woman complains of severe itching of her perineum, wrists, and breasts. The symptoms worsen at night. Examination reveals excoriation in all the above areas. No hives are visible. The most likely diagnosis is**

   A. allergy
   B. scabies
   C. molluscum contagiosum
   D. lice
   E. pityriasis rosea

4. **A 26-year-old woman from the British Virgin Islands is found to have several painless beefy-red ulcers on the vulva. A biopsy is taken and depicted in Figure 22–1. The diagnosis is**

   A. syphilis
   B. chancroid
   C. herpes simplex
   D. lymphogranuloma venereum
   E. granuloma inguinale

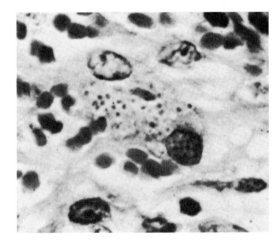

FIGURE 22–1 (From Hart, G: In Holmes KK, Mårdh PA, Sparling PF, et al., eds: Sexually Transmitted Diseases. New York, McGraw-Hill, 1984, p 394.)

5. **After injection of lidocaine (Xylocaine) as an anesthetic, the correct needle-handling procedure is to**

   A. break or bend the needle so it cannot be reused
   B. dispose of the needle and syringe separately
   C. recap the needle before disposal
   D. drop the needle in a bleach solution
   E. place the needle and syringe in a puncture-proof container

6. **A patient with severe toxic shock syndrome is most likely to have**

   A. total lymphocytes greater than 1000/mL
   B. polymorphonuclear cells less than 80%
   C. aspartate aminotransferase less than 30 U/L
   D. Blood urea nitrogen (BUN) greater than 20 mg/dL
   E. platelets greater than 300,000

7. **The basic underlying pathophysiologic disturbance in a patient with AIDS is**

   A. an infection with opportunistic organisms such as *Pneumocystis carinii*
   B. a cancer that affects the cell-mediated immune system
   C. a decrease in the number and function of T_4 lymphocytes
   D. a decrease in serum immunoglobulin G (IgG) and IgA
   E. thrombocytopenia

8. **How many different species of bacteria are found in the vagina of a normal asymptomatic woman when culturing is carefully performed?**

   A. 2–3
   B. 6–10
   C. 12–15
   D. 17–29
   E. more than 30

9. **The most specific test commonly used to detect human immunodeficiency virus (HIV) infection is**

   A. enzyme-linked immunosorbent assay (ELISA)
   B. Southern blot
   C. polymerase chain reaction (PCR)
   D. Northern blot
   E. Western blot

10. **A young woman complains of a bad odor from the vaginal area after sexual intercourse and during menses. She has very little discharge, but it is irritating. The direct reason for the odor is most likely**

    A. breakdown of blood or protein in semen
    B. increased number of anaerobes
    C. *Escherichia coli*
    D. normal vaginal secretions
    E. release of amines in an alkaline milieu

11. **A 26-year-old woman complains of a vaginal discharge associated with itching and burning. The pH of the discharge is 5.5. Which of the following is the *most likely* diagnosis?**

    A. *Chlamydia* cervicitis
    B. gonorrhea cervicitis
    C. yeast vaginitis
    D. *Trichomonas* vaginitis
    E. bacterial vaginosis

12. **A young woman whose partner is an IV drug abuser feels well but wishes to be tested for HIV antibodies. Both the ELISA and the Western blot test results are positive. Her CD4 count is 380/μL. Into which Centers for Disease Control and Prevention (CDC) group of HIV infections should she be classified?**

    A. A2
    B. B1
    C. B2
    D. B3
    E. C1

13. **Clue cells are often visible in the wet mount of the vaginal secretions of a patient with bacterial vaginosis. A clue cell is a(n)**

    A. white blood cell with phagocytized bacteria
    B. epithelial squamous cell covered with bacteria
    C. epithelial columnar cell covered with bacteria
    D. white blood cell containing gram-negative paired cocci
    E. squamous cell epithelium containing macrophages

14. **After *Candida albicans*, the yeast most often found in the vagina is**

    A. *Trichophyton rubrum*
    B. *Candida glabrata*
    C. *Microsporum canis*
    D. *Candida tropicalis*
    E. *Pityrosporum orbiculare*

15. A 21-year-old woman is seen in the emergency department with hypotension, fever, diarrhea, headache, myalgia, red eyes, and a skin rash. She states that she has felt ill for 2 days and the symptoms are now worse. She is sexually active and uses barrier contraception. She denies abdominal pain, vaginal discharge, or ingestion of any drug except aspirin. Her periods are regular. Her last normal period began 4 days ago. The most likely diagnosis is

    A. Rocky Mountain spotted fever
    B. scarlet fever
    C. toxic shock syndrome
    D. meningococcemia
    E. leptospirosis

16. A 28-year-old woman complains of severe pubic itching. On examination, a few small brown spots are seen on the suprapubic skin. The most likely diagnosis is

    A. junctional nevi
    B. scabies
    C. yeast
    D. *Trichomonas* infection
    E. lice

17. Bartholin duct infection is usually due to

    A. *Gonococcus*
    B. *Chlamydia trachomatis*
    C. polymicrobial flora
    D. *Bacteroides*
    E. *Escherichia coli*

18. Which of the following women is most likely to have a Bartholin gland carcinoma?

    A. 13-year-old prepubertal girl
    B. 22-year-old sexually active woman
    C. 31-year-old prostitute
    D. 39-year-old monogamous married woman
    E. 52-year-old virginal woman

19. A urine culture need not be obtained in which of the following female patients? Symptoms of cystitis are present and pyuria has been identified by a leukocyte esterase urine dipstick.

    A. 32-year-old woman with repeated episodes of cystitis
    B. 24-year-old newlywed with her first episode of cystitis
    C. 48-year-old woman with a history of renal stones
    D. 23-year-old diabetic woman
    E. healthy, active 67-year-old woman

20. A 32-year-old afebrile woman experiences a sudden onset of dysuria, frequency, and urgency. She also complains of suprapubic discomfort. Which of the following is the most likely diagnosis?

    A. vaginitis
    B. cervicitis
    C. cystitis
    D. urethritis
    E. pyelonephritis

21. A woman is most likely to have more than 10 white blood cells per high-powered field in a specimen of cervical mucus if she has a positive test result for

    A. yeast
    B. *Trichomonas*
    C. *Chlamydia trachomatis*
    D. gonorrhea
    E. bacterial vaginosis

22. A patient asks for the most effective short-term treatment for her vulvar warts. Of the following, the best choice is

    A. electrocautery
    B. laser therapy
    C. interlesional interferon
    D. excision
    E. cryotherapy

23. In asymptomatic women, *Candida* species are most prevalent on the epithelium of the

    A. vagina
    B. rectum
    C. mouth
    D. skin

24. A 23-year-old woman has had an irritating and smelly vaginal discharge for 5 to 6 days. On examination, she has evidence of a homogeneous yellow-gray discharge at the introitus and a slightly red vagina. On wet-mount slide, the pH is 5.5 and an amine odor, numerous clue cells, and motile *Trichomonas* organisms are evident. The best choice of treatment is

    A. fluconazole orally
    B. clotrimazole intervaginally
    C. metronidazole orally
    D. metronidazole intervaginally
    E. clindamycin orally

25. A sexually active asymptomatic woman with no abnormal physical findings had a positive rapid plasma regain (RPR) test result. A specific text for syphilis (FTA-ABS) also yielded positive results, and she was treated with 2.4 million units of benzathine penicillin. You would expect

   A. the FTA-ABS result to become negative
   B. a rash to develop on her hands and feet
   C. her RPR result to become negative
   D. a chancre to develop
   E. tabes to develop

26. Which of the following is most likely to give a false-negative result for syphilis?

   A. malaria
   B. anticardiolipin antibody
   C. infectious mononucleosis
   D. systemic lupus erythematosus
   E. chronic liver disease

27. A 16-year-old examined during her menstrual period has hypertension, skin rash, fever, and myalgia. She is found to have *Staphylococcus* in her vaginal culture. The girl's mother asks you to explain her daughter's illness and asks about a proposed treatment plan. You should tell her that

   A. the symptoms are due to *Staphylococcus aureus* bacteremia
   B. almost all cases are sexually transmitted
   C. antibiotic treatment is of no help
   D. she should stop using tampons
   E. she should use a diaphragm or a cervical cap for contraception

28. A 24-year-old woman has had several sexual contacts in the last 20 days, but she had no sexual contact for several months before this time. She has a small, tender ulcer of 3 days' duration on her vulva. She also has firm, slightly tender inguinal nodes. She has no other signs or symptoms. At this visit, you should obtain a culture specimen for herpes simplex virus and

   A. give 1 week of oral cephalosporin
   B. aspirate the lymph node
   C. obtain a Frei test
   D. perform a dark-field study
   E. perform a biopsy for cancer

29. Approximately what percentage of persons infected with genital herpes are unaware of their infection?

   A. 5%
   B. 20%
   C. 50%
   D. 80%
   E. 95%

30. Oral fluconazol treatment for yeast vaginitis has which of the following characteristics?

   A. has multiple interaction with other drugs
   B. requires multiple doses
   C. is not a imidazole
   D. has a short duration of action (6–8 hours)
   E. causes more liver damage than ketoconazol

31. Which of the following rapid tests for detecting *Chlamydia trachomatis* is equivalent in efficacy to standard tissue culture?

   A. slide tests
   B. Pap smears
   C. ligase chain reaction (LCR)
   D. ELISA
   E. DNA hybridization

DIRECTIONS:

for Questions 32–39: For each numbered item, select the one heading most closely associated with it. Each lettered item may be used once, more than once, or not at all.

32–35. Match the causative organism with the disease or lesion.

   (A) *Calymmatobacterium*
   (B) *Chlamydia trachomatis*
   (C) spirochete
   (D) *Mycobacterium*
   (E) *Haemophilus ducreyi*

32. **Gumma**

33. **Granuloma inguinale**

34. **Chancroid**

35. **Condyloma latum**

36–39. Match the disease with the figure.

   (A) primary herpes
   (B) molluscum contagiosum
   (C) condyloma acuminatum
   (D) lymphogranuloma venereum
   (E) invasive cancer

36. Figure 22–2

37. Figure 22–3

38. Figure 22–4

39. Figure 22–5

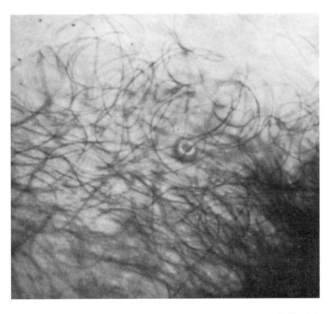

FIGURE 22–2 (From Brown ST: In Holmes KK, Mårdh PA, Sparling PF, et al., eds: Sexually Transmitted Diseases. New York, McGraw-Hill, 1984, p 394.)

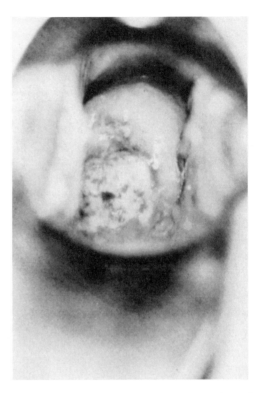

FIGURE 22–4 (From Kaufman RH, Faro S: Clin Obstet Gynecol 28:154, 1985.)

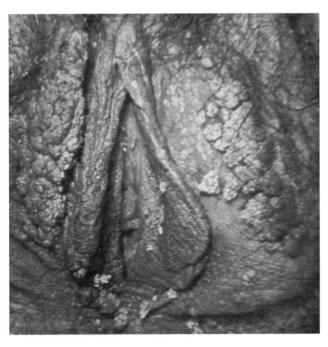

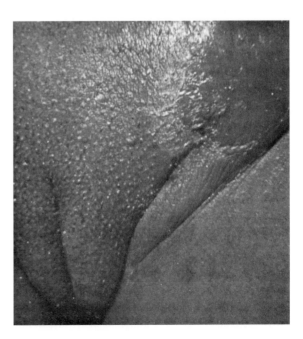

FIGURE 22–3 (From Friedrich EG: Vulvar Disease, 2nd ed. Philadelphia, WB Saunders, 1983, p 25.)

FIGURE 22–5 (From Friedrich EG: Vulvar Disease, 2nd ed. Philadelphia, WB Saunders, 1983, p 229.)

DIRECTIONS:

for Questions 40–41: Match the described case with the appropriate HIV classification:

(A) A-1
(B) A-3
(C) B-2
(D) C-1
(E) C-2

40. A 20-year-old asymptomatic Caucasian woman who has a positive HIV test result and a CD4 T cell count of > 500 μL.

41. A 24-year-old woman who has cervical dysplasia and a positive HIV test result with a CD4 T cell count of 340/μL.

ANSWERS

1. **A,** Pages 642–643. Resistance to many antibiotics is growing among bacteria causing urinary tract infections. Ampicillin, which was very effective in the 1980s, is now not effective in approximately 40% and trimethoprim-sulfamethoxazole is not effective in approximately 20% of cystitis cases. One should check regional health departments for local resistance patterns.

2. **E,** Page 679. The repetitive and cyclic nature of the symptoms makes flu and Lyme disease unlikely. Lyme disease is due to a spirochete carried by a tick and may cause similar early symptoms. Later, it often causes significant arthritis. Lyme disease is not repetitive and has a classic skin lesion, erythema migrans. Weil disease is the sequela of a severe infection with leptospirosis, which is a rare condition and much more severe than the symptoms outlined. However, it is one of the differential diagnoses in cases of severe toxic shock syndrome. The premenstrual syndrome occurs before menses. A mild form, or "forme fruste," of toxic shock syndrome is likely with the use of tampons. Vaginal cultures for *Staphylococcus aureus* should be taken, and the use of tampons should be discontinued until the bacteria are eradicated. Tampons should then be used for no longer than 6 hours.

3. **B,** Page 648. The distribution, with increased itching at night, makes scabies the most likely diagnosis. This diagnosis can be proven by an India ink test to identify the burrows or by making a slide of the scrapings from the affected skin and using mineral oil to prevent loss of specimen. Treatment is with premethrin cream, sulfa, or lindane. Lindane resistance has been reported, and lindane should not be used in pregnancy or in children under the age of 2 years. Ivermectin is a new topical treatment. Allergies are unlikely to have a concomitant genital, wrist, and breast distribution and are often associated with hives.

Molluscum contagiosum has classic umbilicated papules, and lice tend to be located in hair-bearing areas. Pityriasis rosea has a truncal and upper-extremity distribution, often with a history of a herald patch.

4. **E,** Page 660; Figure 22–1. Granuloma inguinale is due to gram-negative, nonmotile encapsulated rod, *Calymmatobacterium granulomatis*. The pathognomonic Donovan bodies are clusters of dark-staining, bipolar-appearing (safety pin–like) bacteria in large mononuclear cells. The disease is found in subtropical areas and is rare in the United States. Treatment is with tetracycline. The differential diagnoses are discussed under Questions 32–35. Treatment of sexually transmitted disease can be found on the CDC website www.cdc.gov.

5. **E,** Page 688. Because of the danger of hepatitis and HIV infection from a needle-stick exposure, the safest technique is to dispose of both needle and syringe in a puncture-resistant disposable container. Any manipulation of the needle, including capping, breaking, or removal, increases the risk of inadvertent skin puncture and contamination.

6. **D,** Page 680. A patient with severe toxic shock syndrome usually has fewer than 860 lymphocytes/mL, polymorphonuclear cells more than 90%, platelets less than 150,000, aspartate aminotransferase greater than 40 units/dL, and a BUN greater than 20 mg/dL. The last two measurements indicate liver and kidney involvement, which occurs in severe disease. An elevated creatine phosphokinase level is also common because of muscle damage.

7. **C,** Page 681. AIDS victims often acquire the disease from contact with homosexuals or from sharing of IV drug needles. They may suffer infection with opportunistic bacteria, viruses, or parasites; experience thrombocytopenia or Kaposi sarcoma; or have increased immunoglobulins.

The basic problem is infection of the T lymphocytes with a CD4 marker by HIV RNA. This causes a decrease in function of these T_4 lymphocytes, resulting in breakdown of cell-mediated immune responses that allows the secondary infections or Kaposi sarcoma to occur.

8. **D,** Page 669. The most common bacteria in the vagina are the lactobacilli, found in 60% to 80% of healthy women. Other facultative aerobes include diphtheroids, streptococci, staphylococci, *Gardnerella vaginalis,* and *Escherichia coli.* Anaerobes can be cultured in the vagina of approximately 80% of healthy women. These include *Peptostreptococcus, Peptococcus,* and *Bacteroides* organisms. Healthy asymptomatic women harbor 17 to 29 species of bacteria. *Candida* is also commonly found. The quantity of the different species varies. Both anaerobes and aerobes are found in significantly increased amounts in patients with bacterial vaginosis.

9. **C,** Page 686. ELISA is a screening test for antibodies against HIV that yields a small, though significant, number of false-positive and false-negative results. This can have a great impact because HIV diagnosis carries such a severe prognosis. The Western blot test is another method of detecting specific antibodies to proteins of HIV. The Southern blot and Northern blot tests use the same methodology to detect DNA and RNA, respectively. PCR is an extremely sensitive and specific method for testing specific types of DNA. It can be used as a test for HIV. Human deficiency viral DNA, if present, documents infection with HIV.

10. **E,** Page 670. Volatile amines are released in an alkaline media. The normal pH of the vagina is less than 4.5, but both blood and semen have a high pH (approximately 7.2 to 7.4). The amines are formed by anaerobic bacteria. When these bacteria are found in greater number, these amines become volatile (and therefore noticeable) when the pH rises above the normal vaginal pH of 4.5. Addition of KOH to vaginal secretion volatizes the amines. This forms the basis for the "sniff test," the fishy smell associated with bacterial vaginosis.

11. **E,** Page 669. The normal pH of the healthy vagina is 3.8 to 4.2. If the pH is greater than 5.0, bacterial vaginosis, trichomoniasis, or some other bacterial infection is likely. Bacterial vaginosis is the most common and therefore more likely than the other bacterial options. A yeast infection or physiologic discharge is more likely if the pH is normal. Testing the pH is quick and easy, and it is good at separating symptomatic vaginal discharge into bacterial infections versus yeast and physiologic discharge. The pH should be measured routinely in patients with complaints of vaginal discharge; it can be done easily by using nitrazine or pH paper.

12. **A,** Pages 682–683; Table 22–12 in Stenchever. HIV infection has been categorized by symptoms into three categories, each of which has three subgroups, based on the CD4-positive T cell counts. Category A patients are those with initial viremia who may have symptoms ranging from nothing to a mononucleosis type of illness. Antibodies to HIV may be absent or low. Category A includes patients with generalized lymphadenopathy. A latent period follows, which may last for 10 or more years, and is by far the most common situation for HIV-positive persons. During the latency period, patients are asymptomatic. Each year, a small number of patients progress to category B. Persons in category B have symptoms. Category C patients have clinical AIDS, which manifests in malignancy (most commonly lymphomas or Kaposi sarcoma), weight loss, diarrhea, central nervous system symptoms, and repeated opportunistic infection. Within each group (A through C), the patients are subclassified by the level of their CD4 counts: subcategory (1) has >500, (2) has 200–499, and (3) has <200/µL CD4-positive T cell counts.

13. **B,** Page 679; Figure 22–24 in Stenchever. A clue cell is a squamous epithelial cell so heavily covered with numerous bacteria that its outline is obscured. Clue cells are found in high numbers in patients with bacterial vaginosis. Columnar cells are rarely visible on wet mount slides. White blood cells with intracellular gram-negative diplococci are indicative of gonococcal infection. Macrophages in the epithelium are visible on histologic specimens, not on wet mounts.

14. **B,** Pages 675–678. *Candida* organisms are found normally in 25% of women. They are opportunistic pathogens that grow in the gastrointestinal tract from the mouth to the anus, even more readily than in the vagina. *Candida glabrata* is occasionally found in the vagina and is said to cause burning rather than itching. It does not produce filaments; therefore, only spores are found. It does not respond well to the imidazoles. Very resistant cases that do not respond to a prolonged regimen of imidazoles may be treated with gentian violet. *Trichophyton rubrum* is the fungus that usually causes tinea cruris (jock itch) or tinea corporis. *Microsporum canis* causes tinea capitis, and *Pityrosporum orbiculare* causes tinea versicolor.

15. **C,** Pages 679–680. The onset and the menstrual period and symptoms make toxic shock syndrome the most likely of the diagnoses listed. The patient has hypotension, rash, fever, and three organ symptom manifestations, thereby meeting the criteria for the diagnosis of toxic shock syndrome. However, it is important to remember that other diseases cause similar symptoms, such as Rocky

Mountain spotted fever, scarlet fever, meningococcemia, leptospirosis, measles, Kawasaki disease, and Lyme disease.

16. **E,** Page 647. A classic finding is a "freckle, that moves slowly." Significant symptoms may be caused by very few lice. Treatment is with permethrin 1% cream or with lindane 1% shampoo in one application. The patient should be reevaluated in 1 week and retreated if lice or eggs are observed. *Trichomonas* organisms do not live on the skin. Junctional nevi do not itch. Yeast causes generalized redness, often with pustules. Scabies usually cause twisted burrows under the skin.

17. **C,** Page 646. Although it was thought that most Bartholin duct infections were due to gonococcus, most infections involve a polymicrobial flora, similar to the bacterial flora found in the vagina. Noninfected cysts are usually asymptomatic. In women younger than 40 years, these asymptomatic cysts require no treatment. For acute abscesses, the treatment is drainage. The abscess may be excised if there is recurrence, persistence, or enlargement. In women older than 40 years, excision or adequate biopsy is important to rule out the rare case of adenocarcinoma.

18. **E,** Page 647. The mean age of discovery of a Bartholin gland carcinoma is 50. Bartholin gland carcinoma is an adenocarcinoma, which is more dependent on age than on sexual activity. Adenocarcinoma must be considered any time enlargement of a Bartholin gland is found in a woman beyond reproductive age.

19. **B,** Page 644. If cystitis with pyuria is uncomplicated, it can be treated without a culture. However, if it occurs repetitively, or if the patient has a complicated renal or medical history or is an older adult, a culture should be obtained. Treatment of uncomplicated urinary tract infection is a 3-day course of trimethoprim-sulfamethoxazole, trimethoprim alone, or one of the quinolones (which are more expensive). Use of the quinolones is preferred with nonpregnant, complicated urinary tract infection or if the local level of resistance to other antibiotics is high, because these agents offer a wider spectrum of coverage. Quinolones are contraindicated in pregnancy.

20. **C,** Page 642. Cystitis commonly has an acute onset with dysuria, frequency, and urgency. It also manifests in suprapubic pain without significant fever. Urethritis usually does not involve suprapubic pain, and pyelonephritis usually causes a fever and flank pain. Vaginitis may cause some dysuria but usually not urgency and frequency, whereas cervicitis alone does not cause urinary symptoms. However, the same organism that causes urethritis may infect any of the other organs; therefore, a physical examination should be completed.

21. **C,** Page 690. Women with a cervical *Chlamydia trachomatis* infection may have mucopus, especially in the follicular phase of the cycle. Yeast and bacterial vaginosis usually do not affect the cervical mucus. Herpes simplex, chlamydia, and gonorrhea can be found in the endocervical canal, but the number of white blood cells is smaller in herpes and gonorrhea than in chlamydia. Most women with either chlamydia or gonorrhea do not have cervical mucopus; therefore, mucopus is of diagnostic importance only if present. When mucopus is present, approximately half of patients have chlamydia. Fortunately, new rapid sampling methods are available to diagnose chlamydia; they include the use of monoclonal antibodies or ELISA as well as DNA and PCR tests. PCR tests can be used to screen low-risk populations and provide treatments before infections become symptomatic.

22. **A,** Pages 651–654; Table 22–5 in Stenchever. Electrocautery or electroexcision has a high initial efficacy but is expensive, as is surgical excision. Electrocautery is generally better than cryotherapy, but it is also more expensive. Topical podofilox, which a patient can apply herself, and trichloroacetic acid are both good for treatment of recently developed warts and are inexpensive. Interferon has been used both systematically and locally to effect some improvement in resolution of visible warts; however, none of these modalities destroys the viable viral DNA in the basal cells or virions in the epithelium, which can be found at a distance from the florid wart. Therefore, close observation and follow-up are required. All treatment methods are associated with a fairly high recurrence rate.

23. **B,** Page 675. *Candida* species are part of the normal vaginal flora in approximately 25% of women. They are more prevalent in the bowel (3 to 4 times) and the mouth (2 times). These organisms are not usually found on intact skin. The prevalence is increased in patients who have been taking antibiotics or are immunosuppressed or diabetic. Symptoms caused by *Candida* often flare up after treatment with antibodies for either genital or nongenital disease. Treatment for *Candida* can be either topical or oral. Fluconazole is an oral medication with a good treatment efficacy after one dose of 150 mg PO. However, it is best reserved for resistant cases because of possible side effects and drug interactions.

24. **C,** Page 674. This patient has a mixed vaginitis with both bacterial vaginosis and *Trichomonas* infection. The treatment of choice for *Trichomonas* is metronidazole given systemically. Administration of 1 g BID for 1 day gives a good cure rate and involves a low incidence of nausea. The 1-day

dose also yields greater compliance than a longer dosage regimen. Fluconazole and clotrimazole are treatments for yeast, which this patient does not have, at least at present. In some patients, a systemic yeast infection develops after management of another type of vaginitis. Clotrimazole helps to treat *Trichomonas* infections, but it is not as effective as metronidazole. Clindamycin can be used to treat bacterial vaginosis, but it is not the best drug for *Trichomonas*. Metronidazole gel works well for bacterial vaginosis, but it is not as effective as oral metronidazole is for *Trichomonas* infections. The male partner also should be treated for *Trichomonas*.

25. **C, Page 616.** The levels with nonspecific tests for syphilis usually decline after adequate treatment and, in fact, should be followed up after therapy to ensure that the titer drops. If it does not, inadequate treatment, reinfection or concurrent HIV infection must be considered. One would not expect the rash of secondary syphilis to develop after adequate treatment. The FTA-ABS result usually remains positive for life. A Jarisch-Herxheimer reaction is likely after penicillin treatment of primary or secondary syphilis, but development of primary chancre, secondary rash, or tertiary neurosyphilis with tabes, paresis, or gumma is rare in cases treated adequately.

26. **B, Page 644.** If a person has excess anticardiolipin antibodies, a false-negative serologic test result for syphilis may occur. This is known as the *prozone phenomenon*. Malaria, infectious mononucleosis, subacute lupus erythematosus, and chronic liver disease may give a false-positive nonspecific serologic test result for syphilis. If a nonspecific serologic test, such as the Venereal Disease Research Laboratories (VDRL) or RPR, is positive, a specific test, such as the *Treponema pallidum* immobilization test, the FTA-ABS, or a micro-hemagglutination assay for antibodies for *Treponema pallidum* is indicated.

27. **D, Page 679.** The symptoms are due to absorption of an exotoxin produced by *Staphylococcus aureus*. Blood cultures are rarely positive. The use of tampons allows *Staphylococcus* to grow and excrete the exotoxin, which is then absorbed through the vaginal mucosa. Sexual transmission is not a common factor because *Staphylococcus* can commonly be cultured from the vagina of sexually inactive women. Treatment with an antistaphylococcal antibiotic prevents recurrent episodes, which occur in approximately one third of untreated women even if they stop using tampons. The 16-year-old should be encouraged to stop using tampons or at least to change them every 6 hours during the day and use sanitary napkins at night. Use of a cervical cap or diaphragm for contraception increases the risk of nonmenstrual toxic shock.

28. **D, Page 656.** In a woman with this history, the primary possibility is herpes simplex virus. However, the differential diagnosis must include syphilis along with several less common possibilities, such as chancroid, granuloma inguinale, and cancer. A herpes simplex virus culture is indicated, as is a dark-field study. A serologic test for syphilis should be obtained in case the woman had syphilis earlier, but it is too soon for test results to be positive from her recent exposure. Approximately 4 to 6 weeks must elapse for a serologic test for syphilis to yield positive results. Cancer is unlikely in this age group, but it could be ruled out by biopsy if the lesion is not healed or markedly improved within 2 weeks. A Frei test for lymphogranuloma venereum is no longer done because better tests are available. Treatment should await diagnosis. Antibiotics do not help a herpes simplex virus infection, which is the most likely diagnosis. The lymph nodes are not fluctuant, and aspiration is not likely to help because the patient is unlikely to have lymphogranuloma venereum or chancroid.

29. **D, Page 655.** Genital HSV is a common affliction. Contrary to popular belief, most infected persons are not aware of their infection. They have had subclinical or unnoticed symptoms. Because they do not know that they have HSV, they may have unprotected sex and continue to spread the disease. For those who know that they have HSV, both episodic and prophylactic treatment are available to treat or decrease occurrences (Table 22–1, Table 22–2.).

30. **A, Pages 676–677.** Fluconazole is usually given as a single oral dose of 150 mg, which results in therapeutic levels in the vaginal epithelium for

---

TABLE 22–1

Recommended Regimens for Episodic Recurrent Herpes Simplex Virus Infection

---

Acyclovir 400 mg orally three times a day for 5 days,

or

Acyclovir 200 mg orally five times a day for 5 days,

or

Acyclovir 800 mg orally twice a day for 5 days,

or

Famciclovir 125 mg orally twice a day for 5 days,

or

Valacyclovir 500 mg orally twice a day for 5 days.

From CDC: 1998 guidelines for treatment of sexually transmitted diseases. MMWR 47:23, 1997.

TABLE 22–2
Recommended Regimens for Daily Herpes Simplex Virus Suppressive Therapy

Acyclovir 400 mg orally twice a day,

or

Famciclovir 250 mg orally twice a day,

or

Valacyclovir 250 mg orally twice a day,

or

Valacyclovir 500 mg orally once a day,

or

Valacyclovir 1000 mg orally once a day.

From CDC: 1998 guidelines for treatment of sexually transmitted diseases. MMWR 47:23, 1997.

approximately three days. This drug is an imidizole, and therefore *Candida* species that are resistant to topical imidizole preparations may require higher doses and longer treatments. Fluconazole causes less hepatic damage than ketoconazole. The major problem is that it interacts with many drugs—for example, it may cause hypoglycemia in patients taking oral diabetic medications, and it increases the effect of coumadin and is contraindicated in patients taking cisapride because of cardiac conduction changes. Carefully check patient medications before prescribing this common drug, which is often used for a common condition.

31. **C**, Pages 692–693. The LCR test is comparable in specificity and sensitivity to tissue culture and is much faster. It can be done in urine with good results, thereby avoiding the requirement of a pelvic examination to obtain intracervical cultures. The other tests lack adequate sensitivity and specificity, although some are used in locations of very high prevalence because of their low cost and greater availability.

32–35. 32, **C**; 33, **A**; 34, **E**; 35, **C**; Pages 660–663. *Chlamydia* is well known to cause cervicitis, nonspecific urethritis, pelvic inflammatory disease, and trachoma. This organism also causes lymphogranuloma venereum, which is not as common. Gummas and condylomata lata are lesions of secondary syphilis, which are not common and are not as well known as the chancre of primary syphilis. Chancroid is a rare disease caused by *Haemophilus ducreyi*, which may form the classic school-of-fish appearance of extracellular streptobacillary chains on a Gram smear. Granuloma inguinale is caused by *Calymmatobacterium granulomatis* and is rare in the United States. Granuloma generally starts as an asymptomatic nodule, which then develops into a painless ulcer. It is hard to remember the signs, symptoms, causative agents, diagnostic methods, and treatment of rare diseases; however, these rare manifestations should be reviewed regularly because they are all included in the differential diagnosis for common genital lesions, such as condylomata acuminata or herpes, and the less common, but serious, condition of vulvar carcinoma.

36–39. 36, **B**; 37, **C**; 38, **A**; 39, **D**; Pages 649, 652, 657, 661. Visual identification of some vulvar lesions is easy, but confirmation by culture or biopsy is usually indicated. Molluscum contagiosum lesions appear umbilicated and have a central core of hyperkeratotic epidermis, which is easily expelled. Microscopically, the lesion contains intracytoplasmic inclusions. Treatment is by curettage. Lymphogranuloma venereum is caused by *Chlamydia trachomatis*. Its secondary stage includes enlarged lymph nodes, which coalesce to form skin depressions between groups of the inflamed nodes, yielding the groove sign. Fluctuant nodes may be aspirated for diagnosis. Treatment includes administration of tetracycline or erythromycin for 3 to 6 weeks. Herpes simplex may form a necrotic ulcer of the cervix with remarkably few systemic symptoms. It must be remembered that the herpes simplex virus is likely in a young woman, and therefore cultures for the herpesvirus should be obtained. In such cases, if culture does not confirm the diagnosis and the ulcer persists, biopsy is indicated to rule out cancer. A course of acyclovir should be given for treatment of a significant herpes infection. Treatment decreases the time and severity of symptoms but does not affect the frequency of recurrence. In the majority of women, condyloma acuminatum can be diagnosed by direct inspection. The warts tend to occur on moist skin. Initial infections usually begin in the vestibule and adjacent areas of the labia. However, all adjacent moist epithelium may be involved with condyloma. Initial lesions are pedunculated soft papules that are approximately 2 to 3 mm in diameter and 10 to 20 mm long. They may occur as a single papule or in clusters. The management of the individual case depends on the location, size, and extent of the condyloma and whether the woman is pregnant. There is a wide range of therapeutic choices, including chemical, cautery, and immunologic therapy. Since all these lesions can be confused with cancer, one should not hesitate to perform a biopsy if there is doubt. Perhaps the only exception to biopsy is the fluctuant nodes of lymphogranuloma venereum, which tend to form draining sinuses after incision.

TABLE 22–3

1993 Revised Classification System for HIV Infection and Expanded AIDS Surveillance Case Definition for Adolescents and Adults*

	Clinical Categories		
CD4 + T-Cell Categories	**(A)** **Asymptomatic, Acute** **(Primary) HIV or PGL**[†]	**(B)** **Symptomatic, Not** **(A) or (C) Conditions**	**(C)** **AIDS-Indicator** **Conditions**
(1) ≥300/µL	A1	B1	C1
(2) 200–499/µL	A2	B2	C2
(3) <200/µL	A3	B3	C3
AIDS-indicator T-cell count			

From *MMWR* 41:1, 1992.

*Persons with AIDS-indicator conditions (Category C) as well as those with CD4+ T-lymphocyte counts <200/µL (Categories A3 or B3) will be reportable as AIDS cases in the United States and territories, effective Jan. 1, 1993.

[†]*PGL*, Persistent generalized lymphadenopathy. Clinical Category A includes acute (primary) HIV infection.

40–41. 40, **B;** 41, **C;** Pages 681–684. The 1993 Revised Classification System categorizes persons with HIV into categories A, B, and C and subcategorizes them depending on the level of their CD4 T cell count (Table 22–3). Group A members are asymptomatic; group B members are symptomatic but do not have persistent generalized lymphadenopathy or any of the AIDS-indicator conditions; and those in group C have AIDS-indicator conditions. A woman with cervical dysplasia is included in group B, whereas a woman with invasive carcinoma is in group C. In the 1993 AIDS Surveillance Case Definition, invasive cervical cancer, pulmonary tuberculosis, and recurrent pneumonia were added to the list of previous indicators defining full-blown AIDS. Subcategories based on the CD4 T cell count are those with (1) more than 500, (2) between 200 and 499, and (3) below 500.

Chemotherapy for AIDS has progressed rapidly. Currently, triple therapy using two reverse transcriptase inhibitors and a protease inhibitor is more effective in decreasing replication and load. All pregnant women should be offered HIV testing because treatment during pregnancy, labor, and delivery may prevent vertical transmission to the infant.

A decrease in the number and quality of CD4 lymphocytes (T_4 lymphocytes with CD4 receptors) allows opportunistic infections to develop because these lymphocytes modulate many of the human immune system functions. Without the protection these lymphocytes offer, organisms that normally would not cause a problem result in serious disease (eg, *Pneumocystis* pneumonia). HIV-infected monocytes migrate into the central nervous system, causing central nervous system symptoms, which are the presenting complaints in one third of AIDS cases and occur in more than 80% of affected patients at some time during the illness. Unfortunately, the treatment medications do not penetrate the central nervous system. Kaposi carcinoma is the best-known associated malignancy, but lymphomas are also common.

Infections of the Upper Genital Tract

DIRECTIONS:

for Questions 1–11: Select the one best answer or completion.

1. In a tuboovarian complex associated with acute pelvic inflammatory disease (PID), the flora is predominantly

   A. group D *Enterococcus*
   B. mixed anaerobes
   C. *Chlamydia trachomatis*
   D. *Neisseria gonorrhoeae*
   E. *Escherichia coli*

2. A 16-year-old nullipara has bilateral lower abdominal pain, a fever of 38°C, and a tender left adnexal thickening. A cervical culture is positive for *Chlamydia trachomatis*. The best treatment would be

   A. outpatient treatment with intramuscular cefoxitin and oral doxycycline
   B. oral doxycycline alone
   C. intramuscular procaine penicillin
   D. hospitalization with parenteral doxycycline and cefoxitin
   E. hospitalization with parenteral cefoxitin alone

3. Empirical antibiotic protocols used to treat acute PID generally provide inadequate coverage for which of the following organisms?

   A. *Neisseria gonorrhoeae*
   B. *Chlamydia trachomatis*
   C. *Bacteroides* species
   D. *Peptococcus* species
   E. *Clostridium* species

4. The most accurate method of diagnosing acute PID is

   A. history
   B. pelvic examination
   C. ultrasonography
   D. leukocytosis
   E. diagnostic laparoscopy

5. Of the following contraceptive methods, the one that is associated with the lowest risk of sexually transmitted disease is

   A. nonoxynol-9 (spermicidal jelly or cream)
   B. an intrauterine device (IUD)
   C. condoms
   D. oral contraceptives
   E. a diaphragm

6. When clinical criteria alone are used to diagnose acute PID, the percentage of false-positives is approximately

   A. 15%
   B. 25%
   C. 35%
   D. 45%
   E. 55%

7. Bacteriologic and immunologic studies suggest that the most prevalent sexually transmitted organism causing upper tract disease in the United States is

   A. the human immunodeficiency virus (HIV)
   B. Herpes simplex virus
   C. *Neisseria gonorrhoeae*
   D. *Chlamydia trachomatis*
   E. *Mycoplasma hominis*

8. A cervical culture from a 27-year-old patient who is hospitalized for treatment of acute salpingitis is positive for *Neisseria gonorrhoeae*. The likelihood of a fallopian tube culture being positive for the same organism is

   A. 5%
   B. 10%
   C. 25%
   D. 50%
   E. 75%

9. The most frequent symptom of acute PID is

   A. vaginal discharge
   B. abnormal bleeding
   C. nausea and vomiting
   D. lower abdominal pain
   E. urinary frequency

10. A 32-year-old multipara with an IUD in place is hospitalized for treatment of acute PID. The IUD should be removed

    A. as soon as the diagnosis has been made
    B. as soon as antibiotics have been started
    C. as soon as adequate levels of antibiotics have been achieved
    D. 24 hours after antibiotics have been initiated
    E. at the conclusion of parenteral antibiotic therapy

11. A 24-year-old nullipara is being treated for bilateral tuboovarian abscesses noted on ultrasonography. Triple antibiotics, including clindamycin, gentamicin, and ampicillin, have been given for 72 hours. Pain and fever persist. The abscess is *not* pointing into the cul-de-sac. The most appropriate next step in the treatment of this patient is

    A. total abdominal hysterectomy with bilateral salpingo-oophorectomy
    B. laparoscope-assisted vaginal hysterectomy
    C. bilateral salpingo-oophorectomy
    D. colpotomy drainage of abscess
    E. transvaginal aspiration of abscess under ultrasound guidance

---

DIRECTIONS:

for Questions 12–17: For each numbered item, select the one heading most closely associated with it. Each lettered heading may be used once, more than once, or not at all.

12–14. **Percentage affected**

   (A) 1%–4%
   (B) 5%–10%
   (C) 20%–25%
   (D) 40%–50%
   (E) >60%

12. Mortality rate associated with ruptured tuboovarian abscess

13. Recurrence rate of PID

14. Percentage of ectopic pregnancies occurring in tubes damaged by previous salpingitis

15–17. **Match the findings with the preferred therapy**

   (A) intravenous doxycycline and cefoxitin
   (B) intravenous clindamycin and gentamicin
   (C) intramuscular cefoxitin plus oral probenecid
   (D) intramuscular ceftriaxone plus 10 days of tetracycline
   (E) intramuscular ceftriaxone plus 10 days of erythromycin

15. Positive *Neisseria gonorrhoeae* culture from cervix, no fever, no tenderness

16. 7-cm abscess, fever, negative cervical culture

17. Bilateral adnexal tenderness, low-grade fever

DIRECTIONS:

for each numbered item 18–26, indicate whether it is associated with

---

   A. only (A)
   B. only (B)
   C. both (A) and (B)
   D. neither (A) nor (B)

18–19. **Match the statements about acute PID with the causative organism**

   (A) *Chlamydia trachomatis*
   (B) *Neisseria gonorrhoeae*
   (C) both
   (D) neither

18. 5–10% are associated with Fitz-Hugh-Curtis syndrome (perihepatic inflammation)

19. Body temperature exceeds 38°C in more than two thirds of patients

20–21. **Match the appropriate antibiotic or antibiotics with the situation**

   (A) ceftriaxone 250 mg
   (B) doxycycline 100 mg twice a day
   (C) both
   (D) neither

20. Acute PID without fever, nausea, or vomiting

21. A pharyngeal culture positive for *Neisseria gonorrhoeae*

22–23. Relationship with upper tract infection or colonization

    (A) ectopic pregnancy
    (B) chronic pelvic pain
    (C) both
    (D) neither

22. At least a fourfold increase in patients with acute PID

23. Related to colonization of endosalpinx by anaerobic bacteria

24–26. Frequency, cause, and effect of two of the more uncommon organisms associated with pelvic infections

    (A) *Actinomyces* infection
    (B) tuberculosis infection
    (C) both
    (D) neither

24. Rare cause of infection of the upper genital tract in the United States

25. Associated with IUD use

26. A cause of infertility

DIRECTIONS:

for Questions 27–31: For each of the questions below, select the one best answer or completion.

---

27. **Acute PID caused by *Neisseria gonorrhoeae* can resist therapy by**

    A. suppressing the antibody response in patients
    B. causing necrotic destruction of tubal epithelium
    C. producing penicillinase
    D. inhibiting local inflammatory response

28. **The most common organism associated with *nonpuerperal* endometritis is**

    A. cytomegalovirus
    B. *Neisseria gonorrhoeae*
    C. *Chlamydia trachomatis*
    D. *Streptococcus agalactiae*

29. **Oral contraceptives protect against sexually transmitted diseases by**

    A. altering bacterial flora of the vagina
    B. altering the cervical mucus
    C. decreasing the volume of menstruation
    D. altering the endometrial lining

30. **A 62-year-old patient is being treated for PID. The differential should include**

    A. hypothyroidism
    B. genital tract malignancy
    C. urinary tract infection
    D. exogenous hormone exposure

31. **Which of the following is associated with a reduction in the risk of PID?**

    A. vaginal douching
    B. IUD use
    C. a history of a tubal ligation
    D. a history of treated pelvic infection in the past

ANSWERS

1. **B,** Page 710. Abscesses caused by acute PID contain a mixture of anaerobes and facultative or aerobic organisms. The environment of an abscess cavity results in a low level of oxygen tension. Therefore, anaerobic organisms predominate and have been reported to be present in 60% to 100% of cases.

2. **D,** Pages 722–725. This question addresses optimal treatment of acute PID. Especially important in this patient are her young age, nulliparity, demonstrable fever, and the presence of a palpable inflammatory thickening. Outpatient therapy does not provide high enough levels of appropriate antibiotics to successfully penetrate a developing tuboovarian complex. The presence of *Chlamydia trachomatis* mandates treatment with doxycycline and the presence of a palpable

inflammatory thickening implicates other opportunistic organisms as pathogens. Cefoxitin is an excellent antibiotic for *Peptococcus* and *Peptostreptococcus* as well as *Escherichia coli*. An alternative to this regimen would include parenteral clindamycin and an aminoglycoside. This combination has an advantage of better coverage for anaerobic infections and facultative gram-negative rods.

3. **E,** Page 724. Empirical antibiotic protocols should cover a wide range of bacteria, including *Neisseria gonorrhoeae*, *Chlamydia trachomatis*, anaerobic rods and cocci, gram-negative aerobic rods, gram-positive aerobes, and *Mycoplasma* species. *Clostridium* species are rarely implicated in acute tuboovarian disease; therefore, treatment for this group of organisms is not indicated initially. Selection of one antibiotic protocol over another often depends on the clinical history and combinations of findings such as those shown in Table 23–6 (from Stenchever and colleagues). Unfortunately, recent epidemiologic studies have shown that most women with acute PID are treated as outpatients and have received only a single antibiotic regimen. Of these, less than one third of patients received tetracycline to treat possible chlamydial infection. This underscores the need for thorough knowledge of the bacteriology of acute PID as a polymicrobial infection.

4. **E,** Page 718. Direct visualization of the pelvic organs is the most accurate method of diagnosing acute PID. Therefore, laparoscopy is the gold standard. The pelvic organs may appear red, with an indurated, edematous oviduct, or purulent material may be obvious. Laparoscopy should be used for patients who are not responding to antimicrobial therapy, or for those patients in whom cultures of purulent material need to be obtained.

5. **D,** Pages 713–715. Using arbitrary risk rating scales in which the risk of acute PID in sexually active women not using contraception is assigned a score of 1, the following observations have been calculated. The corresponding risk of women wearing an IUD is 2 to 4, among women using oral contraceptives 0.3, and is 0.4 among women using a barrier method, including spermicidal preparations. Nonoxynol-9, the material found in spermicidal preparations, is both bactericidal and viricidal, and laboratory tests have demonstrated its effectiveness among all sexually transmitted diseases, including HIV.

6. **C,** Page 716. Patients with acute PID present with a wide range of nonspecific clinical symptoms. Since the diagnosis is usually based on clinical criteria, the false-positive and false-negative rates are high. Laparoscopic studies of women with a

clinical diagnosis of acute PID suggest that this diagnosis is wrong in over one third of patients. Of this approximately 35%, 20% have no identifiable intraabdominal or pelvic disease and approximately 15% have other entities, such as ectopic pregnancy, acute appendicitis, or torsion of an adnexa.

7. **D,** Pages 710–712. *Chlamydia trachomatis* is an intracellular, sexually transmitted bacterial pathogen. This organism has recently become more prevalent than gonorrhea. Antibodies against *Chlamydia trachomatis* are found in 20% to 40% of sexually active women. Among women with acute PID in whom cultures are negative for *Chlamydia*, serial antibody testing shows evidence of acute chlamydial infection in 10% to 30%. Although considered a sexually transmitted organism, herpes is generally not associated with acute upper tract infection and HIV is considered a systemic illness rather than an infection limited to the upper genital tract. *Mycoplasma hominis* appears in direct tubal cultures in approximately 15% of women with acute inflammatory disease; the gonococcus is cultured less than 15% of the time in women with upper tract disease.

8. **D,** Page 710. Approximately 15% of women with cervical infection caused by *Neisseria gonorrhoeae* subsequently experience acute salpingitis. Among women in whom endocervical cultures are positive for this organism at the time of treatment for acute salpingitis, the same organisms are cultured from the fallopian tubes in 50%. If *Neisseria gonorrhoeae* is the only organism cultured from the tubes, a patient should respond rapidly to antimicrobial therapy.

9. **D,** Page 717; Tables 23–10, 23–11 in Stenchever. By far the most frequent symptom of acute PID is pain in the lower abdomen. Over 90% of women present with diffuse bilateral lower abdominal pain, usually described as constant and dull. It is usually of short duration; if the pain has been present for longer than 3 weeks, it is unlikely that the patient has acute PID. Approximately 75% of patients have an associated endocervical infection with vaginal discharge. Abnormal vaginal bleeding occurs in approximately 40% of patients. Nausea and vomiting are late symptoms in the course of this disease. Because of the importance of aggressive antibiotic therapy, current recommendations for treatment suggest that the diagnosis of upper tract infection should be strongly entertained for any patient with lower abdominal pain, adnexal pain, and cervical motion tenderness.

10. **C,** Page 724. Acute PID associated with the presence of an IUD is usually more advanced at the time of diagnosis. This is due to both physician and patient delays in the diagnosis. The patient

misinterprets early signs and symptoms of pelvic inflammation as being related to the presence of the IUD. Patients with an IUD should be hospitalized and given parenteral antibiotics. The IUD should be removed as soon as therapeutic levels of intravenous antibiotics have been obtained.

11. **E**, Page 726. Management of a tuboovarian abscess should be medical; operative intervention should only be undertaken if medical treatment fails. In women who have not completed their families, every effort should be made to conserve reproductive potential. Actions to consider are unilateral removal of the tuboovarian complex or abscess if the disease is unilateral. Similarly, colpotomy is appropriate if the abscess is pointing posteriorly. In a young patient as described, given the clinical circumstances, a new approach that would retain as much reproductive potential as possible is transvaginal aspiration under ultrasound guidance. Laparoscopic aspiration has also been used but does not appear to have any greater benefit than ultrasound-guided aspiration.

12–14. 12, **B**; 13, **C**; 14, **D**; Pages 728–731. Before antibiotic therapy, the mortality rate associated with acute PID was 1% of all patients. Although the death rate has improved with modern treatment, it has been estimated that there still is one death every other day in the United States directly related to PID. Most of these deaths result from rupture of a tuboovarian complex, the mortality rate of which is 5% to 10%. Approximately 25% of patients experience recurrent PID. Younger women become reinfected twice as often as older women. The number of ectopic pregnancies has doubled since the early 1990s and is directly related and proportional to the increase in sexually transmitted diseases. Pathologic studies estimate that approximately one half of ectopic pregnancies occur in oviducts damaged by previous salpingitis.

15–17. 15, **D**; 16, **B**; 17, **A**; Pages 722–724. Patients without evidence of upper tract disease in whom screening cultures are positive may be treated with outpatient antibiotics such as intramuscular ceftriaxone plus 10 days of tetracycline or oral ofloxacin and metronidazole. Treatment with intramuscular cefoxitin plus oral probenecid without a tetracycline account for the likelihood of a coexistent *Chlamydia* infection. Erythromycin has been substituted for tetracycline in patients who are allergic to the latter. This regimen is based on limited data, and the report did not mention a tetracycline allergy. In the presence of an abscess or tuboovarian complex, one assumes the presence of anaerobic organisms and facultative gram-negative rods. Therefore, a regimen of treatment including parenteral clindamycin and

an aminoglycoside is preferable. Cervical cultures are oftentimes negative in the presence of a pyosalpinx. In cases of acute salpingitis without a palpable abscess, doxycycline accompanied by broad-spectrum agents such as cefoxitin is adequate since there is no need to penetrate an abscess cavity.

18–19. 18, **C**; 19, **D**; Page 718. Five to 10% of women with acute PID caused by either *Chlamydia trachomatis* or *Neisseria gonorrhoeae* experience symptoms of perihepatic inflammation—-the Fitz-Hugh-Curtis syndrome. This condition is often mistakenly diagnosed as either pneumonia or acute cholecystitis. The symptoms include right upper quadrant pain, pleuritic pain, and tenderness in the right upper quadrant when the liver is palpated. The syndrome develops from the transperitoneal or vascular dissemination of the organisms causing the acute PID. Only one of three women with acute PID presents with a temperature greater than 38°C as borne out in laparoscopically confirmed cases of acute PID. Whereas the gonococcus survives no more than a few days in the endosalpinx of untreated patients, *Chlamydia* organisms may remain in the fallopian tubes for months after initial colonization of the upper genital tract.

20–21. 20, **C**; 21, **C**; Pages 723–724. Recommended therapy for the ambulatory management of PID includes ceftriaxone, 250 mg intramuscularly, plus doxycycline, 100 mg orally two times per day for 10 to 14 days or oral ofloxacin and metronidazole. Both rectal and pharyngeal gonorrheal infections are difficult to treat. The Centers for Disease Control and Prevention advise the use of ceftriaxone, 250 mg in a single intramuscular dose, along with doxycycline, 100 mg orally twice per day for 7 days, for pharyngeal or rectal gonorrheal infections.

22–23. 22, **C**; 23, **D**; Pages 728–731. Acute PID can be directly related to medical sequelae in 25% of patients. The rate of ectopic pregnancy following acute PID climbs 6 to 10 times, and the chance of chronic pelvic pain increases fourfold. In the United States each year, 26,000 ectopic pregnancies and 90,000 new cases of chronic abdominal pelvic pain are directly related to PID. Neither entity is directly related to species-specific anaerobic colonization of the endosalpinx. The term *chronic PID* should not be used since the majority of cases with sequelae of chronic pelvic infection are bacteriologically sterile, including a hydrosalpinx. Chronic pelvic pain may exist with minimal visual anatomic changes and in the absence of positive endosalpingeal cultures.

24–26. 24, **C**; 25, **A**; 26, **B**; Page 731. Both *Actinomyces* and tuberculosis are rare causes of infection of the upper genital tract. Tuberculosis, however, is a frequent cause of chronic PID and infertility outside the United States. Most cases of *Actinomyces* infection have occurred in women wearing an IUD. In fact, there is controversy as to whether an IUD should be removed from a woman in whom *Actinomyces* is found on Pap smear. If *Actinomyces* is part of a polymicrobial infection, "sulfur granules" constitute histologic evidence of this organism. The usual primary site of infection for tuberculosis is the lung. The bacteria are spread hematogenously, and the infection becomes located in the fallopian tube. From there, it spreads to the endometrium and to the ovaries. Primary symptoms are infertility and abnormal bleeding.

27. **C**, Page 710. Acute PID caused by *Neisseria gonorrhoeae* can resist therapy by producing penicillinase. These strains of gonorrhea become resistant to penicillin by acquiring a resistance factor plasmid. By 1989, 6% of gonorrhea strains were resistant to penicillin. Resistance is not caused by suppressing the antibody response, as antibodies against the outer membrane of the gonococcus develop in 70% of women with severe pelvic infection. By its natural course, the gonococcus produces an intense inflammatory reaction in the tubes, which causes the tubal lumen to swell with necrotic debris and purulent material.

28. **C**, Page 708. Nonpuerperal endometritis is an obscure chronic infection of the lining of the uterus. Although research about this entity is scant, it probably represents an intermediate state of ascending infection that is spreading through the canaliculi, which connect the lower genital tract to the upper genital tract. There is a correlation between serum antibody levels against both *Mycoplasma hominis* and *Chlamydia trachomatis* with the prevalence of nonpuerperal endometritis. Organisms commonly found associated with nonpuerperal endometritis include *Chlamydia trachomatis, Neisseria gonorrhoeae, Streptococcus agalactiae*, cytomegalovirus, and herpes simplex.

29. **B**, Page 713. Oral contraceptive use is associated with a lower incidence of acute PID and a milder form of infection of the upper genital tract when it does occur. The decrease in incidence of upper tract disease is thought to be secondary to a thicker cervical mucus, which is caused by the progestin component of oral contraceptives. The decrease in duration of menstrual flow theoretically creates a shorter interval for bacterial colonization of the upper tract.

30. **B**, Page 713. Spontaneous PID is extremely unusual in woman who are not sexually active or who are amenorrheic. If PID is found in a postmenopausal woman, genital malignancies, diabetes, or a concurrent intestinal disease is also usually present.

31. **C**, Pages 713–715. Frequent vaginal douching increases the risk of PID 3.6 times over women who douche less than once a month. In addition, despite criticism of the epidemiologic studies, the risk of acute pelvic inflammation in women who wear an IUD appears to be two to three times greater during the first 4 months after the IUD is inserted over those women who do not use any contraception. Salpingitis does occur after tubal ligation, although infrequently. In one series, salpingitis of the proximal stump of previously ligated fallopian tubes was 1 in 450. Patients who have had one episode of PID are at increased risk because of both the tubal damage and the behaviors related to the original episode.

Preoperative Counseling and Management

Select the one best answer or completion.

1. The part of the preoperative evaluation most likely to reveal medically important information is the

    A. medical history
    B. laboratory evaluation
    C. physical examination
    D. nursing evaluation

2. Of the following, the cephalosporin with the longest half-life is

    A. cephalothin
    B. cefazolin
    C. cefoxitin
    D. cefotaxime
    E. moxalactam

3. An intravenous pyelogram is ordered for a 48-year-old woman scheduled to have a hysterectomy for large uterine myomata. The risk of mortality from the imaging procedure is

    A. 1 in 1000
    B. 1 in 10,000
    C. 1 in 100,000
    D. 1 in 1 million

4. A 35-year-old woman with heart disease, who has difficulty walking one block without becoming short of breath, needs an emergency laparotomy for a suspected ectopic pregnancy. According to the DRIPPS American Society of Anesthesiology risk classification, her condition is class

    A. 1
    B. 2
    C. 3
    D. 4
    E. 5

5. Which of the following antihypertensive medications should be discontinued before a surgical procedure?

    A. β-blockers
    B. diuretics
    C. clonidine
    D. calcium channel blockers
    E. monoamine oxidase (MAO) inhibitors

6. If an abnormality is found during routine chest radiography performed before surgery on an asymptomatic patient, the finding is most likely to be

    A. false-positive
    B. false-negative
    C. true-positive
    D. true-negative

7. A 37-year-old obese woman with stage 1B carcinoma of the cervix is scheduled for a radical hysterectomy and node dissection. She has been taking birth control pills for contraception and has a history of varicose veins. Which of the following factors places her at the greatest risk for postoperative thromboembolism?

    A. obesity
    B. carcinoma of the cervix
    C. varicose veins
    D. age
    E. estrogen use

8. A 42-year-old woman with diabetes is taking 28 units of insulin each day and has fasting blood sugar levels ranging between 105 and 180 mg/dL. She also has urinary stress incontinence that is amenable to surgical repair. The next appropriate step is to

   A. schedule the surgery as soon as practical
   B. refuse to operate
   C. set up appointments to evaluate and control her diabetes better
   D. admit her to the hospital for diabetic control
   E. increase her insulin 5 units a day and schedule the surgery

9. The most likely allergy to cause an anaphylactic reaction during elective surgery in children is

   A. prophylactic antibiotics
   B. eggs
   C. latex
   D. mold
   E. opioids

10. A 23-year-old healthy woman is being evaluated for an exploratory laparotomy for a possible unruptured ectopic pregnancy. She has no cardiac symptoms. A midsystolic click over the mitral area is heard with no other extraneous sounds or murmurs. This is most likely the result of

    A. hypovolemia
    B. increased cardiac output of pregnancy
    C. endogenous catecholamines
    D. pulmonary hypertension
    E. mitral valve prolapse

11. An asymptomatic patient is undergoing hysterectomy for markedly enlarged leiomyomata. If a postoperative complication were to arise, it would be most likely in the

    A. gastrointestinal system
    B. central nervous system
    C. cardiovascular system
    D. musculoskeletal system
    E. respiratory system

12. The current recommended protocol for antibiotic prophylaxis for bacterial endocarditis is

    A. penicillin VK, 250 mg PO every 6 hours
    B. cephalothin, 1 g every 8 hours × 3 doses
    C. tetracycline, 500 mg, and metronidazole, 1 g, 1 hour before surgery
    D. ceftriaxone, 250 mg IM every 6 hours × 3 doses
    E. ampicillin, 2 g, and gentamicin, 1.5 mg/kg, 30 minutes before surgery

13. A 35-year-old woman who smokes heavily has severe urinary stress incontinence with coughing. She is scheduled for surgical repair. For the best results in her postoperative recovery, she should be told

    A. to stop smoking the day before surgery
    B. to stop smoking 5 days before surgery
    C. to stop smoking 10 days before surgery
    D. to stop smoking 8 weeks before surgery

14. Pulmonary complications following surgery are most likely in a patient who

    A. weighs 30% more than her ideal weight
    B. is a smoker
    C. has asthma
    D. has experienced a myocardial infarction within 3 months
    E. has uncontrolled diabetes mellitus

15. Two days after a vaginal hysterectomy, a patient who otherwise is doing very well complains of continuing pain in her left knee. The knee hurts when flexed, and there is pain on pressure in the lateral joint area. The most likely cause is

    A. septic arthritis from bacteremia
    B. an anterior cruciate ligament tear
    C. gouty arthritis
    D. improper positioning during surgery
    E. thrombophlebitis

16. During a preoperative physical examination of a patient scheduled for abdominal hysterectomy, asymptomatic bacterial vaginosis is found. The most appropriate management is to

    A. add anaerobic coverage to any prophylactic antibiotics used during surgery
    B. use an iodine-based antiseptic preparation of the vagina at the time of surgery
    C. advise the use of an antibacterial douche the night before surgery
    D. delay surgery for 2 weeks while the infection is treated
    E. make no change in management

17. The method of mechanical bowel preparation that has the greatest efficacy and patient compliance is

    A. 3 days of liquid diet
    B. oral polyethylene glycol in balanced salt solution (GoLYTELY or Colyte)
    C. clear water enemas
    D. oral sodium phosphate

18. A 58-year-old patient who is scheduled for total abdominal hysterectomy and bilateral salpingo-oophorectomy is taking several medications. Which of the following should be discontinued several days to several weeks before the procedure?

    A. cortisol
    B. warfarin
    C. ibuprofen
    D. nicotine transdermal patch
    E. MAO inhibitors (eg, Nardil)

19. A 28-year-old woman has been scheduled for exploratory surgery to evaluate an anterior pelvic cystic mass palpated in clinic. Before the procedure, a bowel "prep" and bladder catheterization were performed. On examination with the patient under anesthesia, no mass is palpated. A possible explanation is that

    A. a loop of bowel was mistaken for an adnexal cyst
    B. bladder distention now obscures the mass
    C. increased abdominal wall tone has made evaluation more difficult
    D. juxtaposition of the mass and the uterus has occurred

20. A 63-year-old woman with a long smoking history is scheduled for exploratory laparotomy. Indicated tests of pulmonary function are

    A. arterial partial oxygen pressure (Po_2)
    B. residual capacity
    C. forced expiratory volume at 1 second (FEV_1)
    D. functional reserve capacity

21. You wish to decrease the risk of thromboembolic disease in a healthy 60-year-old woman who is undergoing oral replacement estrogen therapy and is scheduled for an anterior vaginal repair. You should

    A. discontinue her replacement estrogen therapy
    B. order prophylactic heparin
    C. begin low-dose aspirin therapy 1 week before surgery
    D. begin ambulation early

22. A 52-year-old woman with diabetes and an elevated creatinine level (1.9 mg/dL) has an $8 \times 9 \times 10$ cm pelvic mass for which you are planning exploratory surgery. This patient has no known allergies. The safest method to determine the location of the ureters in relation to the mass is to perform

    A. an intravenous pyelography
    B. magnetic resonance imaging
    C. ultrasonography of the kidneys
    D. operative evaluation
    E. computed tomography with contrast

23. A hypertensive 63-year-old woman with procidentia experienced a myocardial infarction 2 months ago. She is mildly hypertensive and has had angina for several years. The procidentia is becoming ulcerated and is creating care problems. She wants surgical repair. The factor in this patient's history that most directly predicts the risk of an adverse outcome is

    A. stable angina
    B. myocardial infarction within 3 months of surgery
    C. hypertension
    D. pelvic organ prolapse
    E. ulceration and infection of the cervix

24. A history of which of the following should result in the delay of elective surgery until further evaluation is obtained?

    A. moderate hypertension
    B. treated hypothyroidism
    C. renal insufficiency
    D. asthma

25. Compared with the cost of an allogeneic blood transfusion, the cost of an autologous blood transfusion is

    A. more than $50 less
    B. roughly the same
    C. more than $50 more

26. Based on recent work, after what age is it cost-effective to obtain routine preoperative electrocardiography for an asymptomatic woman?

    A. 40
    B. 45
    C. 50
    D. 55
    E. 60

27. Based on ^{125}I fibrinogen scanning techniques, the percentage of women undergoing elective surgery for benign disease who have evidence of thrombophlebitis is approximately

    A. 4%
    B. 8%
    C. 15%
    D. 22%
    E. 36%

28. Recent studies indicate that patients may be allowed clear liquids up to

    A. 12 hours before surgery
    B. 8 hours before surgery
    C. 6 hours before surgery
    D. 2 hours before surgery

29. **Abrupt withdrawal of β-blocking antihypertensive agents before surgery may induce**
    A. hyperkalemia
    B. increased blood pressure
    C. abrupt cardiac arrest
    D. asthma-like bronchospasm

30. **Meta-analysis of studies indicates that the use of an incentive spirometer or deep breathing exercises can result in a decreased risk of pulmonary complications of about**
    A. 20%
    B. 30%
    C. 40%
    D. 50%
    E. 60%

ANSWERS

1. **A,** Pages 742–743. A careful history is the most valuable portion of any evaluation, but its importance tends to be overlooked. Instead, laboratory tests or imaging techniques giving numerical or written data are often overemphasized by both the patient and the physician. An adequate history should include questions regarding the major organ systems, medications, allergies, habits, and family and social history. A thorough history and physical examination form a rational basis for further laboratory assessment and other diagnostic aids.

2. **E,** Page 749; Table 24–3 in Stenchever. The half-life of a medication determines how long that drug will be active. Of the first- and second-generation cephalosporins, moxalactam has the longest half-life (120 minutes) and cefazolin has the next longest (100 minutes). Cefazolin reaches high peak serum levels (80 µg/mL after a 1-g dose), but it has rather high protein binding (80%, which leaves 20% free in the tissues). Moxalactam is only 50% protein-bound.

3. **C,** Page 755. An allergic reaction to the contrast medium used in intravenous pyelography occurs in 5% to 8% of women. This is often an allergy to the iodine in the contrast. Of these reactions, approximately 1% to 2% are life-threatening, with an estimated mortality rate of 1 in 100,000. An intravenous pyelogram should be considered for significant reasons such as large pelvic masses or pelvic malignancies, but it should not be obtained routinely.

4. **C,** Page 748. The DRIPPS–American Society of Anesthesiology anesthesia risk classification is shown in Table 24–2 in Stenchever. In this patient with severe, but not incapacitating, disease, the condition is class 3. Because of the emergency nature of the surgery, her anesthetic risk is doubled.

5. **E,** Page 748. MAO inhibitors should be stopped 2 weeks or more before surgery because they can augment the effects of sympathetic amines to produce severe increases in blood pressure.

Sympathetic amines are given to prevent hypotension during surgical procedures. There is a concomitant release of catecholamines from the stress of surgery. Other antihypertensive medications should be maintained during surgery.

6. **A,** Pages 745–746. The most likely abnormality to be discovered during routine preoperative chest radiography performed on an asymptomatic patient is not an abnormality at all, but a false-positive finding. Studies indicate that, when performed on asymptomatic patients, preoperative chest radiography is more likely to yield a false-positive result and lead to additional, often invasive tests than it is to uncover a finding that will alter the management or course of surgery.

7. **B,** Pages 751–753; Table 24–6 in Stenchever. All the factors—obesity, carcinoma of the cervix, varicose veins, age, and use of birth control pills—increase this patient's risk of thromboembolism. However, the greatest risk in this patient is the malignancy. Adding to her high risk are the problems of longer surgery, immobilization after surgery, and risk for postoperative infection. Ideally, the birth control pills should be stopped for at least 4 weeks before the surgery. She is a candidate for minidose heparin or intermittent-pressure leg wraps as prophylaxis against thrombosis.

8. **C,** Pages 757–758. No elective surgery should be scheduled for this patient until her diabetes has been evaluated and is under better control. Her cardiovascular, renal, and neurologic systems should be evaluated with appropriate tests. Maintenance of a postprandial serum glucose level of less than 140 mg/mL should be achieved and controlled at that level over several weeks before elective surgery is scheduled. Frequent monitoring of diet, exercise, insulin, and blood sugars is necessary to maintain good control.

9. **C,** Pages 759–760. Latex allergies are responsible for 12% of the perioperative anaphylactic reactions in adult patients and for 70% of such reactions in children. For this reason, a careful history aimed at

uncovering a possible latex sensitivity should be a part of every preoperative evaluation.

10. **E,** Page 761. Mitral valve prolapse is not uncommon in young women and is most often diagnosed by the characteristic midsystolic click heard over the mitral area. Mitral valve prolapse with no evidence of other cardiac disease does not contraindicate surgery, nor does it require prophylactic antibiotics, although some authorities suggest that they be given. If antibiotics are used, ampicillin, 2 g IM or IV, and gentamicin, 1.5 mg/kg IM, should be given 1 hour before surgery.

11. **E,** Pages 755–757. Mild chronic obstructive pulmonary disease (COPD) is a frequent finding, especially in obese patients or patients who smoke. Anesthesia, postoperative pain, abdominal distention, and relative immobility combine to produce symptomatic atelectasis in many patients, and this effect is intensified in those with preexisting pulmonary disease. Such patients need definite preoperative instructions in deep breathing, coughing, movement, and pulmonary ventilatory exercises to prevent severe pulmonary complications.

12. **E,** Page 761. The suggested regimen for bacterial endocarditis prophylaxis is ampicillin, 2 g, and gentamicin, 1.5 mg/kg, 30 minutes before surgery. If the patient is allergic to penicillin, vancomycin, 1 g IV, may be substituted for the ampicillin.

13. **D,** Page 756. Smoking causes a sixfold increase in the risk of postoperative pulmonary complications. Smoke deposits particulate matter in the lungs and paralyzes respiratory cilia, preventing normal removal of these particles. Coughing is increased. This places additional stress on the surgical repair. Therefore, it is best if the patient can stop smoking for a prolonged time, but even her willingness to stop smoking for a few days will decrease sputum production and aid the postoperative course.

14. **B,** Pages 755–757. Common conditions can cause a marked increase in surgical risk. Obesity greater than 30% of average doubles the risk of surgery. Current smoking increases the risk of pulmonary complications sixfold even if the amount of smoking is small. Asthma increases the risk of pulmonary complications fourfold. Diabetes and cardiovascular disease may cause problems because of increased cortisol, catecholamines, glucagon, and antidiuretic hormone released by the patient during the perioperative period in addition to the potential stress of changing blood volumes or possible infections that may occur. Patients with diabetes also have poor wound healing and an increased infection rate. A myocardial infarction within 3 months of surgery increases the mortality rate from recurrent infarction 30%

if noncardiac surgery is performed during this time.

15. **D,** Pages 751–752, 762. Pressure on the joint by the stirrup or by a surgeon leaning on the supported leg is most likely. In the absence of heat or fever, a septic process is unlikely. The location and timing are wrong for thrombophlebitis. The position is also wrong for an anterior cruciate ligament tear. This is an unusual site for gout. Remember to check for pressure points after positioning any patient at the time of surgery.

16. **D,** Page 749. Multiple reports have documented a linear relationship between the presence of bacterial vaginosis and postoperative pelvic infections. Studies also indicate that the only effective way to reduce this risk is to actively treat the infection and allow the vaginal ecosystem to return to normal before proceeding with elective surgery.

17. **D,** Pages 753–754. Randomized trials indicate that the most effective, best tolerated method of clearing the bowel prior to surgery is oral sodium phosphate (90 mL). Other oral preparations require very large volumes (4 L), resulting in poor compliance and patient acceptance. Diet modifications are generally ineffective at producing the required decompression of the bowel needed. Enemas may result in fluid or electrolyte disturbances, though the use of a sodium phosphate enema (Fleets) may be appropriate when emptying of the distal colon is all that is required.

18. **E,** Page 748. MAO inhibitors should be stopped. Anticoagulants and corticosteroids may be continued with adjustment in type and dosage before and during surgery. If anticoagulation is needed, it is better to use heparin than warfarin. Cortisol should be increased if a patient is taking adrenal-suppressive doses for other systemic disease. Thyroid replacement therapy in its usual dosage should be continued until the day of surgery. The insulin requirement must be carefully adjusted, with reliance on frequent serum glucose determinations during the perioperative period. Although aspirin produces an irreversible change in clotting by way of altered platelet function, ibuprofen is a competitive inhibitor of platelet function, making discontinuation of the medication several days in advance desirable but unnecessary. Nicotine patch therapy may be continued through the surgical and postoperative periods.

19. **A,** Page 762. Most surgeons have discovered that a suspected pelvic pathologic condition has disappeared or that a previously unsuspected pathologic condition was present when they performed an examination under anesthesia just before surgery. Therefore, this examination should be routinely performed on patients who are undergoing surgery for suspected pelvic masses.

Rupture of the cyst before the time of surgery and a full bladder may easily be mistaken for an adnexal mass in the office setting, resulting in the absence of findings at the time of surgery. Examination with the patient under anesthesia, when the abdominal wall is relaxed and the bowel and bladder are emptied, allows for a more reliable examination, permitting identification even of masses close to the uterus.

20. **C,** Page 756. In an older patient in whom respiratory problems are suggested by the history or physical examination, an extensive evaluation of the pulmonary function is warranted. The vital capacity should be greater than 50% of the predicted normal for the patient's age and body size, and the Po_2 should be greater than 65 mmHg. The FEV_1 should be greater than 75% of the predicted normal volume. A chest radiograph should also appear normal. If any of these findings is abnormal, further evaluation and treatment should be done before surgery. Residual and functional reserve capacity may be established through formal pulmonary function testing, but these data are of limited value as isolated measures.

21. **D,** Pages 751–752. This healthy woman is undergoing a short procedure that has no high-risk factors dictating the use of subcutaneous doses of heparin for prophylaxis. Her low-risk status also means that the risks of aspirin therapy in a surgical patient exceed the potential benefits that might theoretically be associated with the inhibited platelet function induced by the therapy. Replacement estrogen is not associated with increased thrombosis. However, a younger woman taking birth control pills should stop them several weeks before major elective surgery. Birth control pills decrease the concentration of coagulating inhibitors (antithrombin) and elevate several clotting factors. Early ambulation is one of the best preventive measures.

22. **D,** Pages 754–755. A patient with both renal insufficiency and diabetes is at significantly increased risk for acute renal insufficiency after an intravenous pyelogram. The risk of allergic reaction from an intravenous pyelogram is 5% to 8% in any patient. Most of these reactions are mild. Pretreatment with corticosteroids decreases this risk. However, this risk is not a major contraindication. Knowing the position of the ureters does not guarantee safety during surgery. The best way to prevent injury during surgery is to identify the ureters during surgery. An intravenous pyelogram is the best way to demonstrate a double ureter, which is uncommon; ultrasonography occasionally reveals a double ureter, particularly if the ureters are distended. In this patient,

ultrasound evaluation might give the needed information without the risks inherent in intravenous pyelography, but ultrasonography is neither cost-effective nor sufficient to guarantee safety at surgery.

23. **B,** Page 760. Angina of recent occurrence (within 3 months) is a high risk factor, but stable angina is not. The recent myocardial infarction is of serious concern. Patients with recent myocardial infarction should wait at least 6 months before undergoing any elective surgery. The risk of repeat myocardial infarction persists for several days postoperatively, and about one third occur on the third or fourth postoperative day. Therefore, the patient should be followed up closely in the immediate postoperative period. No clinical tests predict the degree of risk for these patients. While tissue integrity leading to uterine prolapse may increase the risk of recurrent pelvic floor problems, the greatest threat to this patient is a recurrent myocardial infarct.

24. **C,** Pages 759–760. Moderate hypertension that is not complicated by angina does not require specific consultation before elective surgery. Although stable angina is not a contraindication to surgery per se, any patient who has angina of any duration or has signs of renal insufficiency should be evaluated by a cardiologist before elective surgery. Neither treated hypothyroidism nor stable asthma is a contraindication to surgery. Evidence of incomplete treatment or unstable pulmonary function, however, should prompt an evaluation before elective surgery.

25. **C,** Page 743. Studies indicate that autologous blood transfusions cost between $68 and $4783 more than standard (allogeneic) blood transfusions.

26. **E,** Page 746. In the past, routine preoperative electrocardiograms were recommended for asymptomatic women after the age of 50. Recent studies by Callahan and coworkers suggest that this figure should be raised to age 60.

27. **B,** Page 751. Thrombophlebitis develops in approximately 15% of women undergoing surgery for benign disease and 22% of patients undergoing surgery for malignancies. About 40% of those women with thrombophlebitis have asymptomatic pulmonary emboli. As a result, roughly 40% of deaths following gynecologic surgery are directly or indirectly related to pulmonary embolism.

28. **D,** Page 747. Although it is traditional to ask patients not to eat or drink anything during the 6 hours preceding surgery, recent studies indicate that patients may safely be allowed to maintain fluid intake up to 2 hours before the planned procedure.

29. **C,** Page 760. Abrupt withdrawal of α-blocking antihypertensive agents before surgery has resulted in myocardial infarct, ventricular tachycardia, or abrupt cardiac arrest. For this reason, the agents should be either continued throughout the perioperative period or gradually withdrawn well in advance of the planned surgery.

30. **D,** Page 757. Meta-analysis of studies indicates that the use of either an incentive spirometer or deep breathing exercises can result in a 50% decrease in the risk of pulmonary complications. Effective pain control, such as that offered by epidural analgesia, also reduces the risk of pulmonary complications.

Postoperative Counseling and Management

1. The initial management of moderate superficial thrombophlebitis at the site of an intravenous catheter includes all the following *except*

   A. heat
   B. elevation
   C. rest
   D. ibuprofen
   E. heparin

2. The most cost-efficient modality in preventing and treating atelectasis is

   A. chest physical therapy
   B. bedside incentive spirometer
   C. intermittent positive pressure breathing
   D. aerosol therapy
   E. bronchoscopy

3. On the fifth postoperative day a patient has a fever of 102°F (38.9°C) but does not feel sick. She does not appear as sick as her temperature would imply. The patient has been receiving intravenous cephalothin (Keflin) for a suspected urinary tract infection for 5 days. The most likely diagnosis is

   A. atelectasis
   B. urinary tract infection
   C. wound infection
   D. drug fever
   E. pneumonia

4. A 45-year-old woman underwent vaginal hysterectomy 12 hours ago. She is now showing evidence of intraabdominal hemorrhage. The best test to confirm the diagnosis is

   A. magnetic resonance imaging (MRI)
   B. ultrasonography
   C. Kidneys, ureter, bladder radiography
   D. computed tomography (CT)
   E. angiography

5. The most likely sign of pulmonary emboli is

   A. tachycardia
   B. tachypnea
   C. rales
   D. cyanosis
   E. accentuation of pulmonic closure

6. Three weeks after a vaginal hysterectomy and posterior repair, a 47-year-old patient complains of 10 days of involuntary passage of gas and small amounts of fecal material from the vagina and a foul-smelling vaginal discharge. On physical examination, a 0.5-cm dark-red area of what appears to be granulation tissue is seen in the lower third of the posterior vagina. At this point, you would

   A. place the patient on a low-residue diet
   B. perform a sigmoidoscopy
   C. perform a barium enema
   D. schedule the patient for immediate repair
   E. schedule the patient for a diverting colostomy

7. The currently preferred method for detecting deep vein thrombophlebitis is

   A. physical examination
   B. venography
   C. fibrinogen ^{125}I scan
   D. duplex ultrasonography
   E. impedance plethysmography

8. Of the symptoms listed, the *least* common in cases of a documented pulmonary embolus is

   A. dyspnea
   B. chest pain
   C. apprehension
   D. hemoptysis
   E. cough

9. A 35-year-old patient has just undergone a difficult abdominal hysterectomy for large leiomyomata. During surgery, it was estimated that she lost 2000 mL of blood. Records indicate that the patient was given 2000 mL of 5% dextrose in Ringer's lactate as intravenous fluid. Currently, her blood pressure is 90/60 and her pulse is 115. Preoperatively her blood pressure was 135/85 and during surgery it was about 100–150/70–100. Urine output has been 25 to 30 mL/hr. The patient's current problem is probably due to the

   A. sedative effect of anesthesia
   B. inadequate fluid replacement
   C. inadequate hemostasis and continued blood loss
   D. myocardial infarction
   E. physiologic release of aldosterone and antidiuretic hormone

10. The test with the greatest efficacy in detecting pulmonary emboli is

   A. pulmonary angiography
   B. ventilation-perfusion lung scan
   C. arterial blood gas determination
   D. electrocardiography
   E. chest radiography

11. Three hours after a total abdominal hysterectomy for large leiomyomata, a 35-year-old patient experiences increasing tachycardia and decreasing blood pressure. The operative blood loss is estimated at 800 mL, and the patient received 1500 mL of 5% dextrose in Ringer's lactate during the operation. Initial management should include

   A. having the patient void to estimate urinary output
   B. insertion of a central venous pressure line
   C. infusion of a crystalloid solution, 3 mL for each milliliter of estimated blood loss
   D. immediate exploratory surgery
   E. sedation to allay anxiety

12. The most reliable early sign of hypovolemia caused by postoperative intraperitoneal hemorrhage is

   A. shoulder pain
   B. cold, clammy extremities
   C. muscle rigidity
   D. decreased urine output
   E. skin pallor

13. Factors that contribute to the development of wound infection include all the following *except*

   A. inappropriate prophylactic antibiotics
   B. obesity
   C. use of cautery
   D. presence of a hematoma
   E. increased duration of preoperative hospitalization

14. A nurse calls you on the phone about an obese 40-year-old patient who underwent a total abdominal hysterectomy 18 hours ago. She reports that the vital signs are a temperature of 100.4°F (38°C), a blood pressure of 80/40, a pulse of 110, and respiration of 30. The nurse raises the possibility of postoperative atelectasis. The findings that support her hypothesis include all the following *except*

   A. temperature
   B. pulse
   C. respiratory rate
   D. blood pressure
   E. number of hours since surgery

15. The typical conditions associated with the development of femoral neuropathy following an abdominal operation are

   A. short stature, thin body habitus, transverse incision, self-retaining retractors
   B. short stature, fat body habitus, transverse incision, large Richardson retractors
   C. short stature, fat body habitus, vertical incision, self-retaining retractors
   D. tall stature, thin body habitus, vertical incision, large Richardson retractors

16. For symptomatic leiomyomata, you are planning to perform a total abdominal hysterectomy and bilateral salpingo-oophorectomy on a 50-year-old markedly obese, hypertensive, insulin-dependent patient with diabetes. Methods to reduce the risk of deep vein thrombophlebitis in this patient include the combination of

   A. subcutaneous low-dose heparin and intravenous dextran
   B. subcutaneous low-dose heparin and intraoperative and postoperative intermittent leg compression
   C. intraoperative and postoperative intermittent leg compression and intravenous dextran
   D. intraoperative and postoperative intermittent leg compression and dihydroergotamine mesylate
   E. dihydroergotamine mesylate and subcutaneous low-dose heparin

17. The most accurate statement concerning the postoperative use of urinary tract catheters is that

    A. a Foley catheter is associated with earlier spontaneous voiding than is a suprapubic catheter
    B. suprapubic catheters are less comfortable than Foley catheters
    C. infections are more common after Foley catheter use than after intermittent straight catherization
    D. prophylactic antibiotics are recommended if urinary catheters are used
    E. symptoms associated with a catheter-acquired infection are more pronounced than cystitis unrelated to a catheter

18. Three days after a total abdominal hysterectomy and bilateral salpingo-oophorectomy, a 35-year-old patient is found to have a hematocrit of 18%. Her preoperative hematocrit was 31%. Blood loss at surgery was estimated at 1200 mL. Vital signs are stable. The patient has mild lower abdominal tenderness and a 5-cm tender fluctuant midline mass at the apex of her vaginal cuff. Given the most likely diagnosis, you would

    A. order an intravenous pyelogram
    B. order an endovaginal ultrasound scan
    C. order a barium enema
    D. begin a transfusion of packed red blood cells
    E. plan an exploratory laparotomy

19. A 30-year-old patient develops a fever to 102.2°F (39°C) 3 weeks after a vaginal hysterectomy. Based on the timing of the onset of fever, the most likely cause of the fever is

    A. pneumonia
    B. cuff cellulitis
    C. an ovarian abscess
    D. deep vein thrombophlebitis
    E. a urinary tract infection

20. Which of the following complications is a consequence of pelvic node dissection?

    A. cuff cellulitis
    B. granulation tissue
    C. prolapsed fallopian tube
    D. lymphocyst
    E. ovarian abscess

21. Which of the following is associated with fatal intraperitoneal rupture?

    A. cuff cellulitis
    B. dermoid cyst
    C. endometrioma
    D. lymphocyst
    E. ovarian abscess

22. An obese patient underwent a longer-than-usual surgical procedure through a lower abdominal incision. The operating time was prolonged by mild intraoperative hypotension, which responded to fluids and oxygen, and by bleeding at the wound site, which was controlled by a pressure dressing. Because of the blood lost at surgery and the patient's late return to the hospital floor, she is asked to remain in bed. During the first 24 hours after surgery this patient is at increased risk for

    A. pneumonia
    B. atelectasis
    C. pulmonary embolism
    D. decreased pulmonary blood shunting

23. Which of the following is indicated for nonmassive pulmonary emboli?

    A. heparin therapy
    B. thrombolytic (streptokinase-urokinase) therapy
    C. sodium warfarin (Coumadin)
    D. aspirin

24. A patient who recently underwent an abdominal hysterectomy for benign disease is suspected of having either a vesicovaginal or a ureterovaginal fistula. Which of the following bedside tests or observations would be used to differentiate between these two types of fistula?

    A. intermittent loss of urine
    B. intravenous administration of indigo carmine causes staining of a vaginal tampon
    C. transurethral instillation of methylene blue causes staining of a vaginal tampon
    D. uninfected urine obtained by transurethral catheter

25. You are called to evaluate a postoperative patient with nausea and vomiting. You entertain the possibility of either a bowel obstruction or an ileus. Which of the following would most favor the diagnosis of ileus over bowel obstruction?

    A. progressively severe crampy pain
    B. nausea and vomiting
    C. absence of bowel sounds
    D. air-fluid levels on abdominal radiograph

26. Postoperative factors contributing to the development of atelectasis include all the following *except*

    A. incisional pain
    B. bulky abdominal dressings
    C. anorexia
    D. high-concentration oxygen therapy

27. All the following causes of shock are classified as cardiogenic *except*

    A. cardiac tamponade
    B. ischemia
    C. an anaphylactic reaction
    D. pulmonary embolism

28. Wound dehiscence is associated with

    A. an incision through an area of previous incision
    B. the use of synthetic absorbable suture
    C. a vertical abdominal incision
    D. a single-layer through-and-through closure

29. Sequelae of deep vein thrombophlebitis include all the following *except*

    A. muscle atrophy
    B. pain on exercise (claudication)
    C. skin ulceration
    D. chronic edema

30. Of clinically recognized pulmonary emboli, what proportion is multiple?

    A. 10%
    B. 25%
    C. 50%
    D. 75%
    E. 90%

31. You are called to evaluate a patient with diabetes who was thought to have a Bartholin gland abscess that was drained 36 hours earlier. Your inspection of the wound reveals a wound with dark edges with crepitance and bulla formation. The areas adjacent to the wound are not tender to the touch, with anesthetic area up to several centimeters away. The patient has previously reported significant wound pain. She has moderate tachycardia and a temperature > 102°F (38.8°C). These findings suggest a diagnosis of

    A. folliculitis
    B. cellulitis
    C. adenitis
    D. necrotizing fasciitis

32. What medical condition lowers the negative predictive value of the D-dimer test?

    A. diabetes
    B. hypertension
    C. cancer
    D. hyperthyroidism
    E. hepatitis

33. Which of the following is *least* effective in preventing postoperative nausea and vomiting?

    A. use of inhalation anesthetic agents
    B. minimal use of narcotics
    C. hydration
    D. restricting movement in the immediate post-operative period

34. Which of the following antibiotics is most likely to induce *Clostridium difficile*–associated diarrhea and colitis?

    A. clindamycin
    B. tetracycline
    C. erythromycin
    D. metronidazole
    E. vancomycin

ANSWERS

1. **E, Pages 781–782.** Superficial thrombophlebitis is most commonly associated with intravenous catheters. Although the inflammation does not necessarily cease when the catheter is removed, it is recommended that removal be completed as soon as the diagnosis is made. Mild cases of superficial thrombophlebitis should be treated with rest, local heat, and elevation. A nonsteroidal anti-inflammatory agent such as ibuprofen may be used in cases that are more severe. The use of heparin and antibiotics is reserved for the rare case of proximal progression of inflammation.

2. **B, Pages 774–776.** The basis for preventing atelectasis consists of simple activities that are, unfortunately, more difficult for the postoperative patient. These include taking deep breaths, walking, coughing, turning from side to side, and not lying supine. If necessary, an incentive spirometer can be used effectively to prevent or treat atelectasis. If these methods do not clear the atelectasis, the patient should be managed with chest physical therapy, intermittent positive pressure breathing, or aerosol therapy. Bronchoscopy may be required to remove large mucous plugs.

3. **D**, Page 733. Drug fever is often a diagnosis of exclusion. It may be suspected if eosinophilia is discovered or if the patient feels and looks better than the temperature course might suggest. Presumptive evidence of drug fever is a fever that disappears when a drug is discontinued.

4. **D**, Page 778. The gold standard of imaging studies to identify abdominal and pelvic hemorrhage is a CT scan performed without either intravenous or oral contrast material. An unenhanced CT scan rapidly identifies the exact location of the hemorrhage. In an emergency situation, the use of a helical scanner facilitates an even more rapid acquisition of images.

5. **B**, Page 788. In a national study of documented pulmonary emboli conducted by Blinder and Coleman (Blinder RA, Coleman RE: Evaluation of pulmonary embolism. Radiol Clin North Am 23:392, 1985), tachypnea was found in more than 90% of the patients, rales in 58%, tachycardia in 44%, cyanosis in 20%, and accentuation of pulmonic closure in 53%. Shock and syncope were associated with massive pulmonary emboli.

6. **A**, Page 798. The patient described has the classic symptoms of a rectovaginal fistula: involuntary loss of gas and stool and a foul-smelling vaginal discharge. This condition is more commonly associated with obstetric than with gynecologic complications. Initial therapy includes a low-residue diet and diphenoxylate with atropine (Lomotil). One in four rectovaginal fistulas heals spontaneously. If a corrective operation must be performed, a 2- to 3-month delay is appropriate. Preoperative evaluation should include visualization of the entire vagina and sigmoidoscopy of the rectal mucosa to discover if there is more than one opening. A barium enema or flexible endoscopy is needed if the coexistence of inflammatory bowel disease is suspected. A diverting colostomy should be used for all radiation-induced fistulas; the majority of fistulas associated with inflammatory bowel disease; and some large postoperative fistulas at the apex of the vagina, which lie above the peritoneal reflection.

7. **B**, Pages 782–787; Table 25–4 in Stenchever. Although signs and symptoms of deep vein thrombophlebitis depend on the severity and extent of the process, 50% of patients are asymptomatic. Physical examination of the legs results in false-positive findings 50% of the time. In cases in which signs and symptoms suggest deep vein thrombophlebitis, the diagnosis should be confirmed with an imaging technique. Venography is the most accurate current method for detecting deep vein thrombophlebitis. The diagnostic accuracy is 95% for iliofemoral thrombophlebitis. Scanning with fibrinogen ^{125}I is an excellent method to screen women for occult thrombi.

This test has been used extensively in research protocols. However, its clinical use is being replaced by duplex ultrasonography. Duplex ultrasonography is a noninvasive screening test for deep venous thrombosis. Real-time ultrasound imaging provides visualization of the larger veins, whereas simultaneous sensitive Doppler is focused on the suspect vessel. The technology depends on changes in venous flow for a positive diagnosis. The advantages of this method are that it is not invasive and is easy to use, highly accurate, objective, simple, and reproducible. The main disadvantage of duplex diagnosis is that the accuracy is limited when investigating small vessels in the calf. Impedance plethysmography is another noninvasive screening method used to detect deep venous thrombosis. This method has at least a 15% false-negative rate and a 20% false-positive rate. As with Doppler studies, the accuracy of this method to detect thrombi of small vessels is limited.

8. **D**, Page 788; Table 25–8 in Stenchever. Signs and symptoms of a pulmonary embolus are nonspecific. Chest pain, dyspnea, and apprehension are the most common symptoms. In a national study conducted by Blinder and Coleman (Blinder RA, Coleman RE: Evaluation of pulmonary embolism. Radiol Clin North Am 23:392, 1985), only 30% of patients with documented pulmonary embolus had hemoptysis. Cough was found in 53%.

9. **B**, Pages 776–780. This patient has significant hypotension and tachycardia. Her reaction is more than an effect of anesthesia, although hypotension in the immediate postoperative period may be secondary to the residual effects of anesthesia, oversedation, or hypothermia. The physiologic release of aldosterone and antidiuretic hormone is a response to the stress of surgery. The higher level of aldosterone produces an increase in both sodium and water retention, whereas increased levels of antidiuretic hormone promote free water retention. Depending on the type and amount of intraoperative and postoperative intravenous fluids, the hematocrit on the first postoperative day may be misleading and may reflect fluid changes rather than postoperative hemorrhage. There is nothing in this history to suggest either myocardial infarction or continued blood loss, although both are certainly possible. Tachycardia and decreased urine output are two early signs of hypovolemia. Actual measurement of intraoperative blood loss is imprecise, even with extensive use of suction equipment. Studies have demonstrated that 15% to 45% of surgical blood loss is absorbed on surgical drapes, laparotomy pads, and other areas. Thus the blood loss was probably underestimated. Even if this were a

correct estimate, the three-to-one rule suggests a replacement ratio of 3 mL of crystalloid solution for every 1 mL of blood loss. This patient received 1 ml of crystalloid solution for every 1 mL of blood loss.

10. **B**, Pages 789–790. Table 25–9 and Figure 25–7 in Stenchever. Pulmonary angiography is the most definitive test in the detection of emboli. This test is not ordered routinely because of the potential morbidity (hypotension and cardiac arrhythmias) and the risk of death associated with its use. Most deaths are directly related to pulmonary hypertension and right ventricular dysfunction. Because of potential morbidity (5%) and mortality (0.2%) associated with angiography, the ventilation-perfusion lung scan is the first imaging technique usually used to diagnose a pulmonary embolus. A negative scan essentially rules out an embolus. Findings on blood-gas determination, chest radiography, and electrocardiography are helpful but not diagnostic.

11. **C**, Pages 776–780. The goals in initially treating the patient who has presumed postoperative hemorrhage should be replacement of circulating blood volume and establishment of cellular perfusion and oxygenation. Crystalloid solution should be infused rapidly, with 3 mL being used for each 1 mL of blood loss. A Foley catheter is used in all cases to monitor urinary output. One should not rely on the patient's ability to void. The urinary output should be greater than 30 mL/hr. The pulmonary wedge pressure should be between 10 and 15 mm Hg. Thus, a Swan-Ganz catheter should be inserted if rapid changes in fluid status and blood pressure continue. This is preferable to a central venous pressure line. Studies have demonstrated that with the patient in the supine position, the volume of intravascular depletion is severely underestimated by a central venous pressure measurement. Exploratory surgery should be performed promptly if there is evidence of postoperative bleeding, but only after adequate volume replacement has been accomplished. Although sedation may help to relieve the patient's anxiety, it is apt to make the problem worse.

12. **D**, Page 777. Tachycardia and decreased urine output are two early signs of hypovolemia resulting from hidden internal bleeding. Tachycardia is caused by the body's adrenergic response to hemorrhage, and the decreased urine output is a result of poor perfusion of the kidneys. With further loss of blood the patient becomes agitated, appears weak, and experiences skin pallor and cold, clammy extremities. Muscle rigidity of the abdominal wall is a late sign of intraperitoneal hemorrhage and is not due to hypovolemia.

13. **A**, Page 800. Many factors contribute to the development of wound infection. Most significant are local factors, which include the presence of foreign bodies, necrotic tissue, hematomas, dead space, use of cautery, and decreased tissue perfusion. Systemic factors include malnutrition, obesity, diabetes, liver disease, immunosuppression, age, and increased duration of preoperative hospitalization. Prevention is the foundation of any approach to the management of wound infections. Prophylactic antibiotics, especially in high-risk cases, definitely decrease the incidence of wound infection. The use of inappropriate antibiotics would neither decrease the incidence nor be a source of infection. Such medication might be responsible for the overgrowth of endogenous bacteria.

14. **D**, Pages 774–776. The classic triad of atelectasis is marked by fever, tachypnea, and tachycardia, appearing in the first 72 postoperative hours. These findings must, however, be evaluated along with the other clinical factors. In the case described here, the marked hypotension of 80/40 in an obese patient should also suggest other causes, such as postoperative bleeding and a pulmonary embolus.

15. **A**, Page 805. Factors that contribute to the development of femoral neuropathy are thinness, long retractor blades, prolonged operative times, and systemic diseases such as diabetes mellitus, gout, alcoholism, and malnutrition. However, the classic patient who experiences this complication is a short, thin, athletic woman who has a transverse incision in which a self-retaining retractor is used.

16. **B**, Pages 782–783. Women who are at high risk for deep vein thrombophlebitis should be treated with both low-dose heparin and pneumatic compression devices. Embolex (dihydroergotamine mesylate plus heparin) has also been shown to be effective; however, because of its listed contraindications of sepsis, hypertension, and atherosclerotic heart disease (ASHD), this agent would not be advisable for this patient. Dextran is expensive, and anaphylaxis occurs in approximately 1 in 3500 patients. The method of action of dextran is not understood. It may decrease platelet adhesion, or it may decrease blood viscosity. The cost for external pneumatic compression is nearly the same as that of low-dose heparin, and either is about 50% of the cost of prophylatic dextran.

17. **C**, Pages 791–793. Compared with intermittent straight catheterization and suprapubic catheterization, the use of a Foley catheter delays spontaneous voiding, is more uncomfortable, and predisposes the patient to urinary tract infection. Although systemic prophylactic antibiotics decrease the initial incidence of infection, the

effect is only short-lived. The use of prophylactic antibiotics also promotes the emergence of antibiotic-resistant bacteria. As a result, antibiotics are not recommended for a catheterized patient unless the patient is immunocompromised. In fact, catheter-related infections are not treated with antibiotics unless the patient is febrile. The signs and symptoms associated with a catheter-acquired lower tract urinary infection are less pronounced and less specific than cystitis that develops unrelated to catheter use.

18. **D,** Page 780. Most young healthy women without a complicating medical illness tolerate hematocrits of about 20% to 22% without needing a transfusion. The patient described has probably experienced a postoperative cuff hematoma. The hematoma is usually the result of slow venous oozing and is self-limited. Even if the hematoma is not infected, a low-grade fever is common because of inflammation surrounding the hematoma. The diagnosis of a retroperitoneal hematoma is usually possible by physical examination. Imaging studies are rarely necessary in this situation. Both a barium enema and ultrasonography would not contribute to either the diagnosis or the management. You might consider ordering an intravenous pyelogram if the position of the hematoma suggests that a ureter might be obstructed. Hematomas less than 5 cm in diameter may be treated conservatively. Surgical management is usually not recommended unless there is evidence of persistent blood loss or infection. If needed, the operative procedure is usually done by way of the extraperitoneal route (transvaginally).

19. **C,** Page 773; Table 25–1 in Stenchever. Only 20% of postoperative fevers are directly related to infection. It is not unusual for hysterectomy to cause a mild temperature elevation during the first 72 postoperative hours with no identifiable infection. Atelectasis is the cause of more than 90% of fevers occurring in the first 48 hours. Pneumonia, cuff cellulitis, phlebitis, and urinary tract infections tend to cause fever after the first 48 hours. Chronologically, most ovarian abscesses appear later in the postoperative course than do other retroperitoneal abscesses. Ovarian abscesses usually appear 2 to 3 weeks postoperatively, but cases have been reported as late as 3 to 4 months after surgery.

20. **D,** Page 804. A lymphocyst is a local collection of lymphatic fluid found most frequently after a pelvic node dissection. Conditions that predispose the patient to formation of a lymphocyst are previous radiation and anticoagulation. Small cysts regress spontaneously, whereas larger ones require intermittent aspiration or insertion of an indwelling catheter. Traditional surgical management involves removing a large segment of the wall of the lymphocyst and placing a tongue of omentum in the cavity.

21. **E,** Page 804. An ovarian abscess is a potentially fatal complication of hysterectomy. If the diagnosis is not made, intraperitoneal rupture may ensue. Ovarian abscesses arise from bacterial colonization of the ovarian cortex. This may occur either through disruption of the ovarian capsule by the presence of a corpus luteum or via an operative disruption such as cystectomy. Initial therapy is parenteral administration of broad-spectrum antibiotics, although most patients require surgical removal of the affected adnexa.

22. **B,** Page 774. Although this patient is at increased risk for eventual pneumonia, in the first 24 hours her greatest risk is that of atelectasis. Risk factors for this problem include her weight, the prolonged surgery, the use of high-concentration oxygen therapy, incisional pain, inactivity, and a restrictive dressing. If symptoms ensue, it is critical to be able to differentiate postoperative atelectasis from pneumonia. The two conditions are commonly associated, and the treatments are the same except for the addition of parenteral antibiotics for the patient with pneumonia. Patients who are obese are at risk for both conditions. Atelectasis is commonly associated with tubular breathing, decreased breath sounds, and moist inspiratory rales, especially over the base of the lungs. With both pneumonia and atelectasis, fever and tachycardia are present. An important difference is that pneumonia also typically involves productive, purulent sputum. The classic physical finding of pneumonia is coarse rales over the infected area. The patient usually has a higher temperature and more systemic toxicity than does a woman with atelectasis. A patchy infiltrate visible on a chest radiograph is compatible with either condition. Both pneumonia and atelectasis result in increased pulmonary blood shunting. Prolonged immobility and obesity are both risk factors for pulmonary embolism, but these tend to occur after the first 24 hours. The risk may be minimized by early ambulation and use of leg-compressing stockings.

23. **A,** Page 790. The management of most cases of pulmonary emboli includes full-dose intravenous heparin. One method of administration is to give an initial loading dose of 5000 IU followed by an hourly infusion of 1000 to 1500 IU. Recently, some women have been treated with thrombolytic (streptokinase-urokinase) therapy or recombinant human tissue–type plasminogen activator. However, this therapy is more expensive and more dangerous than heparin. Thrombolytic therapy is strictly reserved for cases of massive embolus.

A thrombolytic agent is used only in the first 24 hours of therapy. Heparin is continued for 7 to 10 days. All patients with pulmonary emboli should undergo warfarin therapy for 3 to 6 months. Neither heparin nor thrombolytic therapy is indicated for long-term therapy. Although aspirin has anticoagulant action, through its inhibition of platelet aggregation, and may be effective in reducing the long-term risk of some clotting-related processes such as recurrent heart attack, it is not indicated for the initial treatment of a pulmonary embolism.

24. **C**, Pages 793–794. The classic symptom of a vesico-vaginal fistula is painless and almost continuous loss of urine. If this loss is intermittent and related to position, a ureterovaginal fistula should be suspected. Unfortunately, this distinction is not always present and is insufficient to establish the location of the fistula. Intravenous injection of 1 to 2 mL of indigo carmine will result in the blue staining of a vaginal tampon for both ureterovaginal fistula and vesicovaginal fistula. If a vesicovaginal fistula is suspected, methylene blue is instilled into the bladder. A tampon is placed in the vagina. The tampon will be discolored blue if a vesicovaginal fistula exists but not if a ureterovaginal fistula is present. In most cases, both a vesicovaginal and a ureterovaginal fistula are not associated with bladder infections, thus making the absence of infection of little value in establishing either the existence or the location of a possible fistula. The repair of both vesicovaginal and ureterovaginal fistulas should be delayed 2 to 6 months after the initial operation to allow possible spontaneous healing or, if that does not occur, to maximize the integrity and health of the surgical area after it has healed completely.

25. **C**, Pages 794–798; Table 25–15 in Stenchever. Adynamic ileus probably is a result of poorly coordinated motor activity of the small intestine. It is not easily differentiated from small bowel obstruction. The patient with an ileus is uncomfortable, but it is the patient with an obstruction who suffers from progressively severe, crampy abdominal pain. Patients with either an ileus or a small bowel obstruction experience nausea and vomiting. Bowel sounds are hypoactive or absent with an ileus, whereas in obstruction peristaltic rushes and high-pitched tinkles are common. Air-fluid levels on abdominal radiograph may occur in either ileus or obstruction. In the former, they occur infrequently and, if so, at the same levels. In the latter, air-fluid levels are common and demonstrate a step-ladder appearance—multiple air-fluid levels throughout the small intestine with an absence of gas in the colon and rectum.

26. **C**, Pages 774–776. Atelectasis develops in 10% of women who undergo pelvic surgery. It is the most common cause of postoperative fever. Pain, the supine position, and abdominal distention deter the patient from taking deep inspirations. Deep breaths normally expand all areas of the lung, thus preventing atelectasis. Similarly, immobility and binding around the abdomen and chest cause the patient to breathe at lower lung volumes, thus predisposing to atelectasis. Obesity, smoking, age greater than 60 years, prolonged operative time, high-concentration oxygen therapy, and coexisting medical problems such as cardiac disease and pulmonary infection all predispose patients to postoperative atelectasis. Anorexia per se is not known to be a direct cause of atelectasis.

27. **C**, Page 776. Shock is a condition in which circulatory insufficiency prevents adequate vascular perfusion of vital organs. The etiologic complex of shock includes cardiac failure, sepsis, an anaphylactic reaction, and hemorrhage. Shock caused by postoperative hemorrhage usually occurs within the first few hours after surgery. This condition is primarily the result of inadequate hemostasis. In general, it takes a reduction of approximately 20% of the blood volume to produce shock in a woman of reproductive age. Changes in the ability of the heart to provide perfusion, such as those caused by cardiac tamponade or pulmonary embolism, may also result in cardiogenic shock. Anaphylactic reactions result in shock through peripheral vascular effects.

28. **A**, Pages 801–802. Wound dehiscence usually implies disruption of the abdominal wound though the fascia but not through the peritoneum. Wound infection is present in approximately half of women with a wound disruption. As stronger synthetic absorbance sutures have replaced catgut, the incidence of dehiscence has decreased. Whether a vertical or a horizontal incision has been made appears to have little effect on the incidence of dehiscence. Important mechanical factors predisposing to disruption are conditions that increase the tension on the incision line, such as abdominal distention and chronic lung disease. Other factors include obesity, the patient's age, malignant disease, prior radiation, and whether the incision was made through a previous incision. A mass closure with through-and-through monofilament nylon is a commonly used approach for abdominal incisions that have broken down. An alternative is the Smead-Jones closure.

29. **A**, Pages 782–784. Deep vein thrombophlebitis is the process of venous thrombosis formation occurring in any deep vein because of blood

coagulation and fibrin formation in the presence of venous stasis. In addition to pulmonary embolus, major sequelae of deep vein thrombophlebitis include chronic venous insufficiency resulting in damage to the valves of deep veins. This produces shunting of blood to superficial veins, skin ulceration, pain on exercise, and chronic edema. Deep vein thrombophlebitis has not been shown to be associated with muscle atrophy.

30. **C**, Page 788. Although the most common location of pulmonary emboli is the lower lobe of the right lung, of clinically recognized pulmonary emboli, roughly 50% are multiple.

31. **D**, Page 801. Necrotizing fasciitis is a life-threatening complication of any soft tissue infection. More common in patients with compromised resistance or microvascular disease, such as that associated with diabetes or alcohol abuse, this complication must be suspected in any patient with a rapidly progressing infection. Symptoms of excessive fever or pain and findings of dark wound edges, crepitance, and bulla formation in the anesthetic area up to several centimeters away are suggestive of necrotizing fasciitis. Emergency treatment with wide debridement is required, but even with aggressive surgical therapy mortality rates approaching 50% are not uncommon.

32. **C**, Pages 788–789. The rapid measurement of plasma D-dimer levels is useful in screening women with a suspected pulmonary embolus. There is no need to perform angiography when the level of D-dimer is below 500 ng/mL and the level of clinical suspicion is low. The negative predictive value is 99% in these cases. A negative D-dimer result in women with cancer does not reliably exclude venous thrombosis or pulmonary embolus because the negative predictive value is lower in patients with cancer.

33. **A**, Page 794. Approximately 25% of women experience postoperative nausea and vomiting. Certain preventive measures may be used to minimize postoperative nausea and vomiting, including adequate hydration, minimizing use of inhalation agents and narcotics, avoiding nitrous oxide, and avoiding excessive movement in the immediate postoperative period. Drugs that may be used for prevention and treatment include droperidol, phenothiazines, metoclopramide, and 5-HT3 antagonists.

34. **A**, Page 799. Virtually all antibiotics have been associated with *C. difficile* diarrhea. The highest risk is associated with second- and third-generation cephalosporins, ampicillin, amoxicillin, and clindamycin. Symptoms usually appear 5 to 10 days after the initiation of antibiotic therapy.

PART FOUR

Gynecologic Oncology

Principles of Radiation Therapy and Chemotherapy in Gynecologic Cancer

DIRECTIONS:

for Questions 1–14: Select the one best answer or completion.

1. The growth phase in which a cell is most sensitive to radiation damage is

   A. mitosis
   B. protein synthesis
   C. DNA duplication
   D. RNA synthesis
   E. the resting phase

2. Three months ago, a 60-year-old woman completed a nine-course treatment with cyclophosphamide (Cytoxan), cisplatin, and doxorubicin (Adriamycin) for stage III serous cystadenocarcinoma of the ovary. At a "second look" operation 1 year after the onset of treatment, there is no microscopic or macroscopic evidence of the disease. This response is best called a(n)

   A. cure
   B. complete response
   C. objective response
   D. stabilization
   E. partial remission

3. Energy (such as that used to treat cancers) transmitted from a source to a target area

   A. converges as it approaches target tissue
   B. diverges as it approaches target tissue
   C. travels parallel as it approaches target tissue— that is, neither converges nor diverges
   D. converges or diverges, depending on the energy source
   E. is transmitted as a wave form

4. Each of the following improves the effectiveness of a chemotherapeutic agent *except* a

   A. small original tumor burden
   B. more frequent administration of the chemotherapeutic agent
   C. higher dose of chemotherapeutic agent
   D. smaller percentage of cells in G_o (resting) phase
   E. decreased mitotic activity of tumor cells

5. The major advantage of high-energy particulate radiation, such as accelerated neutrons, is that it

   A. can kill the cell directly
   B. has low linear energy transfer (LET)
   C. is most effective in well-oxygenated tissue
   D. can be administered from both external and internal sources
   E. does not decrease proportional to the distance traveled

6. Radiation therapy complications occur in the treatment of cervical cancer. The one that is *least* problematic when it occurs is

   A. compromise of the bone marrow in the sacrum and lower vertebrae
   B. endometrial fibrosis with secondary amenorrhea
   C. intestinal mucosa necrosis and fistula formation
   D. radiation cystitis
   E. vaginal mucosa with vaginal obliteration

7. The following statements are true regarding bowel complications with radiation therapy *except*

   A. Diarrhea is common during the acute phases of treatment.
   B. If enteric fistulas are going to form, they usually have occurred by 6 months.
   C. Proctitis is rare with a median dose of 6300 cGy.
   D. Small bowel injuries are more common in patients with previous pelvic surgery.
   E. Decreased vitamin B_{12} and bile salt absorption may occur as a result of large bowel damage (sigmoiditis).

8. An example of an agent used to diminish the toxicity of chemotherapeutic agents is

   A. interferon
   B. interleukin
   C. T-cell activator
   D. erythropoietin
   E. tumor necrosis factor

9. Ifosfamide has marked antitumor effects, but it also is highly toxic to the

   A. liver
   B. gastrointestinal tract
   C. central nervous system
   D. heart
   E. genitourinary system

10. Each of the following potentiates the effects of radiation therapy on tumor growth *except*

    A. hyperthermia
    B. hyperfractionation
    C. cisplatin
    D. decreasing the size of the field

11. Paclitaxel (Taxol), which was originally derived from the bark of the Western yew, is used in the treatment of ovarian cancer. The following statements about paclitaxel are true *except*

    A. Bradycardia can occur but rarely is severe.
    B. It disrupts the function of microtubules.
    C. Neutropenia is a major side effect.
    D. Peripheral neuropathy may occur that is synergistic with platinum.
    E. Severe hypersensitivity reactions and hypotension may occur.

12. Which of the following has *minimal* bone marrow suppression toxicity when used to treat gynecologic malignancies?

    A. doxorubicin
    B. cisplatin
    C. cyclophosphamide
    D. methotrexate
    E. vinblastine

13. Which of the following chemotherapeutic agents is especially neurotoxic?

    A. doxorubicin
    B. carboplatin
    C. 5-FU
    D. methotrexate
    E. vincristine

14. Which of the following chemotherapeutic agents is highly toxic to the lungs and may cause pneumonitis and pulmonary fibrosis?

    A. doxorubicin
    B. bleomycin
    C. cisplatin
    D. methotrexate
    E. paclitaxel

DIRECTIONS:

for Questions 15–21: For each numbered item, select the one heading most closely associated with it. Each lettered heading may be used once, more than once, or not at all.

15–18. Chemotherapeutic agent characteristics

   A. doxorubicin
   B. cyclophosphamide
   C. methotrexate
   D. vincristine
   E. cisplatin

15. Positively charged alkyl groups react with negatively charged portion of DNA

16. Plant alkaloid that attacks the cell spindle during mitosis

17. Enzymatic inhibitor in the synthesis of purine nucleotides

18. May cause cardiomyopathy

19–21. Match a phase of the cell cycle with each statement (see Figure 26–1).

   A. mitosis (M)
   B. resting cell (G_0)
   C. protein synthesis (G_2)
   D. DNA synthesis (S)

19. Resistant to cytotoxic drugs

20. Most affected by antimetabolites (methotrexate)

21. Most affected by *Vinca* alkaloids (vincristine)

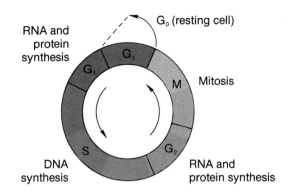

FIGURE 26–1 Phases of the cell
(From Stenchever MA, Droegemueller W, Herbst AL, Mishell DR Jr: Comprehensive Gynecology, 4th ed. St. Louis, Mosby, 2001.)

DIRECTIONS:

for Questions 22–34: Select the one best answer or completion.

22. In brachytherapy various isotopes are used. Which one of the following may be placed within the patient and left there permanently?

   A. cesium-137
   B. cobalt-60
   C. gold-98
   D. iridium-192
   E. radium-226

23. The following statements are true regarding teletherapy *except*

   A. High-energy (short-wavelength) radiation is used for deeper tissues.
   B. Isotopes used are chosen on the basis of defined half-life.
   C. It refers to the placement of the radiation source at a distance from the patient.
   D. It uses the concept of source axis distance (SAD).
   E. It uses the concept of source-to-skin distance (SSD).

24. The following statements regarding the effects on the radiation dose delivered to a gynecologic tumor by external means are true *except*

   A. A 6-MeV (million electron volts) machine is very useful for treating obese patients.
   B. The distance of the source of the radiation to the tumor affects the dose because of the inverse square law.
   C. High-energy machines are particularly useful in treating deep tumors.
   D. A larger field of treatment leads to a greater dose at a given depth.

25. Use of brachytherapy in gynecologic malignancies typically involves the following techniques or principles *except*

   A. afterloading to reduce radiation exposure to medical personnel
   B. allows the treatment of deeper malignancies with less subcutaneous fibrosis
   C. avoids the problem with the inverse square law regarding dose delivery
   D. placement of a tandem in the cervix/uterus and ovoids in the lateral vaginal fornices
   E. use of interstitial implants with the use of radioactive needles

26. Refer to Figure 26–2. In determining the ideal radiation dosage, the point on this figure to achieve is

   A. point *A*
   B. point *B*
   C. point *C*
   D. none of the above

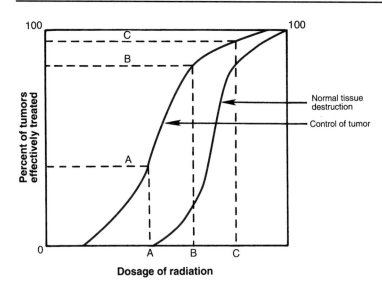

FIGURE 26–2
(From Stenchever MA, Droegemueller W, Herbst AL, Mishell DR Jr: Comprehensive Gynecology, 4th ed. St. Louis, Mosby, 2001.)

27. **Although each agent has unique considerations and toxicities, the following are general principles regarding chemotherapy complications** *except*

    A. Body surface area is typically used to calculate dosage.
    B. Hepatitis or renal dysfunction typically requires a decreased dosage.
    C. Malnourished patients have an increased toxicity rate
    D. Most complications have a component of bone marrow toxicity.
    E. Use of sulfonamides or salicylates typically requires increased dosage of the chemotherapeutic agent to achieve the same effect.

28. **The following statements are true regarding the growth fraction (GF) for a given tumor** *except*

    A. It determines the doubling time.
    B. It increases with maturity.
    C. It is faster after chemotherapy.
    D. It is faster in sites of metastases.
    E. It is faster in smaller tumors.

29. **Ionizing radiation causes cell death by the following means** *except*

    A. directly altering the localized host immune response
    B. leading to the formation of peroxide in tissues
    C. negatively charged electrons affect the DNA of the cell
    D. producing free hydroxyl radicals

30. **Characteristics of electromagnetic ionizing radiation used for tumor therapy include all the following** *except*

    A. It has no mass.
    B. It has no electric charge.
    C. It is produced in discrete quanta.
    D. Higher energies are transmitted at a low frequency of electromagnetic radiation.

31. **The resistance of large tumors to chemotherapy is due to their having the following qualities** *except*

    A. being more likely to contain cells resistant to a cytotoxic agent
    B. heterogenous cell population
    C. increased DNA synthesis
    D. lower growth fraction

32. **The Fletcher suit applicator is used in**

    A. intracavitary brachytherapy
    B. teletherapy
    C. induction chemotherapy
    D. neoadjunctive chemotherapy

33. **Which of the following drugs has been used to protect normal tissue from radiation damage?**

    A. amifostine
    B. vincristine
    C. methotrexate
    D. bleomycin
    E. paclitaxel

34. **All of the following are toxicities associated with the use of 5-fluorouracil** *except*

    A. diarrhea
    B. alopecia
    C. dermatitis
    D. hand-foot syndrome
    E. pulmonary fibrosis

ANSWERS

1. **A,** Page 827; Figure 26–2 in Stenchever. During mitosis, the cell is most sensitive to radiation. Thus, rapidly dividing cells are the most radiosensitive. Dividing radiation into a number of smaller doses (fractionation) allows for effective treatment of the tumor without increasing the complications of irradiation to the normal surrounding tissues that have a rapid turnover, such as the bone marrow and the intestine.

2. **B,** Page 834. In assessing the effect of chemotherapeutic agents, a number of definitions are used to describe the response of the tumor being treated. A cure implies a permanent absence of disease for a period of 5 years or longer. A complete remission or response is total disappearance of the tumor for at least 1 month. An objective response is a 50% or greater reduction in the size of the tumor for at least 1 month. Stabilization is used to indicate that the tumor has not changed in size. The phrase *partial remission* is no longer used in lieu of the term *objective response.*

3. **B,** Page 826. Regardless of the source of electromagnetic or photon radiation, the transmitted energy from the source diverges as the distance it travels from the source increases. This divergence causes a decrease in energy, and the relationship is described by the inverse square law. For example, the dose of radiation 2 cm from a point source is only one-fourth the value of the dose at 1 cm.

4. **E,** Page 833; Figures 26–8 and 26–9 in Stenchever. One of the reasons that chemotherapy appears to affect cancer tissue more than normal tissue is that malignant tumor cells have a higher growth fraction in comparison to normal cells. The ability of a chemotherapeutic agent to destroy a greater number of cancer cells more effectively is enhanced if the agent can be given more frequently or in larger doses per unit time. However, dose and frequency are limited by tolerance of normal tissue. A higher percentage of cells in the G_0, or resting, phase will limit chemotherapeutic effectiveness. Increased, not decreased, mitotic activity of tumor cells will render them more susceptible to successful chemotherapy.

5. **A,** Page 827. With particulate radiation involving the use of heavy particles such as neutrons, the ionization is known as *high linear energy transfer*; that is, the rate of energy loss as it traverses a unit length of tissue is greater than with photon irradiation. This form of radiation produces high-energy recoil protons, which kill the cell directly on impact and are independent of oxygenation. Currently systems are being developed that use neutron generators as a form of external beam therapy. This type of energy cannot be generated by internal sources. Even though this is a high-energy source, the principle of the inverse square law still applies with this type of radiation.

6–7. 6, **B;** 7, **B;** Pages 831–832. In the treatment of gynecologic malignancies, the main sites of radiation damage are the bladder, rectum, large bowel, small bowel, and the remaining reproductive organs. As a rule, complications of the bladder can occur in the form of radiation cystitis, which can lead to complaints of dysuria and frequency. Hematuria may also occur. Fistulas between the vagina and the bladder or between the vagina and the rectum may develop when there has been extensive radiation damage to the intervening tissues. As a general rule, such complications occur 6 months to 2 years after treatment. In addition, the bone marrow of the sacrum and lower vertebra is compromised by pelvic radiation, an important consideration if the patient is to receive subsequent chemotherapy. Obliteration of the vaginal vault is common. This is why surgical treatment of early cancers is often preferred in sexually active women. Also, the endometrial tissue is destroyed, although this is beneficial because the cervix is usually scarred closed, preventing menstrual flow (if it should occur). In actuality, this situation is uncommon because in addition to endometrial damage there is destruction of the ovarian follicles, resulting in ovarian failure.

   The risk of proctitis and cystitis is dose-related. Such complications were not observed in patients whose median dose was 6500 cGy or 6300 cGy but were noted in patients receiving doses of 6750 cGy. Patients with bowel complications not requiring operative intervention frequently have decreased absorption of vitamin B_{12} and bile acid. The small bowel also receives irradiation during external therapy for pelvic tumors. In the acute phase of treatment, this often leads to bowel irritability and diarrhea. Small bowel injuries are more common in patients who have had a previous operation, particularly pelvic surgery that predisposed to adhesions and decreased bowel motility and thus increased radiation damage.

8. **D,** Page 839. Stimulators of the hematopoietic system are being used to diminish the toxicity of chemotherapeutic agents. This includes the use of erythropoietin (EPO) to overcome the chronic anemia that often occurs with chemotherapy. T cells are cells that confer cell-mediated immunity. Interferon and interleukin are forms of cytokines that release humoral factors, which enhance tumor cell damage.

9. **E,** Page 835. Ifosfamide is highly toxic to the bladder and uroepithelium, with reports of severe hemorrhagic cystitis. This drug is a relative of cyclophosphamide, which has long been known to be associated with hemorrhagic cystitis. A urinary metabolite, acrolein, causes the damage. This can be prevented by the prophylactic administration of MESNA, which binds to acrolein and prevents urotoxicity.

10. **D,** Page 829; Figure 26–6 in Stenchever. Larger fields of radiation contain more scattered radiation, which leads to a greater dose at a given depth. Recent experimental work has evaluated hyperfractionation, which involves smaller multiple doses given more frequently—two or three times per day rather than the traditional once-a-day exposure. Multiple chemotherapeutic agents have been used to sensitize cells to radiation. These include 5-fluorouracil, cisplatin, paclitaxel, hydroxyurea, actinomycin D, and topotecan, among others. The mechanism of radiosensitization is different among the various agents. Hyperthermia is also being explored to potentiate the therapeutic effectiveness of radiation.

11. **D,** Page 838. Paclitaxel use has increased markedly since the drug was synthesized. It disrupts the function of microtubules and thereby inhibits cell division. It is a potent agent, and its administration can be accompanied by severe hypersensitivity reactions and hypotension. Neutropenia is the major toxic side effect, but sensory peripheral neuropathy is also a serious problem. As noted by Warner, the distribution of neurotoxicity of paclitaxel is similar to that of cisplatin, but these agents do not appear to be synergistic, which allows them to be used together effectively. Bradycardia can also occur, but it is rarely severe.

12–14. 12, **B;** 13, **E;** 14, **B;** Pages 835–839. Each of the groups of chemotherapeutic agents has its mode of action and typical side effects. It is important to consider these factors when developing multidrug therapies. There are five main groups, as outlined in Table 26–1.

Alkylating agents (cyclophosphamide and ifosfamide). These agents cause major problems of bone marrow depression, gut mucositis, and hemorrhagic cystitis.

Antitumor antibiotics (doxorubicin, bleomycin, mitoxantrone, and actinomycin D). Actinomycin D causes severe myelosuppression, affects the gastrointestinal mucosa, and produces skin toxicity, including alopecia. Adriamycin also causes myelosuppression and commonly results in complete alopecia. Furthermore, it causes a cardiomyopathy that leads to congestive heart failure and can be life-threatening. Bleomycin does

not have significant myelosuppressive effects. It is, however, highly toxic to the lungs, and pneumonitis and pulmonary fibrosis may occur.

Antimetabolites (5-FU and methotrexate). These also are bone marrow–suppressing agents, and they cause gut mucositis. The side effects can be modified or avoided by using a citrovorum factor rescue.

Vinca (plant) alkaloids (vinblastine, vincristine, and etoposide (VP-16)). Vincristine is severely neurotoxic and can produce numbness, motor weakness, and constipation as a result of its autonomic effects. There is little myelosuppression. Vinblastine is myelotoxic, and this tends to be a dose-limiting factor; however, it has less neurotoxicity than vincristine.

Synthetic and miscellaneous compounds (cisplatin, carboplatin, hexamethylmelamine, taxol, and hydroxyurea). Cisplatin is very toxic to the kidneys. It also induces mild myelosuppression, is associated with high-frequency ototoxicity, produces a severe peripheral neuropathy, and causes severe nausea with vomiting. Carboplatin is not toxic to the kidneys but appears more suppressive to the bone marrow. Paclitaxel causes neutropenia but also sensory peripheral neuropathy.

15–18. 15, **B;** 16, **D;** 17, **C;** 18, **A;** Pages 835–839. This series of questions addresses characteristics of commonly used cytotoxic agents in gynecologic malignancy. They represent different causes of drugs with generally different mechanisms of action. Although a single drug characteristic in itself may not seem important, a general knowledge of the classes of cytotoxic agents is important in determining rational therapy for gynecologic malignancy. The alkylating agents, of which chlorambucil and cyclophosphamide are examples, interfere directly with DNA replication and function. Crosslinking of DNA also occurs. These agents may be administered either intravenously or orally, and they are particularly toxic to bone marrow. Vinblastine and vincristine are plant alkaloids. They attack the cell during mitosis and cause toxic destruction of the mitotic spindle. However, this can result in synchronization of the cell cycle for those cells surviving therapy, and therefore these agents are often given as part of a combination treatment to cause a greater sensitivity to other agents. There is little bone marrow suppression with this group of drugs, but they can be severely neurotoxic. Methotrexate has been used longer than any of the other chemotherapeutic agents listed and is an enzyme inhibitor. Metabolic transfer of one carbon unit is prevented, thereby inhibiting the synthesis of thymidylic acid and different purine nucleotides. Side effects of this treatment may be

TABLE 26-1
Side Effects of Drugs Often Used in Gynecologic Oncology

	Bone Marrow	Phlebitis Sclerosant	Neurologic	Skin	Pulm.	Renal	Hepatic	Cardiac	Endo.	Bladder	Gut Mucositis	Allergic	Alopecia	Metabolic	Nausea Vomiting
Antimetabolites															
Methotrexate	***	*	*	*	*	*	**				***		*		*
5-Fluorouracil	***	*	*	*							**		*		*
Alkylating agents															
Cyclophosphamide	***		*	*			*	*	*	**	**		**	*	**
Ifosfamide	**		**							**			**		*
Antitumor antibiotics															
Actinomycin D	***	*	*	*				**			**		**	*	**
Mitoxantrone	***		*					**			**		*		*
Adriamycin	***	**	*								**		**		**
Bleomycin	*		**	***	***		*					*			**
Mitomycin C	***	*		*							*				**
Vinca alkaloids															
Vinblastine	***	*											*		
Vincristine	*	*	***				*						*	*	
Etoposide (VP-16)	***						*				*		**		
Synthetic and miscellaneous compounds															
Hexamethylmelamine	*		*								***				
Cisplatin	*		*			***					*				**
Carboplatin	**		*			*					*				**
Taxol	***	*	**	*				*			*	**	**		*
Hydroxyurea	***		*	*							*	*	*		

Modified from Tattersall MHN: Pharmacology and selection of cytotoxic drugs. In Coppleson M, ed: Gynecologic Oncology, 2nd ed. Edinburgh, Churchill-Livingstone, 1992, p 180.
***indicates dose limiting; **indicates common; *indicates rare.

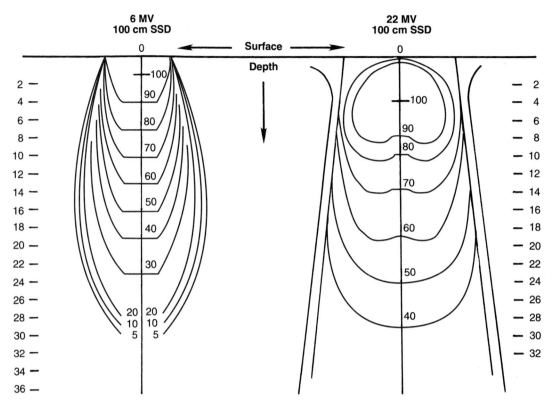

FIGURE 26–3 Comparison of isodose curves and depth-dose distribution for 6-mV and 22-mV beatrons. (Redrawn from DiSaia PJ, Creasman WT: Clinical Gynecologic Oncology, 4th ed. St. Louis, Mosby-Year Book, 1993.)

overcome by administration of folinic acid (citrovorum factor), which replenishes the tetrahydrofolate. The antitumor antibiotics most commonly used in gynecologic malignancy are doxorubicin (Adriamycin) and actinomycin D. Myelosuppression occurs regularly with both of these agents; they are often used as part of multiple-agent protocols. Adriamycin in particular can cause cardiomyopathy, so cardiac function should be monitored by ultrasound evaluation or radionuclide scans. Other chemotherapeutic agents include the heavy metal derivatives, such as cisplatin, and hormones such as progesterone derivatives.

19–21. 19, **B**; 20, **D**; 21, **A**; Pages 832–833, including Figure 26–1 in Stenchever. This series of questions refers to the use of chemotherapy relative to its mechanism of action in the cell replication cycle. Knowledge of cell kinetics is important in understanding the rational use of various chemotherapeutic agents. Knowledge of cell type, size of tumor, and previous treatment is important in determining chemotherapeutic agents. A problem with larger tumors is that they contain a higher proportion of cells in the resting, or G_o, phase of the cell cycle. These cells are resistant to cytotoxic drugs and may become a source of future growth when they leave the G_o phase to enter the cell replication

cycle. Thus smaller tumors, those with a higher growth fraction, and those with a shorter doubling time are the most sensitive to cytotoxic agents.

22. **C**, Page 828. In brachytherapy, various radioisotopes are used for treatment. Which ones are chosen depends on the half-life of the radionuclide. In general, those with a short half-life (eg, gold-198) may be placed within the patient and left permanently, whereas those with a long half-life (eg, cesium-137) are placed temporarily within the patient and then removed after a prescribed dose of irradiation has been administered.

23–24. 23, **B**; 24, **A**; Pages 828–829. Teletherapy refers to the placement of the radioactive source at a distance from the patient; the machine delivers external radiation to the tumor. With external therapy the source of radiation is located at a distance 5 to 10 times greater than the depth of the tumor being irradiated to deliver a uniform dose to the tumor and thus avoid the large dose changes that result because of the inverse square law. This distance is referred to as SSD.

More recently, the concept of SAD has been introduced: it denotes the distance from the radiation source to the central axis of the machine rotation. The patient is positioned so that this axis passes through the center of the tumor, and treatment ports are arranged around this axis to minimize the dose to vital structures.

In general, the higher the energy source of the radiation, the deeper the beam penetrates the tissue. Thus high-energy (short-wavelength) radiation has its predominant effect in deeper tissues and spares the surface or the skin of radiation effects. Whereas a 6-MeV machine achieves maximum dosage at about 0.5 cm beneath the skin, the higher energy machine reaches a depth of 5 cm beneath the skin (Figure 26–3).

In addition to the energy of the beam, the energy of radiation absorbed at various depths is affected by the size of the field being treated. Larger fields contain more scattered radiation, which leads to a greater dose at a given depth.

25. **C,** Page 828. For brachytherapy, the radiation source is placed within or adjacent to the target tissue. This avoids much of the skin damage caused by teletherapy. In the treatment of gynecologic cancers, radioactive needles may be implanted directly into the tissue to be irradiated, or a tandem containing radioactive sources may be placed within the cervix and uterus accompanied by two vaginal ovoids that also contain radioactive material. In such an arrangement, the dose delivered to the tissues is determined by the inverse square law. In practice, the radioactive sources are placed in the devices after the apparatus has been properly placed. This afterloading technique reduces radiation exposure to the personnel treating the patient.

26. **B,** Page 831. It has been observed clinically that the response of the tumor to radiation treatment follows a sigmoid curve, with increasingly effective tumor control associated with increasing dosage (see Figure 26–2). A similar dosage effect exists for normal tissues. The ability of radiation therapy to control tumors depends on the greater tolerance of normal tissues to radiation exposure. Thus, if the level of radiation that causes no normal tissue damage were used, only a small proportion of tumors would be controlled (point *A*). Conversely, if a dosage that could control almost all tumors were used, massive damage to normal tissue would occur and an unacceptable series of complications and even patient death could follow (point *C*). The optimal goal is to achieve maximum tumor control with as little risk of damage to normal tissues as possible (point *B*).

27. **E,** Page 833. The dosage of an anticancer agent is usually calculated in body surface area, which provides a better measure of potential toxicity than body weight, in part because body surface area more closely reflects cardiac output and blood flow. A major problem with most agents is bone marrow toxicity. This is why they are

given cyclically to allow recovery. An additional consideration in toxicity relates to hepatic metabolism or renal excretion. It may be necessary to modify (decrease) the dosage of the drug administered when either renal or hepatic function is compromised. Methotrexate and cisplatin are also bound to albumin; this binding is decreased in patients who are taking sulfonamides or salicylates, both of which increase the toxicity and effects of the chemotherapy. In general, low serum albumin leads to an increase in free circulating chemotherapeutic agent, one reason that malnourished patients have heightened toxicity to chemotherapy.

28. **B,** Page 832. The proportion of cells actually involved in the proliferation of a tumor is known as the growth fraction (GF). It is this proportion that determines the doubling time of a given tumor. In general, smaller tumors and metastatic lesions grow more rapidly than larger tumors. An increase in the growth rate also appears to be operative after the administration of cytotoxic agents. These agents reduce the mass of the tumor, but cell replication then appears to proceed at a faster rate. The nondividing tumor cells may have reached a mature stage, may lack essential nutrition, or may be anoxic.

29. **A,** Page 827. Ionizing radiation causes cell death by dislodging orbital electrons from the atoms of the medium or tissue through which they pass. This produces secondary electrons and free hydroxyl radicals, which damage the cell and the normal DNA replication process. In addition, free hydroxyl radicals may react with molecular oxygen to form peroxide in the tissues. This adds to the lethal effect of radiation. Although there may be a change in the host immune responses based on extensive radiation therapy, there is no known change in local immune response of the target tissues. Furthermore, whereas oxygen is important for the tissue effects of photon irradiation, the oxygen tension of target tissue is not increased. In fact, since cancerous tissue frequently has decreased oxygenation, the effects of photon irradiation in these relatively hypoxic areas are often diminished.

30. **D,** Page 827. One form of ionizing radiation is electromagnetic, which refers to x-rays or gamma rays. These sources of energy have no mass and no electrical charge. They are produced in discrete quanta or photons, and their energy is proportional to their frequency; that is, higher energies are transmitted at a higher frequency of electromagnetic radiation. Since the frequency of a photon is inversely proportional to the wavelength, electromagnetic radiation with shorter wavelengths has a higher frequency and thus

higher energy. Examples of these types of energy sources used to treat tumors includes both external beam therapy and radiation caused by decay of radioactive isotopes. Examples of the use of isotopes are internal systems, such as cesium applicators.

31. **C,** Page 833. Although some tumors may have their origins in a single (stem) cell, clinically evident malignancies are composed of a heterogenous population of cells with different cell cycle lengths and varying growth fractions. Larger tumors are more likely to contain cells resistant to a single cytotoxic agent. An additional problem with larger tumors is their lower growth fraction, meaning a larger proportion of cells in their resting (G_0) phase of the cell cycle. These cells are more resistant to cytotoxic drugs. Because a larger proportion of these cells are in the resting phase, during which there is decreased DNA and RNA synthesis, they do not respond to chemotherapy.

32. **A,** Page 828. In general, there are two techniques used in radiation therapy: internal (brachytherapy) and external (teletherapy). Intracavitary brachytherapy is performed with the aid of specialized applicators, the best known of which is the Fletcher Suit applicator, which is useful for treating cervical tumors or tumors located near the cervix.

33. **A,** Page 831. Recently, drugs have been used as radioprotectors to protect normal tissue from radiation damage while reportedly not affecting tumor radiosensitivity. The best known radioprotector is amifostine, a free-radical scavenger. After administration, this drug penetrates normal tissue, but only slowly into tumors, thereby preferentially protecting normal tissue.

34. **E,** Page 836. 5-FU is a pyrimidine analogue with the ability to inhibit biosynthesis of pyrimidine nucleotides. Although myelosuppressive, it is less so than many other drugs used in gynecologic cancer treatment. Side effects include diarrhea, ulceration of oral mucosa, dermatitis, cardiac toxicity, alopecia, nail changes, acute cerebellar syndrome, hyperpigmentation over the vein used for infusion, and hand-foot syndrome. The drug is used for ovarian carcinomas, endometrial adenocarcinomas, and some cases of squamous cell carcinoma of the cervix.

Immunology and Molecular Oncology in Gynecologic Cancer

DIRECTIONS:

for Questions 1–6: Select the one best answer or completion.

1. When T cells are activated and then enter into the immune response, becoming cytotoxic to tumor cells, they produce a number of soluble immune mediators known as

   A. natural killers
   B. tumor anti-growth factor
   C. immunoglobulins
   D. cytokines
   E. β-activators

2. As a cytokine, tumor necrosis factor (TNF) provides a theoretical advantage over standard chemotherapeutic agents because

   A. its cytotoxicity is greater for malignant cells than for normal cells
   B. it has lower incidence of systemic side effects
   C. it can be used as a replacement for potentially toxic interferons
   D. it stimulates a higher proportion of tumor cells in the replicating phase

3. Which portion of the immunoglobulin molecule allows binding to the phagocyte?

   A. Fab
   B. Fc
   C. hypervariable region
   D. heavy-chain variable region

4. Which of the following cells produce interferon in response to viral infection?

   A. eosinophils
   B. basophils
   C. plasma cells
   D. monocytes
   E. fibroblasts

5. The genes for human leukocyte antigens (HLAs) are located on the

   A. body of chromosome 6
   B. short arm of the X chromosome
   C. long arm of chromosome 13
   D. long arm of chromosome 16
   E. short arm of chromosome 17

6. The immune factor most closely associated with endotoxic shock is

   A. TNF
   B. interleukin
   C. immunoglobulin G (IgG)
   D. IgM
   E. interferon

DIRECTIONS:

for Questions 7–11: For each numbered item, select the one heading most closely associated with it. Each lettered heading may be used once, more than once, or not at all.

7–11.

(A) IgA
(B) IgD
(C) IgE
(D) IgG
(E) IgM

7. Associated with hypersensitivity and parasitic infections

8. Found in saliva, milk colostrum, and genitourinary secretions

9. Most common antibody in the human

10. Most efficient in activating complement

11. Crosses the placenta

DIRECTIONS:

for Questions 12–16: Select the one best answer or completion.

12. T cells differentiate in the

    A. lymph nodes
    B. spleen
    C. Peyer's patches
    D. bone marrow
    E. thymus

13. Which of the following cytokines holds the most promise as an antitumor agent in gynecologic malignancies?

    A. interleukin-1 (IL-1)
    B. IL-2
    C. IL-3
    D. IL-4
    E. IL-5

14. Protooncogenes fall into each of the following groups *except*

    A. growth factors
    B. nonreceptor kinases
    C. cytoplasmic proteins
    D. signal transducers
    E. transcription factors

15. The p53 gene is responsible for

    A. continued cell growth
    B. activation of oncogenes
    C. a protein that promotes cellular proliferation
    D. apoptosis

16. Clusters of differentiation (CD) are cell surface markers that characterize T cells. Which CD is associated with suppressor T cells?

    A. CD2
    B. CD3
    C. CD4
    D. CD8
    E. CD16

DIRECTIONS:

for Questions 17–18: Select the asked-for number of correct answers.

17. Which two of the following are tumor suppressor genes?

    A. p53
    B. HER-2/neu
    C. myc
    D. rb
    E. ras

18. Choose three genes that have been cloned *and* for which the protein can be mass-produced to aid patients.

    A. erythropoietin
    B. BRCA1
    C. granulocyte colony-stimulating factor (G-CSF)
    D. granulocyte-macrophage colony-stimulating factor (GM-CSF)
    E. angiogenesis

ANSWERS

1. **D,** Pages 845–847; Figure 27–2 (in Stenchever). T lymphocytes are cells that confer cell-mediated immunity, whereas B lymphocytes are cells associated with antibody production (immunoglobulins) and humoral immunity. Macrophages also act directly on tumor cells; when activated, they can enter into the immune response and become cytotoxic to tumor cells. This activation process produces a number of soluble immune mediators known as *cytokines* or *lymphokines.* With the development of recombinant DNA technology, these substances can be synthesized and a number of them are being evaluated for their potential in tumor therapy.

2. **A,** Page 848. TNF is a cytokine that induces necrosis of tumor cells in vitro and appears to act synergistically with interferons. TNF appears to be selective for tumor cells, and this provides a theoretical advantage over classic chemotherapeutic agents because approximately 100 to 10,000 times the concentration of TNF is needed to affect normal cells compared with malignant cells in vitro. However, administration of TNF has also been accompanied by severe toxicity, including shocklike symptoms, fever, and hypotension.

3. **B,** Page 845; Figure 27–1, *B* (in Stenchever). The Fc region of the immunoglobulin molecule is responsible for biologic activity and binding to the phagocyte. The Fab, hypervariable region, and heavy-chain variable region are all part of the molecule that specifies the antigen for which the molecule is specific.

4. **E,** Page 848. Interferon and interleukins are types of cytokines produced in response to infection. Interferon is produced by leukocytes, macrophages, epithelial cells, and fibroblasts in response to viral infection. Monocytes, macrophages, and lymphocytes secrete interleukins.

5. **A,** Page 844. The human leukocyte antigens are encoded by a cluster of genes located on the body of chromosome 6. These are the same group of genes that have been called *transplantation antigens* in the past because of their importance in inducing tissue rejection from a host or transplant recipient.

6. **A,** Page 848. TNF is a cytokine that mediates endotoxic shock and is capable of inhibiting tumor cell growth. It also acts synergistically with some chemotherapeutic agents.

7–11. 7, **C;** 8, **A;** 9, **D;** 10, **E;** 11, **D;** Page 845. The most common immunoglobulin, accounting for approximately 70% of serum globulins, is IgG. This is the only immunoglobulin that crosses the placenta, and it is this group of globulins that confers passive immunity to the newborn. IgA makes up about 20% of total immunoglobulins. It is found in saliva, milk colostrum, and genitourinary secretions. IgM makes up 10% of globulins and is most effective in activating complement. IgE is associated with hypersensitivity and parasitic infections. IgD is found on the surface of B cells and may play a role in B-lymphocyte activation, but the exact role of IgD is not understood.

12. **D,** Page 845. T cells originate in the bone marrow and then differentiate in the thymus. From the thymus, T cells migrate to the blood, lymph nodes, spleen, and intestines (in Peyer's patches).

13. **B,** Page 848. IL-2 is produced by T cells and has a primary role in cell-mediated immunity. Studies indicate that IL-2 may be useful in treating ovarian carcinomas. IL-1 is released by macrophages in response to cell damage and stimulates T-cell and IL-2 production. IL-3 stimulates myeloid stem cells. IL-4 and IL-5 stimulate B cells.

14. **C,** Page 849. Protooncogenes are normal cellular components that become altered in a way that permits transformed cell growth. Protooncogenes are involved in cell division. As a group, they are generally placed into six classes: growth factors, receptors with protein kinase activity, nonreceptor kinases, signal transducers, transcription factors, and nuclear proteins.

15. **D,** Page 851. The p53 gene is located on the short arm of chromosome 17. It is critical in the regulation of cell death and suppression of oncogenes. The protein made by the p53 gene is important in inhibiting cell growth through its binding to DNA. This DNA-protein binding results in the expression of several genes that inhibit cell growth. The p53 gene is also important for the suppression of certain oncogenes. When the gene is damaged or deleted, its protein either becomes ineffective or is not made at all, resulting in loss of the normal suppression action and allowing the development of neoplasia.

16. **E,** Page 846. T cells are characterized by CDs. More CD markers are constantly being recognized. T cells, in general, have the CD2 surface marker, whereas CD3 is linked to the T-cell receptor. T-helper/inducer cells have the CD4 surface marker, and it is this marker that is used to assess the impact of HIV infections. CD8 surface markers are associated with suppressor/cytotoxic cells.

17. **A and D,** Pages 849–851. Rb was the first defined gene that restrained tumor proliferation. Usually, two normal gene copies are inherited; in some persons, one copy is defective. If the other gene copy is inactivated, retinoblastoma develops. This

sequence gave rise to the two-hit theory of tumor suppression gene action. P53 suppresses onco-genes and its loss allows neoplasms to develop. Ras genes are transforming genes that alter cell-to-cell relationships. When they mutate, malignant change can occur. Myc is a nuclear oncogene in which overexpression can lead to self-proliferation in the absence of other usually required factors. HER-2/neu is a cell membrane growth factor receptor gene, which when overexpressed is associated with poor prognosis in breast and ovarian cancer.

18. **A, C,** and **D,** Pages 848, 851–853. G-CSF, and GM-CSF are genes that have been cloned and the protein mass produced to stimulate the neutro-phils, other granulocytes, and red blood cell production, especially in chemotherapy-induced bone marrow suppression. BRCA1 is a gene on chromosome 17, which when mutated increases the risk of breast and ovarian cancer. Angiogenesis is the formation of new capillary blood vessels, which may be initiated by growth factors secreted by tumor cells. Finding inhibitors to angiogenesis is a promising area of research because angiogenesis inhibitors may suppress tumor growth by decreasing tumor blood supply without causing toxic side effects.

CHAPTER 28

Intraepithelial Neoplasia of the Cervix

for Questions 1–28: Select the one best answer or completion.

1. In a 35-year-old patient, two Pap smears have been consistent with severe dysplasia, and a colposcopically directed biopsy has shown cervical intraepithelial neoplasia type I (CIN I). Endocervical curettage (ECC) results are negative. The management of choice is
   A. repeating the Pap smear every 3 months
   B. conization
   C. repeating the colposcopy and directed biopsy
   D. cryocautery
   E. laser ablation

2. The difference between leukoplakia and acetowhite epithelium is that
   A. acetowhite epithelium is white, and leukoplakia is not
   B. leukoplakia appears white without acetic acid
   C. leukoplakia is a clinical description, and aceto-white epithelium is a histologic description
   D. leukoplakia is precancerous, and acetowhite epithelium is not
   E. acetowhite epithelium is a clinical diagnosis, and leukoplakia is a histologic diagnosis

3. The risk of cervical cancer for a woman marrying a man whose first wife had cervical cancer compared with the risk for a woman who is marrying a man whose first wife did not have cervical cancer is
   A. 0.3
   B. 0.5
   C. 1.0
   D. 2.0
   E. 3.0

4. The purpose of routine ECC is to
   A. identify which part of the cervical canal has cancer
   B. rule out an endocervical human papilloma virus infection
   C. ascertain with high reliability whether a neoplasm exists in the endocervical canal
   D. document chlamydial cervicitis
   E. detect accurately tubal or ovarian carcinoma

5. In a 32-year-old woman, colposcopically directed excisional biopsy reveals a single focus of microinvasive carcinoma with clear margins. ECC results are negative. The woman should have
   A. no further treatment
   B. a cervical conization
   C. a vaginal hysterectomy
   D. a radical hysterectomy
   E. cryocautery

6. After multiple directed cervical biopsies have resulted in a diagnosis of CIN II, the best technique of cryotherapy with a patient in whom ECC results are negative is a
   A. single 1-minute freeze
   B. single 3-minute freeze
   C. single 5-minute freeze
   D. double 1-minute freeze
   E. double 3-minute freeze

7. A 24-year-old gravida 1 has undergone cervical conization for CIN III. On pathologic review, the proximal margins of the cone were involved with CIN III. The patient wants to retain her childbearing capability. The best immediate course of action is

A. electrocautery
B. cryocautery
C. laser treatment
D. to repeat the cervical conization
E. to follow with Pap smears and colposcopy

8. A 24-year-old woman at 10 weeks of gestation is found to have an abnormal Pap smear consistent with CIN III. Immediate management should include

A. conization
B. colposcopy and biopsy
C. suction dilatation and curettage (D&C)
D. repeat Pap smear
E. hysterectomy

9. Punctation is

A. the area between the squamous cell epithelium of the cervical portio and the columnar cell epithelium of the endocervix
B. a colposcopic pattern that contains white epithelium with stippling caused by blood vessels seen on end
C. a name for cells with perinuclear cavitation
D. a colposcopic pattern that reveals acetowhite areas outlined by blood vessels
E. the pattern of native squamous cell epithelium

10. Which of the following human papillomavirus (HPV) types has low oncogenic potential?

A. 6
B. 16
C. 18
D. 31
E. 52

11. A polymerase chain reaction (PCR) is a(n)

A. enzyme that reproduces itself
B. method of amplifying DNA
C. atomic reaction
D. standard step in performing Southern Blot analysis
E. test limited to finding HPV 16 and 18

12. The greatest risk of cervical cancer is predicted by

A. first coitus at age 17
B. an atypical Pap smear
C. CIN II at the margin of a cervical cone
D. HPV 16 found on cervical smear
E. persistent abnormal cytologic findings after cryocautery for dysplasia

13. According to the Bethesda system for reporting a Pap smear result, a patient who is found to have a result consistent with an HPV infection would be classified as having a(n)

A. high-grade squamous intraepithelial lesion
B. low-grade squamous intraepithelial lesion
C. reactive inflammatory change
D. atypical type undetermined
E. infection

14. In a 50-year-old woman, cervical biopsy shows CIN III, colposcopy results are inadequate, and ECC reveals dysplastic fragments. The cervix sounds to 2 cm. How long should the cone be?

A. 5 mm
B. 7 mm
C. 10 mm
D. 15 mm
E. 18 mm

15. The most common complication of conization is

A. infertility
B. cervical stenosis
C. bleeding
D. an incompetent cervix
E. an infection

16. The characteristic listed below that is of greatest help in identifying HPV infections of the cervix is

A. development of white epithelium with acetic acid
B. atypia on Pap smears
C. koilocytosis on Pap smears
D. Lugol's nonstaining areas on the ectocervix
E. a history of ungual warts

17. To be called *koilocytosis*, the cells must demonstrate which of the following?

A. HPV on polymerase chain reaction
B. both central clearing and atypical nuclei
C. central clearing only
D. atypical nuclei only
E. evidence of gross warts

18. Which of the following is the *lowest* risk factor for squamous cell neoplasia of the cervix?

A. multiple sexual partners
B. lupus erythematosus
C. gonorrhea
D. HPV
E. human immunodeficiency virus (HIV)

19. The finding that is most suspicious for significant dysplasia during a colposcopic examination is

   A. wide intercapillary distances
   B. abnormal vessels
   C. a large transformation zone
   D. an irregular surface pattern
   E. inability to see the transformation zone

20. The requirements for adequate colposcopy include

   A. ECC
   B. demonstration of significant white epithelium
   C. visualization of the entire transformation zone
   D. use of both green and white light
   E. use of ×16 magnification

21. A 35-year-old patient has extensive CIN III on multiple colposcopically directed biopsies and ECC. The transformation zone has not been completely visualized. What is the most appropriate initial management for this patient?

   A. laser ablation
   B. cold-knife conization
   C. cryocautery
   D. electrocautery
   E. hysterectomy

22. A relatively inexpensive outpatient method of obtaining cervical biopsy in the clinic that may cause necrosis of the surgical margins is

   A. cold-knife conization
   B. loop electrosurgical excision procedure (LEEP)
   C. punch biopsy
   D. laser
   E. cryocautery

23. In the Bethesda classification, high-grade squamous intraepithelial lesion (SIL) corresponds to

   A. invasive cancer
   B. CIN II or III
   C. CIN I
   D. atypia
   E. koilocytosis

24. The theory that is currently most accepted for how HPV infection may play a part in cervical neoplasia is that HPV infection causes

   A. a direct malignant change
   B. loss of normal tumor suppression function
   C. interaction with other sexually transmitted diseases to result in malignant change
   D. the development and maintenance of an enlarged transformation zone
   E. eversion of the endocervix

25. A patient with biopsy-proven CIN II asks you about the risk of her lesion's progressing to invasive cancer. You can accurately tell her that the progression rate of the lesion is

   A. <1%
   B. about 5%
   C. about 15%
   D. about 30%
   E. about 60%

26. In a 28-year-old patient, an AGCUS Pap smear has resulted in a question of neoplasia. Your next step in management is based on the possibility that

   A. AGCUS smears are more likely to be false-positive than ASCUS smears
   B. one third of these patients may have a malignant or premalignant lesion
   C. atypical glandular cells are easier to detect than squamous cells
   D. the lesion from which the cells arose is probably in the tube or ovary
   E. this type of cell usually comes from intraperitoneal structures that are not of the reproductive tract

27. A 33-year-old woman has undergone cervical cone biopsy for CIN III. Pap smears should be repeated every 3 to 6 months until how many smears have been negative?

   A. one
   B. two
   C. three
   D. four
   E. five

28. Women with no prior evidence of cervical neoplasia who become infected with HIV have which of the following risks of experiencing biopsy-proven CIN within 3 years?

   A. <2%
   B. 5%–10%
   C. 30%–50%
   D. 60%–70%
   E. >80%

for Questions 29–31. Choose the most appropriate interval between Pap smears for the patients listed in Questions 29–31.

(A) annually
(B) annually until two negative tests, then stop
(C) every 3 to 5 years
(D) every 6 to 8 years
(E) testing may be stopped

29. **A sexually active 14-year-old female**

30. **A 42-year-old woman who had a hysterectomy 1 year ago for CIN III**

31. **A 33-year-old woman who had a hysterectomy 1 year ago for leiomyomata**

for Questions 32–35. Match the histologic picture with the correct diagnosis. See Figures 28–1 through 28–5.

(A) Figure 28–1
(B) Figure 28–2
(C) Figure 28–3
(D) Figure 28–4
(E) Figure 28–5

32. **Cervical intraepithelial neoplasia (CIN I)**

33. **Cervical intraepithelial neoplasia (CIN III)**

34. **Moderate dysplasia of the cervix (CIN II)**

35. **Koilocytosis**

ANSWERS

1. **B,** Page 878. Specific indications for cervical conization are (1) unsatisfactory colposcopy, (2) positive results on ECC, (3) cells on the Pap smear that are not adequately explained by histologic findings on biopsy, (4) microinvasive cancer, and (5) clinical uncertainty regarding the presence of invasive disease. It has also been suggested that conization be performed in patients older than 50 if a biopsy shows carcinoma in situ because the incidence of unsuspected invasion is high beyond this age. The purpose of conization in such a case is to rule out invasive cancer.

2. **B,** Pages 857, 873. *Leukoplakia* and *acetowhite epithelium* are both clinical descriptive terms. Leukoplakia is white before the application of acetic acid, whereas acetowhite epithelium looks normal initially and becomes white after application of acetic acid. Neither term defines a precancerous lesion. The histologic findings of either one may be precancerous, but not necessarily so.

3. **E,** Page 810. Epidemiologic studies indicate that a woman whose husband's first wife had carcinoma of the cervix is at three times the risk for cervical cancer compared with a woman whose husband's first wife did not have cervical cancer. This supports the hypothesis that a factor that causes cervical cancer may be sexually transmitted.

Some other factors that increase the risk of cervical cancer are related to sexual activity, such as multiple sex partners and venereal disease. Other factors are smoking, HPV, and early age of first intercourse.

4. **C,** Page 872. ECC is designed to determine whether or not endocervical neoplasia exists. It can detect dysplasia, squamous cell carcinoma, and adenocarcinoma. ECC should be performed whenever a biopsy is taken from the cervix. ECC cannot identify which part of the cervical canal has cancer, rule out endocervical HPV infection, or document chlamydial cervicitis. Although cells from ovarian or other upper abdominal carcinoma can be found on either Pap smears or ECC specimens, neither of these modalities provides an accurate way of making the diagnosis of upper genital tract or other intraabdominal carcinoma.

5. **B,** Page 878. A biopsy diagnosis of microinvasive cancer of the cervix requires conization to rule out invasive disease. A radical hysterectomy may be too much treatment if no invasion exists, and a total hysterectomy is too little treatment if it does. Cryocautery is not indicated for this lesion. Further study and appropriate treatment are mandatory, depending on the eventual diagnosis. If the cone result is negative and the woman

FIGURE 28–1 (From Stenchever MA, Droegemueller W, Herbst AL, Mishell DR: *Comprehensive Gynecology*, 3rd ed. St Louis, Mosby, 1997.)

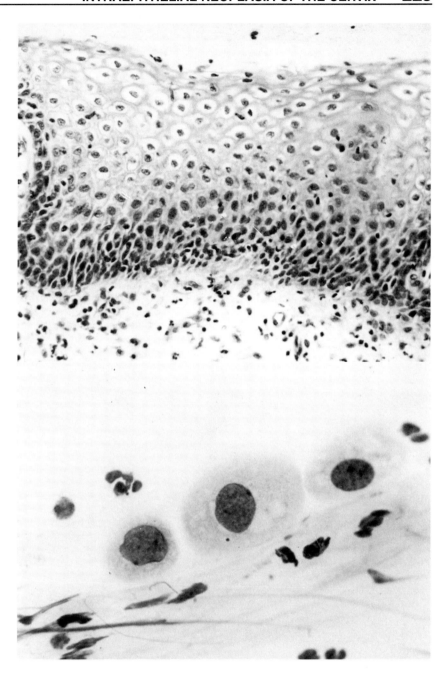

desires more children, the conization can be considered treatment.

6. **E**, Page 877. A double 3-minute freeze cures approximately 90% of CIN lesions in which the initial evaluation is adequate, which it was in this patient. The double freeze destroys most of the transformation zone and cervical crypts. Cryotherapy appears to be less effective for CIN III. For these lesions, excision therapy is preferable. Close follow-up with a Pap smear every 6 months for 1 or 2 years followed by annual Pap smears is needed to ensure that the dysplastic process has been eliminated. Pap smears should be at least annual in patients such as this.

7. **E**, Page 880. Studies have shown that even with positive margins on a cervical conization, up to 70% of these patients have no recurrence at 5 years. With careful follow-up, which includes endocervical Pap smears, most of these patients may retain their fertility.

8. **B**, Pages 880–882. There is no need to terminate the pregnancy for CIN. The first step is to have the patient evaluated by an experienced colposcopist. That physician will perform a biopsy if indicated. Often, the transformation zone and the endocervical canal are seen better because of the cervical eversion that occurs during pregnancy. If invasive cancer is not found, the patient may deliver

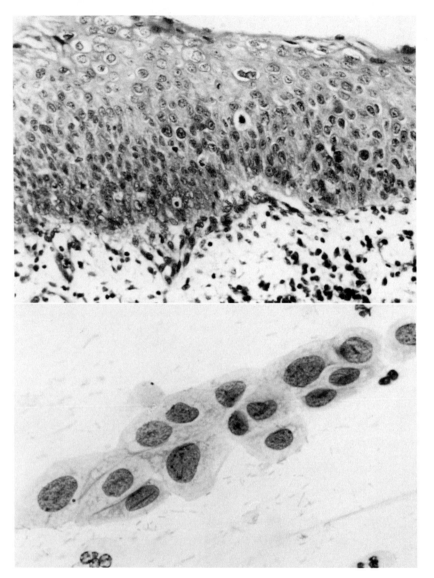

FIGURE 28–2 (From Stenchever MA, Droegemueller W, Herbst AL, Mishell DR: Comprehensive Gynecology, 3rd ed. St Louis, Mosby, 1997.)

vaginally. Conization would be indicated only if there is suspicion of invasion by either cytologic examination or colposcopy that is not confirmed on biopsy. This is a rare situation.

9. **B,** Page 858. *Mosaicism, punctation,* and *transformation zone* are all terms used to describe colposcopic findings. Respectively, they refer to a colposcopic pattern in which acetowhite areas are outlined by blood vessels; a pattern that contains stippling caused by blood vessels seen on end in acetowhite areas; and the expanse of epithelium at the junction between the squamous cell epithelium of the cervix and the columnar cell epithelium of the endocervix. Native squamous cell epithelium is the original squamous cell epithelium found on the portio of the cervix and in the vagina.

10. **A,** Page 868. Type 6 HPV has low oncogenic potential in the cervix but often causes visible warts. Although certain HPV types have been more frequently associated with cervical cancer than others, the use of more sensitive tests has shown a high prevalence of these high-risk types in women in whom cervical cytologic findings are negative. Currently, HPV typing has not proved helpful clinically because of high false-positive rates. Some types, such as HPV 2, have not been associated with cervical carcinoma.

11. **B,** Page 867. PCR is a highly sensitive method of enzymatically reproducing segments of DNA so that very small amounts can be amplified and the segment can be more easily identified and studied. It is a useful technique for many situations because it can detect a single DNA fragment in a million cells. Care must be exercised in its use to prevent amplification of a contaminant, thereby yielding false-positive results. Much current research is seeking a clinically useful method of using HPV detection to help determine the prognosis of CIN.

FIGURE 28–3 (From Stenchever MA, Droegemueller W, Herbst AL, Mishell DR: Comprehensive Gynecology, 3rd ed. St Louis, Mosby, 1997.)

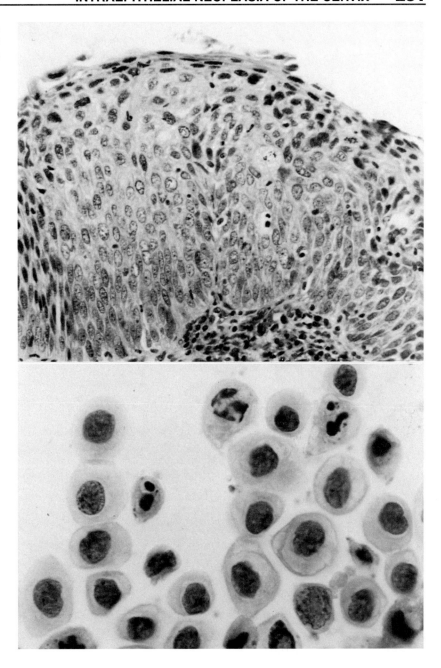

12. **E,** Pages 868–869. Persistent abnormal cervical cytologic findings after treatment for dysplasia is a poor prognostic sign. For this reason, all patients should be followed up with Pap smears after treatment for cervical dysplasia. A finding of positive margins after a cone biopsy carries a low rate of the development of more severe disease, but close follow-up is necessary. Young age of first coitus and mildly abnormal cytologic findings are risk factors, but they are not as significant as persistent positive cytologic findings after treatment. The finding of HPV 16 in the cervix of an otherwise healthy woman requires follow-up smears.

13. **B,** Page 873. The Bethesda system first requires a statement regarding the adequacy of the cytologic preparation for diagnosis. It classifies HPV infection as a low-grade squamous intraepithelial lesion (SIL). Other infections are noted separately. Changes consistent with CIN I are also classified as low-grade SIL. Such smears can be repeated in 6 months.

14. **E,** Page 878; Figure 28–18 in Stenchever. Boonstra's data on 65 specimens showed that approximately 98% of CIN III lesions in younger women had a maximum depth of crypt involvement less than 3.6 mm and extended linearly to the proximal border less than 14.8 mm from the cervical os. In the small number of patients older than 50, the maximum depth of crypt involvement was 4.5 mm and the maximum length of involvement was 17.6 mm.

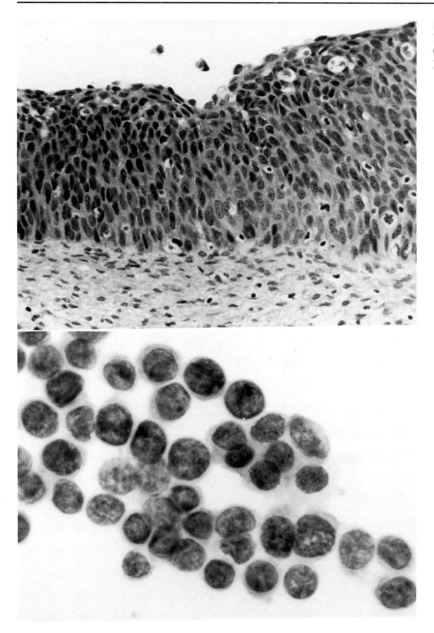

FIGURE 28–4 (From Stenchever MA, Droegemueller W, Herbst AL, Mishell DR: Comprehensive Gynecology, 3rd ed. St Louis, Mosby, 1997.)

The depth and extent of gland involvement increase in older women. As there is a greater risk of cancer in this older group, the cone should remove a greater part of the endocervix. Fortunately, reproduction is no longer an issue in this population. A larger cone is associated with a very small increase in risk in return for a better diagnostic sample. The cone size should be tailored to the patient and the clinical situation.

15. **C,** Page 879. Although infertility and an incompetent cervix may occur, the risk is small; the risk is not an issue in women near or past menopause. Bleeding, both immediate and late (7 to 14 days), is the major complication. Stenosis is rare, and its incidence may be decreased by sounding the cervix at 1 to 3 weeks post conization. Other rare complications are infection, damage to nearby organs, and uterine perforation.

16. **C,** Page 864. Koilocytes are indicative of HPV. They may also be found in areas of dysplasia (CIN), and when so found they imply a concomitant HPV infection. Both CIN and some HPV strains stain acetowhite with the application of acetic acid. Both may result in atypical cells on the Pap smear. For these reasons, colposcopically directed biopsies must be performed to rule out dysplasia when Pap smears or colposcopy yields abnormal findings. It is difficult to distinguish between HPV and mild dysplasia by Pap smear or colposcopy only. If dysplastic cells occur throughout the thickness of the cervical epithelium, the diagnosis is carcinoma in situ, which is included in the term *CIN III.* HPV infection may also be

FIGURE 28–5 (From Stenchever MA, Droegemueller W, Herbst AL, Mishell DR: Comprehensive Gynecology, 3rd ed. St Louis, Mosby, 1997.)

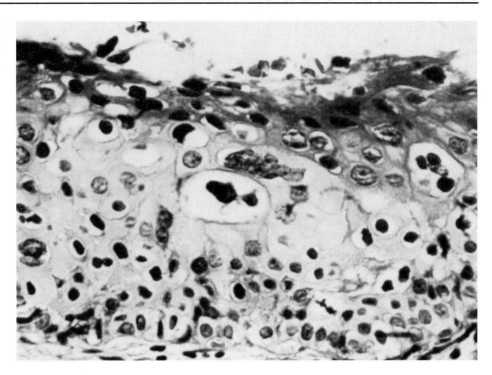

associated with CIN III, but in cases of obvious dysplasia the presence or absence of HPV infection is disregarded for purposes of therapy. Koilocytosis is associated with HPV, as is the finding of asperities or frank wart. White epithelium can be caused by healing, metaplasia, or dysplasia. Atypias are often found with infection or dysplasias as well as with HPV. The finding of Lugol's nonstaining areas is very nonspecific because any cell without glycogen or an erosion where there is an absence of cells will not stain. Ungual warts are not predictive of cervical warts.

17. **B,** Page 857. *Koilocytosis* describes a cellular change associated with HPV infections and should demonstrate both perinuclear clearing and mild nuclear atypia. HPV need not be found by PCR, and gross warts are not necessary for a histologic diagnosis of koilocytosis.

18. **C,** Page 860. Gonorrhea has not been shown to have any direct effect on cervical dysplasia, although all sexually transmitted diseases (STDs) have some association. Some STDs, such as HPV or HIV, are associated with an increased rate of CIN. In HIV-positive patients, the rate of CIN increases as the CD4 count decreases. Multiple partners and smoking are also associated with an increased rate of CIN, although the increased rate associated with smoking may be confounded by the increase in HPV in persons who smoke. Increased incidence is also noted in patients with lupus erythematosus; close cervical surveillance is indicated in these patients.

19. **B,** Pages 873–875. Abnormal vessels with an irregular sausage-like shape constitute the worst colposcopic sign listed. Wide intercapillary distances, irregular surfaces, and a large transformation zone (especially if it is abnormal) are also factors of concern. Inability to see the transformation zone is worrisome because it connotes an inadequate colposcopy, but it does not in itself mean that dysplasia will be found.

20. **C,** Pages 872–873. By definition, adequate colposcopy means visualization of the entire transformation zone. ECC is not required unless there is an additional need for this diagnostic procedure. Any magnification from ×5 to ×20 can be used, although most colposcopic examinations use ×10 to ×16 magnification. Either white or green lights, or both, may be used. A normal cervix may have no significant white epithelium.

21. **B,** Page 878. In this case, with CIN III on both the ECC and the cervical biopsies, the best procedure is a cold-knife cone, which yields tissue for pathologic examination. A hysterectomy should not be performed until invasive cancer has been ruled out. Ablative procedures done by laser, cryocautery, or electrocautery are not appropriate because no tissue remains for pathologic review.

22. **B,** Page 879. The LEEP technique involves the use of a thin electric wire to excise a core of cervical tissue. If it is done too slowly or with the wrong current setting, it may cause heat artifact of the surgical margins, making pathologic interpretation difficult. The laser may also cause heat artifact; it is used mainly in outpatient surgery and

is much more expensive. Cryocautery does not yield a specimen to examine. Neither knife cone nor punch biopsy is likely to cause necrosis of the surgical margin.

23. **B,** Page 859; Figure 28–1 in Stenchever. A diagnosis of high-grade SIL on a Pap smear is an estimate made from a cytologic specimen that a subsequent histologic biopsy will reveal CIN II to III. Low-grade SIL is an estimate that a biopsy will reveal either wart changes (koilocytosis) or CIN I.

24. **B,** Page 869. The current most prevalent explanation of the role of HPV in cervical neoplasia is that the E6 and E7 open reading frames from the HPV genome encode for proteins that suppress normal tumor suppressor genes, such as p53, and retinoblastoma. Because of this assumed association, research is under way to develop vaccines to treat or prevent HPV infection. HPV type-specific antibodies have been developed, and these may provide a way of preventing HPV infection.

25. **B,** Page 869. The higher the grade of dysplasia, the greater the risk of progression to invasive disease. CIN II has a regression rate of about 43%, a persistence rate of about 35%, and a rate of progression to a higher grade of CIN of about 22%. If dysplasia is left completely alone, the rate of progression of CIN II to invasive cancer is approximately 5%. The rate of progression to invasive cancer from CIN I is approximately 1%, and the rate from CIN III can be as high as 12% (Table 28–1).

26. **B,** Page 871. *AGCUS* stands for *a*typical *g*landular *c*ells of *u*ndetermined *s*ignificance. Such Pap smear diagnoses cause even more diagnostic and management confusion than do ASCUS Pap smears. However, particularly in older women, there is a high rate of invasive or in situ adenocarcinoma, usually of the endocervix or endometrium. Rarely, glandular cells can come from higher in the reproductive tract or from cells in the peritoneal cavity. When a comment by the cytopathologist suggests neoplasia on an AGCUS smear, as many as one third of these cervices have been observed to have premalignant or invasive lesions.

27. **C,** Page 882. For patients with high-grade lesions, three negative Pap smears at 4- to 6-month intervals should be obtained before annual smears are resumed. For low-grade lesions, two negative Pap smears are recommended. Studies have shown that most cases of failure to cure CIN (90%) occur in the first two repeat Pap smears. In any event, initial close follow-up and then repeated annual Pap smears are indicated in patients who have had dysplasia because they have already shown their predisposition to form dysplastic change.

28. **C,** Page 861. Women without HIV have been found to have a frequency of CIN of about 4%. If a woman has HIV, the incidence of CIN increases and is between 30% and 56%, depending on the patient's CD4 count. The risk becomes greater as the count becomes lower. Invasive carcinoma of the cervix is now designated as a age case-defining condition in patients infected with HIV.

29–31. 29, **A;** 30, **A;** 31, **C;** Pages 871–872; Table 28–3 in Stenchever. Different reports list different intervals at which Pap smears are recommended. However, all agree that, at minimum, young sexually active women should have Pap smears until at least two smears are negative and then have a Pap smear every year. Most reports also state that high-risk women should continue to have annual Pap smears. High-risk women are those who began sexual intercourse at an early age, have had multiple sexual partners, or have had abnormal Pap smears or HPV or herpes simplex virus infections in the past. A woman who has undergone hysterectomy for dysplastic disease remains at high risk for dysplasia or carcinoma at the vaginal apex. Women who have undergone hysterectomy for benign disease should still have Pap smears, but the interval between them can safely be extended to 3 to 5 years, and some recommend stopping Paps entirely because the yield is extremely low. The pelvic examination done in conjunction with obtaining a Pap smear in any woman is also a good clinical screening tool for such entities as vaginitis, cervicitis, ovarian tumors, and other pelvic pathologic conditions. Examination also brings the patient to the physician for other health maintenance measures such as mammography.

32–35. 32, **A;** 33, **C;** 34, **B;** 35, **E;** Pages 860–865. The concept of dysplastic changes of the cervical epithelium progressing to invasive carcinoma is well established. Various terms have been used to describe the histologic basis of the dysplastic changes in the cervix. Cervical intraepithelial neoplasia (CIN) is designated as I, II, or III. CIN I and II correspond to histologic findings of mild and moderate dysplasia, respectively. CIN III refers to the histologic patterns found in either severe dysplasia or carcinoma in situ. Since the treatment is the same for severe dysplasia or carcinoma in situ, the term *CIN III* has been used to describe both of these entities. Because degrees of CIN or dysplasia lie on a continuum, the distinctions may be interpreted differently by different observers, especially at the less severe end of the spectrum.

Malignant Diseases of the Cervix

for Questions 1–23: Select the one best answer or completion.

1. A patient with a diagnosis of a stage IB adeno-carcinoma of the cervix would have the greatest chance for survival with an initial treatment of

   A. combined radiation and operation
   B. operation
   C. radiation
   D. chemotherapy
   E. operation and immunotherapy

2. In a 49-year-old woman, squamous cell carcinoma of the cervix has been diagnosed by biopsy. On examination with the patient under anesthesia, she is found to have a tumor in the upper third of the vagina and in the parametria. An intravenous pyelogram reveals obstruction of the left ureter. The stage of her tumor is

   A. IB
   B. IIA
   C. IIIA
   D. IIIB
   E. IV

3. Of the following, the most aggressive form of carcinoma of the cervix is

   A. large cell, nonkeratinizing
   B. adenosquamous cell
   C. basaloid
   D. verrucous
   E. glassy cell

4. A 52-year-old patient who underwent supracer-vical hysterectomy in the past now has stage IIB carcinoma of the cervix. The treatment of choice is

   A. external radiation
   B. intracavitary radiation
   C. radical operation
   D. chemotherapy
   E. trachelectomy

5. A 60-year-old woman has a firm nodule above her left clavicle. Her history reveals slight weight loss and mild vaginal spotting for 6 months. She has not had a physical examination or Pap smear for many years. On pelvic examination, she had a large bulky cervix with firm induration extending to the pelvic side walls. A biopsy of the cervix reveals invasive squamous cell carcinoma. The chest radiograph and intravenous pyelogram appear normal. The next step in her care should be

   A. external radiation to 50 Gy
   B. total abdominal hysterectomy and bilateral salpingo-oophorectomy
   C. radical hysterectomy and pelvic lymph node dissection
   D. 500 mg hours of cervical brachytherapy
   E. scalene node biopsy

6. Conization reveals cervical carcinoma. The maximum depth of the tumor from the base of the epithelium is between 6 and 7 mm, and there is no lateral extension greater than 5 mm. There is no parametrial, nodal, or metastatic involvement. According to the 1994 FIGO, the lesion would be staged as

   A. zero
   B. IA1
   C. IA2
   D. IB
   E. II

7. **The proper definition of brachytherapy is**

   A. a surgical procedure that severs nerves to prevent pain
   B. a form of radiation therapy that places the source of radiation near the tumor
   C. a form of radiation therapy that delivers the radiation from a source far from the tumor
   D. a form of chemotherapy that uses local placement of chemotherapeutic agents
   E. a form of chemotherapy that uses systemic placement of chemotherapeutic agents

8. **A hard barrel-shaped cervix is associated most closely with**

   A. multiparity
   B. congenital anomaly
   C. ectopic pregnancy
   D. infection
   E. endophytic cancer

9. **A radical hysterectomy differs from a total abdominal hysterectomy in that it includes surgical removal of the**

   A. paraaortic nodes
   B. pelvic nodes
   C. ovaries
   D. parametrium
   E. base of the bladder

10. **In standard therapy for invasive cervical cancer, point *A* refers to a**

    A. position on the lateral pelvic side wall
    B. point in the pelvis that receives approximately 85 Gy total radiation
    C. surgical landmark that includes nodes
    D. point at the bifurcation of the common iliac arteries marking the upper pelvic nodes
    E. defined anatomic location that, if involved with tumor, changes the dose of chemotherapy

11. **Of the following, the most common complication of radical hysterectomy for cervical cancer is**

    A. hemorrhagic cystitis
    B. stenosis of the vagina
    C. urinary fistula
    D. bladder dysfunction
    E. bowel obstruction

12. **Of the following, the most common complication of radiation treatment for cervical cancer is**

    A. urinary fistula
    B. vaginal stenosis
    C. diarrhea
    D. bone marrow suppression
    E. skin burn

13. **A major advantage of radiation over surgery in the treatment of carcinoma of the cervix stage IB or IIA is**

    A. preservation of ovarian function
    B. less vaginal fibrosis
    C. better cure rate
    D. short duration of therapy
    E. use in extremely ill patients

14. **Effectiveness of treatment of early adenocarcinoma of the cervix appears to be maximized by**

    A. full radiation therapy only
    B. partial radiation and hysterectomy
    C. partial radiation and radical hysterectomy
    D. radical hysterectomy only
    E. radical surgery and chemotherapy

15. **Patients with recurrent carcinoma of the cervix**

    A. have a lesion reappearing within 6 months after therapy
    B. most commonly have recurrences at distant sites
    C. respond well to chemotherapeutic regimens
    D. should undergo periodic evaluation of renal function
    E. rarely have back or sciatic pain

16. **A cervical cancer measuring 4 mm from the basement membrane and extending laterally 6 mm would be staged as**

    A. IA1
    B. IA2
    C. IB1
    D. IB2
    E. IIA

17. **When squamous cell carcinoma of the cervix extends to the endometrium,**

    A. stage II is automatically assigned
    B. staging is increased by one level
    C. it may predispose to distant metastasis
    D. the treatment plan changes
    E. the prognosis is very poor

18. **During pretherapy evaluation of a patient with proven stage IIB invasive cancer of the cervix, a barium enema is most useful to determine**

    A. tumor involvement of the rectum
    B. tumor involvement of the colon
    C. the status of the bowel before radiation therapy
    D. the status of mesenteric and paraaortic nodes
    E. the function of the uterus

19. A stage IB carcinoma of the cervix is treated by radical hysterectomy. The pelvic nodes are found to be infiltrated by the tumor. The patient's 5-year survival rate

    A. remains at about 90% as for all stage I cancer of the cervix
    B. drops to about 75%–80%
    C. drops to about 45%–50%
    D. drops to about 25%–30%
    E. drops to about 5%–10%

20. Radiation therapy to the pelvis is limited by the maximum tolerance of other pelvic organs. The organ that usually limits the radiation dose is the

    A. bladder
    B. large bowel
    C. small bowel
    D. ovary

21. How many centigrays (cGy) are given in the usual dose of external radiation treatment for invasive cervical cancer?

    A. 500–1000
    B. 2500–3000
    C. 4500–5000
    D. 6500–7000
    E. 8500–9000

22. When used to treat advanced stage carcinoma of the cervix, chemoradiation

    A. is most efficacious using multiple chemotherapeutic agents
    B. is most efficacious when the chemotherapy is given after the radiation
    C. has lower survival rates than radiation
    D. is only superior when both pelvic and periaortic nodes are involved
    E. has increased hematologic toxicity

23. A pregnant patient has invasive cervical carcinoma. Which of the following statements is true?

    A. Birth through the cancerous cervix markedly improves the prognosis.
    B. Stage for stage, survival is the same as in a nonpregnant woman.
    C. The tumor is apt to recur in the site of an episiotomy.
    D. Conization is used for diagnosis more liberally.
    E. Treatment is different from that of the nonpregnant woman.

DIRECTIONS:

for Questions 24–37: For each numbered item, select the one heading most closely associated with it. Each lettered heading may be used once, more than once, or not at all.

24–27. Match the patient with the most likely 5-year survival rate.

   (A) 11%
   (B) 39%
   (C) 66%
   (D) 70%
   (E) 85%

24. A 28-year-old woman with stage I squamous cell carcinoma of the cervix

25. A 42-year-old woman with a transected invasive carcinoma of the cervix discovered in an operative specimen after a vaginal hysterectomy for prolapse

26. A 42-year-old woman with stage III carcinoma of the cervix

27. A 28-year-old woman with stage II carcinoma of the cervix discovered during the second trimester of pregnancy

28–30. Match the description with the most likely source of cancer

   (A) vulvar
   (B) cervical
   (C) endometrial
   (D) ovarian
   (E) vaginal

28. Female genital tract cancer causing the greatest number of deaths in the United States

29. Most common female genital tract type of cancer

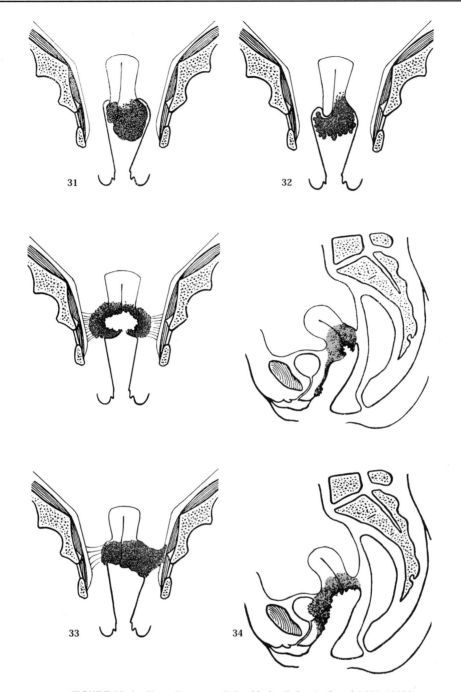

FIGURE 29–1 (From Pettersson F, Bjorkholm E: Semin Oncol 9:289, 1982.)

30. Genital tract cancer whose frequency has shown the greatest decrease as a result of population screening

31–34. Match the stage of cervical cancer with the letter of the illustration depicting it in Figure 29–1.

    (A) stage IVA
    (B) stage IIIA
    (C) stage IIIB
    (D) stage IIB
    (E) stage IB

35–37. Match the following with the entity most closely associated with it.

    (A) adenoma malignum
    (B) verrucous carcinoma
    (C) equal or less than 35 mm^2
    (D) exophytic
    (E) glassy cell

35. Minimal deviation adenocarcinoma

36. Adenosquamous carcinoma

37. Microinvasive carcinoma

ANSWERS

1. **A,** Page 904. Patients with early stages of adenocarcinoma of the cervix experience a better survival rate if treated with partial irradiation by local implants of radium in the cervix and vagina followed by radical operation. The approach of radiation followed by operation is also used in stage IB barrel-shaped squamous cell carcinoma of the cervix. Radiation alone is used for stage IIB or higher cases of carcinoma of the cervix.

2. **D,** Page 897; Table 29–1 in Stenchever. Stage is defined by the greatest extent of tumor spread, which in this case is the ureteral obstruction as demonstrated by the intravenous pyelogram. Currently, in contrast to ovarian carcinoma, cervical cancer is staged by physical examination and a few specialized tests such as an intravenous pyelogram and a chest radiograph. Once the stage is determined, it does not change, even if the operative findings reveal that it is more or less advanced than was determined initially. The staging criteria for cervical cancer should be committed to memory.

3. **E,** Pages 892–893. Glassy cell carcinoma is an aggressive subtype of adenosquamous cell cervical cancer. It is highly malignant and has a predilection for early metastases. Small cell cancer is also quite malignant, whereas verrucous and large cell variants are less so. Other rare cell types include adenoma malignum, adenoid cystic, and basaloid.

4. **A,** Page 909. Currently, supracervical hysterectomies are not often performed. However, they were common in the past. Although radical surgery may be considered for stage I or IIA disease, stage IIB presents a more advanced tumor that is not amenable to surgical therapy. Brachytherapy is difficult because the uterine fundus is removed, which makes it difficult to place intracavitary radiation sources. Therefore, external radiation is the best choice. Chemotherapy as an initial treatment for carcinoma of the cervix is not currently satisfactory, and trachelectomy is inadequate treatment.

5. **E,** Page 898. A patient with a large supraclavicular node, weight loss, and proven invasive carcinoma of the cervix is apt to have metastases via the pelvic and paraaortic nodes to the supraclavicular node. The presence or absence of metastases should be evaluated before any form of therapy is begun because the presence of a positive supraclavicular node would change both the prognosis and the therapy.

6. **D,** Page 897; Table 29–1 in Stenchever. The staging is IB because the tumor exceeds 5 mm in depth. Since there is no parametrial, side wall, ureteral, or metastatic involvement, it would not be stage II or greater. Vascular space involvement should be mentioned separately.

7. **B,** Page 889. Brachytherapy and teletherapy are both forms of radiation therapy. With brachytherapy, the radiation source is placed close to the tumor and interstitial needles, intracervical tandems, or vaginal ovoid applicators are used. A Fletcher-Suit applicator is a specific vaginal ovoid device used to deliver brachytherapy. With teletherapy, the radiation source is at a distance from the patient; it is usually called *external therapy*. An operation in which the lateral spinothalamic tract is severed to prevent pain is called a *cordotomy*.

8. **E,** Pages 889, 898. Cervical carcinoma can develop as an ulcer, a cauliflower-like growth on the outside of the cervix, or a silent penetrating tumor that grows into the cervical stoma. The ulcer or cauliflower (exophytic) type tends to signal its presence with irregular bleeding, whereas the internally growing tumor (endophytic) is asymptomatic for a long time during which metastases often occur. The endophytic tumor often causes a large hard, bulky, barrel-shaped cervix. The cervix may be larger than usual in some patients and in multiparous women. Rarely, the cervix may be swollen with infection, but such a cervix is not commonly regarded as barrel-shaped. Cervical ectopia could also cause a soft enlargement. A hard barrel-shaped cervix should prompt a workup for cervical cancer.

9. **D,** Page 889. A radical hysterectomy removes the entire uterus, upper vagina, and paracervical-parametrial tissue. A total hysterectomy removes only the entire uterus (cervix and fundus). Neither removes the tubes, ovaries, or pelvic or abdominal lymph nodes. If any of these structures is removed, the surgery is identified by stating what is done (eg, bilateral salpingo-oophorectomy, pelvic lymphadenectomy, paraaortic node dissection). Many patients do not realize the difference between these two procedures. Before the operative procedure, the patient should know exactly what is to be done. This requires time for careful counseling to ensure that the patient understands.

10. **B,** Page 906; See Figure 29–2. Points *A* and *B* are defined positions in the pelvis used for calculating radiation dosage. Point *A* is 2 cm cephalad to the vaginal fornix and 2 cm lateral to the cervical canal. Point *B* is 3 cm lateral to point *A* and is on or near the pelvic side wall. Because point *A* is closer to the source of brachytherapy, it receives a

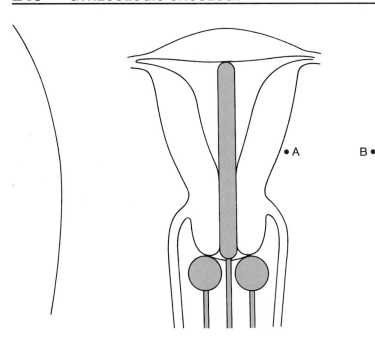

FIGURE 29–2 Points *A* and *B* with central stem (tandem) and two ovoids in place. (From Stenchever MA, Droegemueller W, Herbst AL, Mishell DR: Comprehensive Gynecology, 4th ed. St. Louis, Mosby, 1997.)

higher dose of ionizing radiation (approximately 85 Gy) than point *B* (approximately 50 to 60 Gy) during standard radiation therapy for invasive cervical carcinoma. Neither point *A* nor point *B* is a surgical landmark, nor do these points designate nodes or tumor spread.

11. **D,** Page 904, Surgical complications usually occur soon after the operation. These include bladder dysfunction, which is common and usually temporary. Genital urinary fistula and bowel obstruction may occur but not frequently. Hemorrhagic cystitis and vaginal stenosis are more apt to occur after radiation.

12. **C,** Page 907. Radiation complications can occur during treatment or at any later date, although most appear within 1 or 2 years. Diarrhea is common during treatment. Ulcerations of the vagina and cervix may occur. Postirradiation cystitis (hemorrhagic cystitis) may cause urinary frequency, dysuria, and bleeding. Fibrosis of the vagina or the ureters may be major problems for sexual and urinary function, respectively. Bowel fistulas and rectal bleeding may also occur. Bowel fistulas are more common than urinary fistulas, which may also occur after radiation, but with modern treatment they are rare, occurring most frequently in cases in which there is bulky tumor involvement near the bladder. The risk of radiation complications increases with increased radiation dose. Therefore, as the radiation doses increase to increase the frequency of cure, the rate of complication from the radiation also increases. Attempts are made to achieve an acceptable balance. With modern treatment, skin burn and bone marrow suppression are rare.

13. **E,** Page 902. Radiation can be used in severely ill patients at high risk for major operative procedures. However, in young women with small lesions, operation has the advantage of the preservation of ovarian and sexual function. It also allows for sampling of nodes to test for spread of tumor, which is a distinct advantage in determining the need for further treatment. In stage IB and IIA cervical carcinoma, the cure rate for operation and radiation therapy is similar but radiation treatment takes a longer time. Radiation is better for more advanced disease.

14. **C,** Page 908. There is evidence supporting partial radiation followed by radical hysterectomy within 3 months. For high stage tumors (ie, above IIA), chemoradiation may be best. Women with adenocarcinoma of the cervix tend to be nulliparous and older and are more likely to be diabetic than women with squamous cell cervical carcinoma. Adenocarcinoma of the cervix accounts for about 20% of cervical cancers. One rare type (clear cell) has an increased incidence in women with prior diethylstilbestrol (DES) exposure in utero. Like adenocarcinoma of the ovary, the course of adenocarcinoma of the cervix may be predicted by CA-125 levels.

15. **D,** Page 910. The definition of recurrence of cervical cancer is that it reappears 6 months or more after the time of therapy. If the tumor reappears within 6 months, it is considered persistent. Approximately 50% of recurrences occur in the pelvis. Chemotherapy for recurrent cervical cancer is not very effective, but currently the best response rate occurs with multiple-agent regimens that include cisplatin. These regimens have been

used with an increased survival in patients with positive nodes after radical hysterectomy. Renal function should be evaluated regularly because recurrences may cause ureteral compression or radiation treatment may cause stenosis. Radiation stenosis can occur several years after treatment. Unfortunately, recurrences may also involve nerves in the pelvic area and cause back and leg pain.

16. **B,** Page 895. A cervical cancer that is microscopic and measures between 3 and 5 mm in depth and no more than 7 mm wide is called *microinvasive* and is staged as a I (because it is confined to the cervix) A (because it is microscopic) 2 (because it is greater than 3 mm in depth and has a higher risk of involved pelvic nodes). Treatment may be modified if only microinvasion exists. Any diagnosis of microinvasion must be made by cervical conization; simple cervical punch biopsies cannot be relied on for diagnosis.

17. **C,** Page 901. Involvement of the endometrium by cervical squamous cell cancer does not change the stage but appears to predispose to distant metastasis. Treatment by stage remains the same, and the prognosis is similar stage for stage.

18. **C,** Pages 901–902. Other large bowel pathologic conditions such as diverticulosis may influence radiation therapy. Since the tumor is already known to be stage IIB, by definition it does not involve the bowel or nodes. Neither nodes nor ureters can be well assessed by a barium enema.

19. **C,** Page 904. Finding the positive nodes at surgery does not change the stage, but it does change the likelihood of cure to the range of 45% to 50%. However, the prognosis may be improved if the nodes are removed and the area is irradiated.

20. **C,** Page 906. The damage to tissue caused by radiation depends on the sensitivity of the tissue to radiation, the total dose, and the rate of delivery. The small bowel can be seriously damaged at doses above 50 Gy, especially if adhesions prevent its movement. The bladder and the rectum can usually tolerate 65 Gy or more, although late complications can occur. The ovarian stoma is tolerant, but the eggs are not, being destroyed by doses as low as 5 to 10 Gy. However, ovarian function will be lost anyway and therefore is not the limiting factor in the dose of radiation.

21. **C,** Pages 905–906. Most centers treat invasive cervical cancer with a total of 4500 to 5000 cGy of external radiation. Complications increase with increasing dosage, being about 8% with 4000 to 4500 cGy, 10% with 5000 cGy, and up to 32% with 5500 cGy. Additional local implants increase the total dose to between 50 and 65 Gy at the pelvic sidewall.

22. **E,** Page 906. Several studies have shown both recurrence and survival advantage using chemoradiation to treat advanced cervical carcinoma. There is increased toxicity especially to the hematologic system, but this is least when using one platinum-based agent. The chemotherapy and radiation therapy are given concomitantly. Chemoradiation is a major treatment advance and is more effective in bulky stage IB. This form of treatment may also be more effective in cervical stump cancer and when residual cancer is treated after inadvertent removal of an invasive cancer of the cervix by simple hysterectomy. Although all the reasons given may result in failure of radiation therapy, the most likely is dissemination of tumor outside the field of radiation. Another reason is failure to control the central tumor. The role of concomitant chemotherapy is not clear, but in some studies it seems to be beneficial with large tumors.

23. **B**, Page 910. Pregnant patients with cancer of the cervix have approximately the same stage-for-stage prognosis as nonpregnant patients. Delivery through the cervix does not seem to change the tumor prognosis, but hemorrhage is a serous complication and therefore vaginal delivery is best avoided. Diagnosis may require a cone; however, since this is a dangerous procedure during pregnancy, conization is used only if the diagnosis cannot be made by biopsy. Even microinvasion may wait until delivery for further evaluation. Although tumor in the episiotomy site has been reported, it is not common. Treatment is similar to that of the nonpregnant patient, although it may be delayed to allow delivery of a viable fetus.

24–27. 24, **E;** 25, **D;** 26, **B;** 27, **C;** Pages 901, 909 and Table 29–2 in Stenchever. Although individual reports may give somewhat different figures, the worldwide statistics from FIGO in 1993 showed

TABLE 29–1

Carcinoma of the Uterine Cervix: Distribution by Stage and 5-Year Survival Rates for Patients Treated in 1990–1992 ($n = 11,945$)

Stage	Patients (n)	5-Year Survival
Stage Ia	902	95.01%
Stage Ib	4657	80.1%
Stage II	3364	64.2%
Stage III	2530	38.31%
Stage IV	492	14%

Modified from Pecorelli et al: Annual report on the Results of Treatment in Grnaecological Cancer, XXIII Volume, Milan, 1998. Federation Internationale de Gynecologie et d'Obstetrique.

that the 5-year survival rate for stage I carcinoma of the cervix is approximately 85%; stage II, approximately 66%; stage III, approximately 39%; and stage IV, 11% (see Table 29–1). Patients with carcinoma of the cervix in pregnancy have the same survival rate, stage for stage, as patients who are not pregnant. Overall survival with early carcinoma discovered inadvertently after hysterectomy performed for another reason is approximately 70% whether additional surgery or adjunctive radiation therapy is employed, but it may be as high as 89% if the tumor is small and not transected. The exact percentage (which is different in different studies) is not as important as a general understanding of how the prognosis changes with the stage.

28–30. 28, **D**; 29, **C**; 30, **B**; Pages 890–891. Endometrial carcinoma is the most common of the genital tract cancers, but is causes relatively fewer deaths than either ovarian or cervical cancer because it is often found and treated early. Ovarian cancer is less common, but because of its silent early course, it is often not discovered until it has already metastasized. The incidence of cervical carcinoma has been decreased in part because of early detection of dysplastics lesions by routine Pap smears. However, the incidence rates have increased.

31–34. 31, **E**; 32, **D**; 33, **C**; 34, **A**; Page 899 and Figure 29–10 in Stenchever. A lesion confined to the cervix is stage I. It is stage IA if microscopic and stage IB if grossly visible. If it extends only to the paracervical tissue, it is stage II. If it extends to the distal third of the vagina, it is stage IIIA; if it extends to the pelvic sidewall, it is stage IIIB. Beyond that or if it extends to the bladder or the return, it is stage IV. (See Figure 29–1.)

35–37. 35, **A**; 36, **E**; 37, **C**; Pages 889, 892, 908. *Minimal deviation adenocarcinoma* is another name for adenoma malignum, which is a virulent adenocarcinoma that appears well differentiated. *Glassy cell* is a virulent adenosquamous carcinoma that grows rapidly and metastasizes early. *Microinvasive* is part of the spectrum between carcinoma in situ and invasive cancer. It is found in the cervix and is so small that it is only diagnosed microscopically. By definition, microinvasive adenocarcinoma is not < 5 mm in depth and 7 mm in width, giving a total of < 35 mm^2. *Exophytic* is a descriptive term that means external growth and, when one is referring to the cervix, it means that the tumor is growing on the portio of the cervix and is visible to the eye. *Verrucous* carcinoma looks like a wart, is slow-growing, and metastasizes infrequently.

CHAPTER 30

Neoplastic Diseases of the Uterus

for Questions 1–21: Select the one best answer or completion.

1. A 68-year-old woman complains of vaginal spotting. On examination, she has an atrophic vagina, a clean cervix with a closed os, and a normal-sized uterus. No masses are felt. A Pap smear is obtained from the exocervix. If this patient has endometrial carcinoma, in what percentage of cases will the Pap smear detect it?

   A. 10%
   B. 25%
   C. 50%
   D. 75%
   E. 90%

2. A 53-year-old woman undergoes dilatation and curettage (D&C) for postmenopausal bleeding. The pathology report states that she has a malignant glandular epithelium with areas of squamous metaplasia in the endometrium. What is the most likely diagnosis?

   A. adenocarcinoma
   B. adenoacanthoma
   C. adenosquamous cell carcinoma
   D. atypical adenomatous hyperplasia
   E. endolymphatic stromal myosis

3. A 63-year-old woman undergoes D&C for abnormal vaginal bleeding. On review of the pathology findings from the D&C, you see the pattern shown in Figure 30–1. Many sections appear similar, and no mitotic figures are visible. What is the diagnosis?

   A. clear cell adenocarcinoma
   B. cellular leiomyoma
   C. cystic endometrial hyperplasia
   D. malignant mixed müllerian tumor
   E. atypical adenomatous hyperplasia

4. A 36-year-old woman has undergone D&C for irregular bleeding. The procedure reveals adenomatous hyperplasia without atypia (complex hyperplasia). What can you tell the patient?

   A. Most such cases (more than 50%) progress to carcinoma within 8 to 12 years.
   B. Treatment should be hysterectomy.
   C. Induction of ovulation is contraindicated.
   D. Cyclic progestin therapy should promote monthly withdrawal.
   E. Repeat endometrial sampling is not necessary.

5. A 61-year-old woman with irregular uterine bleeding had complex endometrial hyperplasia with atypia on D&C. The risk of finding carcinoma in her uterus, when the specimen is examined after hysterectomy, is approximately

   A. 1%
   B. 10%
   C. 25%
   D. 50%
   E. 75%

6. A 47-year-old woman has a poorly differentiated endometrial carcinoma and a uterine cavity that measures 10 cm in depth. The endocervix has stromal invasion of endometrial carcinoma, but no other structure is involved. What is the stage of her endometrial cancer?

   A. IA
   B. IB
   C. IC
   D. IIA
   E. IIB

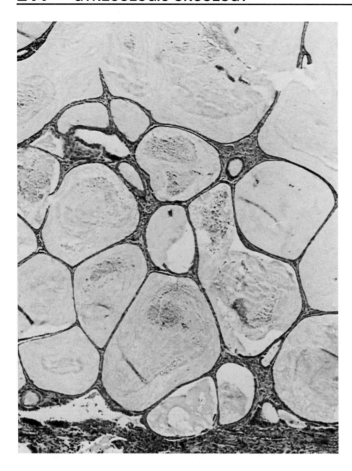

FIGURE 30–1 (From Christopherson WM, Gray LA: In Coppleson M, ed: Gynecologic Oncology. Edinburgh, Churchill-Livingstone, 1981.)

7. A morbidly obese woman undergoes preoperative evaluation for adenocarcinoma of the endometrium. Because of the high risk associated with an abdominal procedure, vaginal surgery is being considered. What tumor marker may be of help in her condition?

   A. human chorionic gonadotropin (hCG)
   B. carcino-embryonic antigen (CEA)
   C. alpha-fetoprotein
   D. CA-125

8. A 52-year-old woman with moderately differentiated endometrial cancer was surgically staged. Her uterus had sounded to 12 cm, and there was no cervical involvement. The cancer was limited to the endometrium. Peritoneal cytologic tests and pelvic and periaortic nodes were negative. According to the most recent (1988) FIGO uterine corpus cancer staging, the stage of this case is

   A. IA
   B. IB
   C. IC
   D. IIA
   E. IIB

9. Which is the most common malignancy of the female genital tract?

   A. endometrial carcinoma
   B. cervical carcinoma
   C. tubal carcinoma
   D. vulvar carcinoma
   E. ovarian carcinoma

10. Which stage III tumor is most likely to respond to progesterone therapy?

    A. carcinoma of the cervix
    B. ovarian carcinoma
    C. endometrial carcinoma
    D. vulvar carcinoma
    E. vaginal carcinoma

11. What dose of medroxyprogesterone therapy has been shown to be effective in the management of recurrent endometrial cancer?

    A. 50 mg/day
    B. 100 mg/day
    C. 200 mg/day
    D. 100 mg/week
    E. 200 mg/week

12. Of the following cytotoxic chemotherapeutic agents, which would be least likely to be used in a patient who has persistence or recurrence of stage III endometrial adenocarcinoma?

    A. cyclophosphamide (Cytoxan)
    B. doxorubicin (Adriamycin)
    C. cisplatin (Platinol)
    D. 5-FU (Adrucil)
    E. mitomycin (Mutamycin)

13. A 57-year-old woman has homologous uterine sarcoma. What is the current recommended primary treatment?

    A. radiation
    B. chemotherapy
    C. operation
    D. operation and chemotherapy
    E. operation and irradiation

14. Ninety percent of adenocarcinomas of the endometrium that recur do so within approximately

    A. 1 year
    B. 3 years
    C. 5 years
    D. 10 years
    E. 20 years

15. Which is the most common sarcoma of the uterus?

    A. endometrial stromal sarcoma
    B. rhabdomyosarcoma
    C. liposarcoma
    D. endolymphatic stroma myosis
    E. leiomyosarcoma

16. A 56-year-old patient is found to have both an endometrial adenocarcinoma and a rhabdomyosarcoma of the uterus. The tumor is best described as a(n)

    A. heterologous sarcoma
    B. endometrial stromal sarcoma
    C. homologous sarcoma
    D. carcinosarcoma
    E. malignant mixed müllerian tumor

17. The World Health Organization has developed terms to classify endometrial hyperplasias. In this system, the term *complex hyperplasia* refers to

    A. atypical adenomatous hyperplasia
    B. cystic hyperplasia
    C. adenomatous hyperplasia
    D. carcinoma in situ
    E. hyperplasia combined with squamous metaplasia

18. During a routine annual examination, a 58-year-old woman asks about the risk of developing uterine cancer. Which of the following is *not* an independent risk factor for endometrial cancer?

    A. age between 55 and 65
    B. late menopause
    C. hypertension
    D. nulliparity
    E. polycystic ovarian disease

19. Tamoxifen therapy has been shown to increase the risk of

    A. endometrial cancer
    B. breast cancer
    C. ovarian cancer
    D. cervical cancer
    E. vulvar cancer

20. In which of the following cases of endometrial adenocarcinoma should paraaortic and pelvic node sampling *not* be done?

    A. endometrial adenocarcinoma, stage I, grade 1
    B. endometrial adenocarcinoma, stage I, grade 2
    C. endometrial adenocarcinoma, stage II
    D. uterine papillary serous carcinoma, stage I

21. A 62-year-old otherwise healthy woman who is not undergoing hormone replacement therapy or taking any other medication comes to the clinic with a concern about possible vaginal bleeding. Pelvic examination reveals an atrophic vagina, a stenotic cervix, and a uterus that is at the upper limit of normal size and mobile without any masses. No bleeding is evident at the time of the examination. An attempt at office endometrial biopsy is unsuccessful because of the cervical stenosis. A transvaginal ultrasonogram reveals an endometrial stripe of 3 mm. Which of the following should be done?

    A. examination and D&C with the patient under anesthesia
    B. repeat attempt to perform endometrial biopsy in clinic
    C. follow-up with ultrasound imaging
    D. total abdominal hysterectomy and bilateral salpingo-oophorectomy
    E. pelvic irradiation

DIRECTIONS:

for Questions 22–35: For each numbered item, select the one heading most closely associated with it. Each lettered heading may be used once, more than once, or not at all.

(A) no further treatment
(B) Provera 10 mg daily on a cyclic basis
(C) Clomid 50 mg on days 1–5
(D) Megace 40–320 mg/day
(E) hysterectomy with bilateral salpingo-oophorectomy

22–24.   Match the following patients with the most appropriate treatment.

22. A 28-year-old woman with complex endometrial hyperplasia found on D&C

23. A 58-year-old woman with atypical complex endometrial hyperplasia

24. A 30-year-old anovulatory woman who wants a pregnancy now but who has atypical complex endometrial hyperplasia

25–29.   Match the photomicrographs with the appropriate diagnosis.

(A) Figure 30–2
(B) Figure 30–3
(C) Figure 30–4
(D) Figure 30–5
(E) Figure 30–6

25. Complex hyperplasia

26. Papillary serous carcinoma

27. Atypical complex hyperplasia

28. Adenocarcinoma with squamous elements (adenoacanthoma)

29. Adenocarcinoma of the endometrium

30–32.   Match each description of a patient with endometrial carcinoma with the correct answer.

(A) grade 1
(B) grade 3
(C) spread only to the endometrium
(D) spread to the middle third of the myometrium
(E) spread to the outer third of the myometrium

30. Greatest risk for node metastasis

31. Greatest risk of recurrence

32. Highest level of estrogen receptors

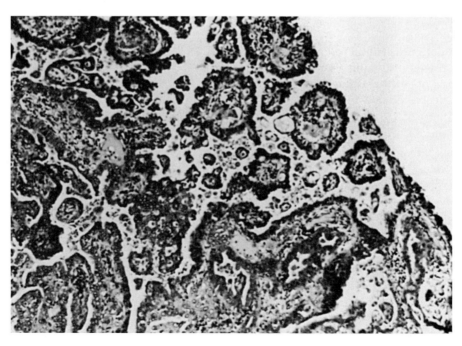

FIGURE 30–2

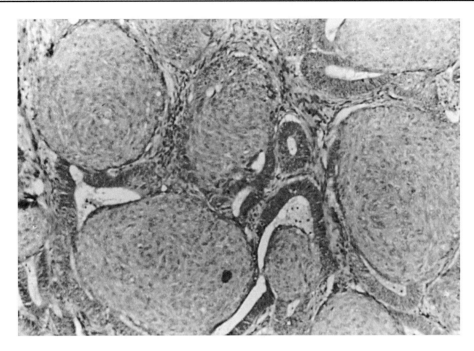

FIGURE 30–3

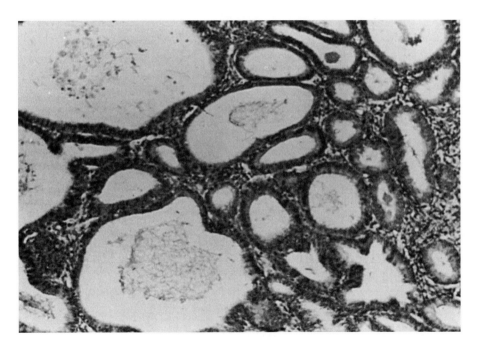

FIGURE 30–4

33–35. Match each pathologic finding with the type of uterine sarcoma.

(A) leiomyosarcoma
(B) benign squamous cells plus adenocarcinoma
(C) rhabdomyosarcoma
(D) squamous cell carcinoma and adenocarcinoma
(E) sarcoma and adenocarcinoma

33. Homologous sarcoma

34. Heterologous sarcoma

35. Malignant mixed müllerian tumor

FIGURE 30–5

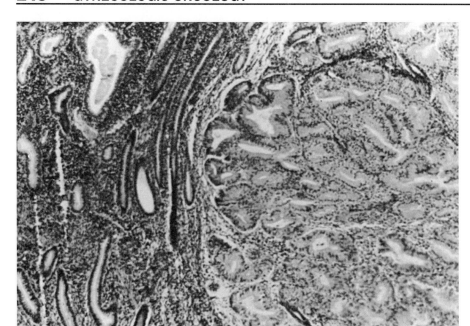

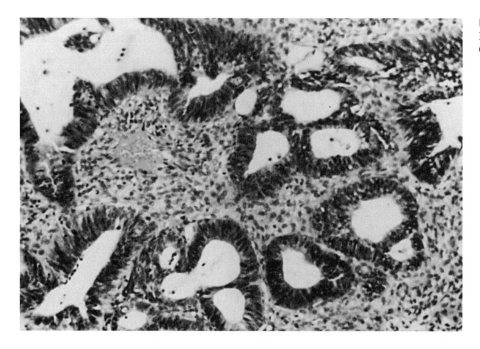

FIGURE 30–6 (Courtesy Robert C. Maier, M.D., Medical College of Georgia.)

ANSWERS

1. **C,** Page 927. A Pap smear has a false-negative rate of about 20% for cervical cancer and at least a 50% false-negative rate for endometrial cancer. Obviously, it is not a good test for endometrial cancer. To rule out endometrial cancer, a thorough sample from the endometrium must be obtained by curettage, preferably with separate samples from the endometrium and the endocervix. The primary symptom of endometrial carcinoma is postmenopausal bleeding.

2. **B,** Page 927. Malignant glandular epithelium in the uterus is adenocarcinoma. A mixture of benign squamous cell epithelium with malignant glandular epithelium is called an *adenoacanthoma*. An adenoacanthoma carries approximately the same prognosis as adenocarcinoma of the same grade and stage and should be treated similarly. If both adenomatous and squamous components were malignant, the tumor would be an adenosquamous cell carcinoma. Atypical adenomatous

hyperplasia is a premalignant lesion in which there is crowding of glands and cytologic atypia. Endolymphatic stromal myosis is a low-grade stromal sarcoma.

3. **C,** Page 922; Figure 30–3 (in Stenchever). The glands are dilated, but the cellular architecture is benign and there is no invasion. A classic benign Swiss-cheese configuration is noted; therefore, the diagnosis is cystic endometrial hyperplasia or simple hyperplasia. Clear cell adenocarcinoma has many malignant cells with clear cytoplasm. A cellular leiomyoma would have whorls of connective tissue cells. A mixed müllerian tumor would have mitotic figures in connective tissue cells. Adenomatous hyperplasia has a crowded glandular architecture with no invasion.

4. **D,** Page 925. Progression of adenomatous hyperplasia is slow and occurs in only a small number of cases. Usually the D&C is therapeutic, but either progestin (if no pregnancy is wanted) or clomiphene (Clomid) for ovulation induction (if pregnancy is desired) is a proven treatment. Hysterectomy is not warranted for adenomatous hyperplasia alone. Repeat endometrial curettage is advised to assess the completeness of the cure.

5. **C,** Page 925. Older women with atypical hyperplasia are at risk both for already having carcinoma (approximately 28%) and for future carcinoma (25%). For this reason, the postmenopausal patient with proven atypical hyperplasia is best treated by hysterectomy.

6. **E,** Page 929; Table 30–4 in Stenchever. The involvement of the cervical stroma by invasive endometrial carcinoma makes the endometrial carcinoma stage IIB. The depth of the uterus does not influence surgical staging, but it is used if only radiation therapy is selected. The reason for doing a fractional D&C during the diagnostic process is to rule out both cervical extension of endometrial invasive tumor and primary cervical carcinoma. Stage IIA would involve only the endocervical glands.

7. **D,** Pages 934–935. Sometimes very obese patients are encountered for whom an abdominal operation is very risky. It has been reported that stage I patients with CA-125 < 20 U/mL have a risk of extrauterine disease of less than 3%, thereby making vaginal hysterectomy a therapeutic option. Another report found that CA-125 levels above 35 U/mL usually predicted extrauterine disease. False-positive cases have been reported, so the results may prove to be a useful guide but are not sufficiently precise to be the sole criterion for performing lymphadenectomy.

8. **A,** Page 929; Table 30–4 in Stenchever. The most recent uterine corpus cancer staging relies on operative evaluation. The older staging is used if irradiation treatment is chosen because the depth of invasion and cytologic washings cannot be evaluated. The depth of the uterine cavity is not a factor in surgical staging, but the extent of proven invasion of the uterus is a factor. In this case, although the uterus was large, the cancer involved only the endometrium and therefore was stage IA. Because the carcinoma was moderately differentiated (G2), node sampling should be done.

9. **A,** Page 920. Although the most common malignancy of the female genital tract is endometrial adenocarcinoma, fewer deaths occur from this disease than from either ovarian or cervical cancer. This is largely because endometrial adenocarcinoma is detected and treated in an early stage. Early detection is possible because irregular uterine bleeding occurs early and is the most common presenting symptom.

10. **C,** Page 941. Progesterone is used in the management of both recurrence and metastasis of endometrial carcinoma. The tumor is more likely to respond if it is well differentiated. Response rates of 10% to 30% have been reported. The rate seems to be higher in patients whose tumors have the largest number of progesterone receptors. Other forms of cytotoxic chemotherapy also have been used. Cytotoxic drugs appear to have a better response rate if the tumor is undifferentiated.

11. **C,** Page 949. Progestin therapy results in responses of 10% to 20% in recurrent endometrial carcinoma. The highest response rates are in tumors with elevated sex steroid receptor levels, well-differentiated tumors, and recurrences at sites not previously irradiated. A dosage of medroxyprogesterone 200 mg/day is effective.

12. **E,** Page 941. The primary chemotherapeutic agent used in endometrial adenocarcinoma is a progestin. Tamoxifen has also been used because it seems to increase the number of progesterone receptors in the tumor tissue. Neither of these agents is cytotoxic, however. In the cytotoxic group, cyclophosphamide, doxorubicin, cisplatin, and 5-FU are frequently used in combination for endometrial carcinoma. Mitomycin has been used primarily in gastric cancer.

13. **C,** Page 944. The treatment for homologous uterine sarcoma is surgical. Metastases or recurrences are usually treated with multiagent chemotherapy. Radiation has not been shown to increase survival significantly, although it appears to decrease the risk of pelvic recurrence. Distant metastases are common and most often occur in the lungs or abdomen. Chemotherapy has been used, but it has not improved survival.

14. **C,** Page 941. Ninety percent of adenocarcinomas of the endometrium that recur do so within 5 years,

but since 10% recur later, prolonged follow-up is important. The most frequent site of recurrence is the pelvis (approximately 50%), followed by the lung (17%).

15. **E,** Page 943. Leiomyosarcomas account for nearly 50% of all uterine sarcomas. They are diagnosed if the tumor contains more than five mitoses per 10 high-power fields. The more mitoses present, the worse the prognosis. Endolymphatic stromal myosis is a more benign form of endometrial stromal sarcoma, both of which are rare. The heterologous rhabdomyosarcoma, liposarcoma, chondrosarcoma, and osteosarcoma are less common than the homologous types. In total, sarcomas account for less than 5% of uterine malignancies.

16. **E,** Pages 946–947. If a uterine sarcoma forms mesenchymal tissue normally found in the uterus, it is called a *homologous sarcoma*. If it forms mesenchymal tissue not normally found in the uterus (eg, bone, fat, striated muscle, and cartilage), it is called *heterologous*. If the heterologous sarcoma is present in combination with adenocarcinoma, it is called a *malignant müllerian mixed tumor (MMMT)*. Prior pelvic radiation therapy is a predisposing factor, having been performed in approximately 12% of patients with MMMT. If an adenocarcinoma and a homologous sarcoma coexist, this tumor may be called a carcinosarcoma. Endolymphatic stromal myosis is a rare low-grade sarcoma made up of cells resembling the endometrial stroma. These are most often found in premenopausal women. Endometrial stromal sarcoma is a more malignant version of the same cell type.

17. **C,** Page 922. Pathologists frequently change terminology. Clinicians must keep abreast of these changes so that the changes will add to, rather than detract from, patient care. Complex hyperplasia refers to adenomatous hyperplasia without atypia.

18. **C,** Page 920. The prevalence of cancer of the endometrium is greatest between the ages of 55 and 65. Other risk factors include unopposed estrogen from any source, such as estrogen-producing ovarian tumors, polycystic ovarian disease, late menopause, obesity, or oral intake of estrogens. Unopposed estrogen, whether from exogenous or endogenous sources, provides a prolonged estrogen effect on the endometrium. Progestins or progesterone decrease formation of estrogen receptors, stimulate the conversion of estradiol to estrone, and promote sloughing of the endometrium when the agent is withdrawn. Hypertension, by itself and unrelated to obesity, is not a risk factor for endometrical carcinoma. African-American women and women with HER-2/NEU oncogene or mutant p53 suppressor gene overexpression experience poorer survival if they have endometrial carcinoma.

19. **A,** Page 921. Women who take tamoxifen for breast carcinoma are at increased risk for endometrial cancer. Tamoxifen is not known to increase the risk of ovarian, cervical, breast, or vulvar cancer.

20. **A,** Page 935. The spread to nodes in stage I, grade 1 adenocarcinoma is less than 2%, and with this low risk of nodal involvement, routine sampling is not warranted. With stage I, grade 2 the risk is approximately 11%; it rises to 25% to 30% in stage I, grade 3 adenocarcinoma. Stage II carries increased risk of pelvic node spread because there is cervical involvement. In papillary serous carcinoma, there is a high rate of extrauterine spread even without myometrial invasion.

21. **C,** Page 924. In cases of questionable uterine bleeding, patients with an endometrial stripe of less than 4 mm have such a low chance of endometrial cancer that they may be followed up with ultrasound examinations unless bleeding was definitely shown to be from the uterus and it persisted. Most likely, the bleeding in this case came from the atrophic vagina. A small amount of estrogen cream may be beneficial. Patients who have been undergoing tamoxifen therapy for breast cancer usually have a thickened endometrial stripe; in the absence of bleeding, this condition can be followed up without endometrial biopsy.

22–24. 22, **B;** 23, **E;** 24, **C;** Page 925. A young woman with benign endometrial hyperplasia could be treated with administration of cyclic progestins (eg, Provera 10 mg for 10 to 14 days each month), which induces monthly withdrawal bleeding. A postmenopausal woman with atypical endometrial hyperplasia (called *carcinoma in situ* by some pathologists) should undergo definitive treatment with removal of the uterus unless medically contraindicated. A young anovulatory woman who desires pregnancy but who has atypical endometrial hyperplasia may be treated with clomiphene citrate to induce ovulation if it is not occurring spontaneously. If successful, this therapy interrupts the continuous unopposed estrogen that had previously stimulated the endometrium.

25–29. 25, **C;** 26, **A;** 27, **E;** 28, **B;** 29, **D;** Pages 922–929. Complex hyperplasia is identified by crowded irregular glands without significant cytologic atypia. Papillary serous carcinoma is a highly malignant form of endometrial carcinoma that has a papillary form resembling papillary serous adenocarcinoma of the ovary. Atypical adenomatous hyperplasia is a premalignant variant of endometrial hyperplasia. It involves cytologic atypia but no invasion. An adenoacanthoma is an endometrical carcinoma that has islands of benign squamous cells. An invasive carcinoma of the endometrium is present on the right side of the figure. It is moderately differential adenocarcinoma and has crowded glands and cellular atypia with stromal invasion.

30–32. 30, **E;** 31, **E;** 32, **A;** Pages 929–931. The highest levels of estrogen receptors usually occur in well-differentiated (ie, grade I) tumors; lower values are noted in grade III tumors. The risk for nodal metastasis is the lowest in grade I tumors with only the endometrium involved. The risk for nodal metastasis rises as the grade of tumor increases and the depth of invasion increases to the outer third of the uterus.

33–35. 33, **A;** 34, **C;** 35, **E;** Pages 942–947. Homologous sarcomas are made up of tissues that are normally found in the uterus, including leiomyosarcomas and endometrial stromal sarcomas. Heterologous sarcomas are those arising from tissues not normally found in the uterus, such as chondrosarcomas, rhabdomyosarcomas, osteosarcomas, and liposarcomas. They may be found alone or mixed with epithelial adenocarcinoma, in which case they are called *malignant mixed müllerian tumors* or *carcinosarcomas*. In uterine sarcomas, the operative stage and the mitotic index are the most important predictors of outcome. A finding of more than five mitoses per 10 high-powered fields justifies a diagnosis of leiomyosarcoma. If there are four mitoses or less than 10 high-powered fields, the course is usually benign. The higher the number of mitoses, the worse the prognosis. Although often discussed, leiomyosarcomas are rare, with the reported incidence being approximately 2 to 4 per 1000 myomas.

Neoplastic Diseases of the Ovary

DIRECTIONS:

for Questions 1–16: Select the one best answer or completion.

1. A 55-year-old woman has an asymptomatic ovarian carcinoma in one ovary. Although her peritoneal cavity is free of tumor, her retroperitoneal nodes are positive for the malignancy. The stage of her ovarian tumor is

   A. IA
   B. IIA
   C. IIB
   D. III
   E. IV

2. The approximate age at which the peak incidence of ovarian cancer occurs is

   A. 40
   B. 55
   C. 65
   D. 75
   E. 85

3. Pseudomyxoma peritonei typically is the result of a rupture of a(n)

   A. mucinous borderline tumor
   B. serous tumor
   C. dysgerminoma
   D. mature teratoma
   E. immature teratoma

4. The cell origin of the most common type of ovarian neoplasm is

   A. germ cells
   B. epithelial cells
   C. stromal cells
   D. lipoid cells
   E. sex cord cells

5. A rare virilizing tumor of the ovary is a

   A. polyembryoma
   B. mucinous cystadenocarcinoma
   C. fibroma
   D. dysgerminoma
   E. Sertoli-Leydig cell tumor

6. A 3-cm right adnexal cyst is noted on routine pelvic examination of a 65-year-old woman. The appropriate management is to

   A. offer reassurance
   B. repeat the examination in 2 to 3 months
   C. suppress the ovary with cyclic estrogen and progesterone
   D. order transvaginal ultrasonography
   E. perform a laparotomy

7. In the patient referred to in Question 6, the additional blood test that might aid in determining management is one for

   A. carcinoembryonic antigen
   B. CA-125
   C. quantitative human chorionic gonadotrophin (β–hCG)
   D. serum estrogen
   E. α-fetoprotein

8. A 67-year-old woman has a breast mass and firm, bilaterally enlarged ovaries. A breast biopsy reveals a mucin-secreting carcinoma. The most likely ovarian diagnosis is

   A. normal ovaries
   B. dysgerminoma
   C. clear cell carcinoma
   D. Brenner tumor
   E. Krukenberg tumor

9. A 30-year-old asymptomatic woman comes to you for a routine gynecologic evaluation and renewal of her birth control prescription. During an otherwise normal pelvic examination, you discover an 8-cm left ovarian cyst. This patient should

A. have her next examination in a year
B. be reevaluated in 2 to 3 months
C. take two birth control pills a day and return in 2 to 3 months
D. undergo computed tomography (CT) of the abdomen and pelvis
E. be scheduled for surgical evaluation

10. The most common type of epithelial tumor is

A. mucinous
B. endometrioid
C. serous
D. clear cell
E. Brenner

11. After complete resection of a stage II ovarian carcinoma, chemotherapy including melphalan (Alkeran) is considered. A major long-term side effect of melphalan is

A. destruction of lymphocytes
B. cardiac toxicity
C. increased risk of leukemia
D. stomatitis
E. pulmonary fibrosis

12. A 60-year-old woman who is not taking any medication experiences postmenopausal bleeding. On pelvic examination, she has a pink, rugated vagina and a 5 × 6 × 4 cm firm right ovarian mass. Office curettage reveals adenomatous endometrial hyperplasia without atypia. The ovarian tumor that would best account for these findings is a

A. serous cystadenoma
B. mucinous cystadenocarcinoma
C. teratoma
D. dysgerminoma
E. granulosa cell tumor

13. A 45-year-old woman who has a mutation in the BRCA-1 gene undergoes prophylactic total abdominal hysterectomy and bilateral salpingo-oophorectomy. Four years later, she experiences a diffuse intraabdominal metastatic carcinoma that is histologically similar to ovarian serous cystadenocarcinoma. The most likely diagnosis of this cancer is

A. pancreatic
B. colon
C. thyroid
D. gastric
E. primary peritoneal

14. The second most common type of ovarian neoplasm is

A. epithelial
B. germ cell
C. stromal
D. lipoid
E. gonadoblastoma

15. In a 22-year-old, the recommended initial treatment of a pure dysgerminoma, 6 cm in diameter and confined to one ovary, is

A. chemotherapy
B. radiation therapy to the pelvis
C. radical hysterectomy and bilateral salpingo-oophorectomy
D. total abdominal hysterectomy, bilateral salpingo-oophorectomy, and omentectomy
E. unilateral salpingo-oophorectomy

16. A 24-year-old gravida 0 is undergoing laparotomy for a 6-cm adnexal mass. The mass is shelled out of the ovary and submitted for frozen section. The latter is not definitive in ruling out a malignancy. The most appropriate next step is to

A. close the ovary and close the abdomen without removing any additional ovarian tissue
B. proceed to a unilateral oophorectomy
C. proceed to a unilateral salpingo-oophorectomy
D. proceed to a total abdominal hysterectomy and bilateral salpingo-oophorectomy
E. proceed to a total abdominal hysterectomy and unilateral salpingo-oophorectomy

DIRECTIONS:

for Questions 17–23: For each numbered item, select the one heading most closely associated with it. Each lettered heading may be used once, more than once, or not at all.

17–19. **Match each photomicrograph with the appropriate ovarian epithelial neoplasm.**

    (A) serous cystadenoma
    (B) mucinous cystadenoma
    (C) endometrioid carcinoma
    (D) clear cell adenocarcinoma
    (E) Brenner cell tumor

17. Figure 31–1

18. Figure 31–2

19. Figure 31–3

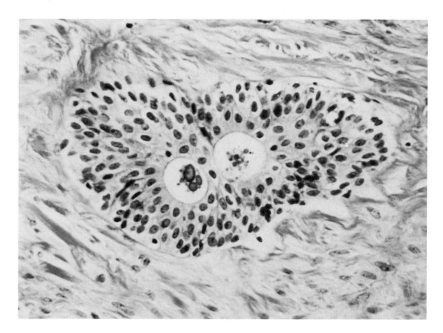

FIGURE 31–1

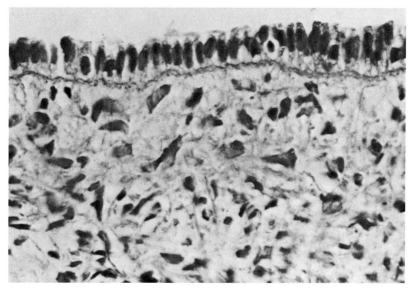

FIGURE 31–2

FIGURE 31–3

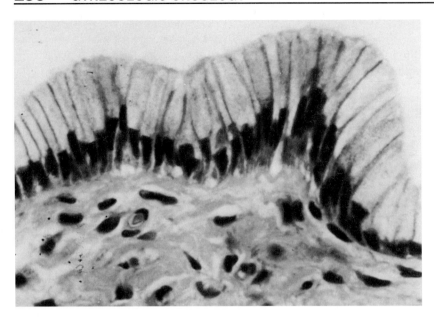

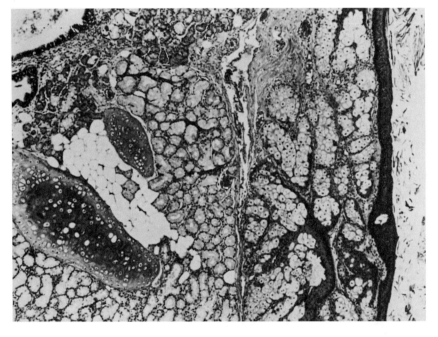

FIGURE 31–4 (From Serov SF, Scully RE and Sobin LH: Histologic typing of ovarian tumors, Geneva, 1973, World Health Organization.)

20–23. **Match each photomicrograph with the appropriate ovarian neoplasm.**

    A. benign cystic teratoma
    B. dysgerminoma
    C. granulosa cell tumor
    D. Krukenberg tumor
    E. endodermal sinus tumor

    20. Figure 31–4

    21. Figure 31–5

    22. Figure 31–6

    23. Figure 31–7

FIGURE 31–5 (From Scully RE: Germ cell tumors of the ovary and fallopian tube. In Meigs JV and Sturgis SH (eds). Progress in gynecology, vol 4. New York, 1963, Grune & Stratton.)

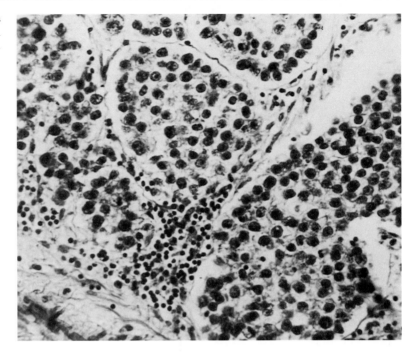

FIGURE 31–6

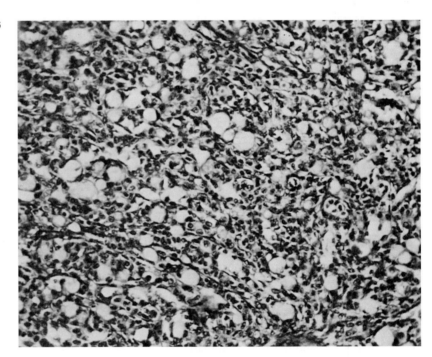

DIRECTIONS:

for Questions 24–27: Select the one best answer or completion.

24. **Which of the following has been shown to be a risk factor for ovarian cancer?**

    A. use of oral contraceptives
    B. pregnancy
    C. breast-feeding
    D. ovulation-inducing drugs
    E. BRCA-2 mutation

25. **The BRCA-1 tumor suppressor gene is on chromosome**

    A. 4
    B. 7
    C. 13
    D. 17
    E. 20

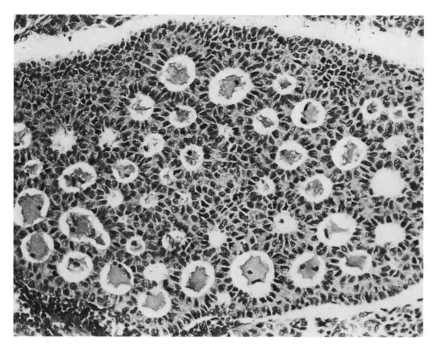

FIGURE 31–7

26. CA-125 is most commonly expressed by what type of ovarian cancer?

    A. epithelial
    B. fibrous stromal
    C. germ cell
    D. lipoid
    E. sex cord stromal

27. Currently, the most usual treatment for advanced ovarian carcinoma includes total abdominal hysterectomy, bilateral salpingo-oophorectomy, debulking, and chemotherapy with a

    A. single alkylating agent
    B. platinum-based agent alone
    C. platinum-based agent plus an alkylating agent
    D. platinum-based agent plus paclitaxel
    E. platinum-based agent plus paclitaxel plus an alkylating agent

DIRECTIONS:

for Questions 28–33: Choose the requested number of correct responses.

28. Which two of the following factors increase the occurrence of ovarian cancer?

    A. increased total number of ovulation
    B. eating vegetables
    C. living in an industrialized country
    D. occluded fallopian tubes
    E. oral contraceptives

29. Surgery for stage II ovarian mucinous adenocarcinoma in a 55-year-old patient includes total abdominal hysterectomy, bilateral salpingo-oophorectomy, and which four of the following?

    A. omentectomy
    B. peritoneal washings for cytologic study
    C. periaortic node biopsy
    D. appendectomy
    E. cholecystectomy

30. In cases of ovarian malignancy, the prognosis is related to which four of the following?

    A. stage
    B. cell type
    C. amount of residual tumor after resection
    D. grade
    E. age at time of surgery

31. The preoperative workup of a 58-year-old patient with a persistent left adnexal mass should always include which two of the following?

    A. history and physical examination
    B. CT
    C. barium enema
    D. informed consent
    E. EKG

32. **Unilateral oophorectomy alone for borderline ovarian tumors is adequate therapy if which four of the following criteria are met?**

    A. The contralateral ovary is normal.
    B. Peritoneal cytologic findings are negative.
    C. Omental and peritoneal biopsies are negative.
    D. Retroperitoneal nodes are found to be negative.
    E. Extensive pathologic sampling shows grade 0.

33. **Which two of the following are descriptive of hereditary ovarian cancer?**

    A. usually are germ cell cancers
    B. are quite lethal
    C. requires prophylactic oophorectomy at menopause
    D. accounts for less than 10% of ovarian cancers
    E. occurs late in life

ANSWERS

1. **D,** Page 966; Table 31–5 in Stenchever. Staging of ovarian cancer is based on the findings of clinical examination and surgical exploration, including the histologic features of the specimen and cytologic aspects of fluids. In this case, the extension of the tumor to the retroperitoneal nodes places the patient in stage III. About 10% to 20% of women with carcinoma apparently confined to one ovary have been found to have retroperitoneal lymph node involvement at the time of surgery. The 5-year survival rate for stage III ovarian carcinoma is approximately 15%.

2. **D,** Page 956; Figure 31–1 in Stenchever. Ovarian cancer causes more deaths in women than any other genital malignancy. This is due to a lack of symptoms early in the disease. Until the tumor is widespread, patients are asymptomatic. Therefore, ovarian malignancies are detected and treated late in the course of their progression. The highest incidence is in patients in their mid to late 70s.

3. **A,** Page 971. The rupture of a borderline mucinous tumor allows the spread of mucin-producing cells in the abdomen. These cells yield a large amount of mucinous material, and their growth often leads to bowel obstruction. The intraabdominal accumulation of mucin is called *pseudomyxoma peritonei.* This condition can cause disability and death, although it is not frankly malignant. Residual cells may respond to cyclophosphamide (Cytoxan), doxorubicin (Adriamycin), and cisplatin combination chemotherapy. Because pseudomyxoma can originate in the appendix, an appendectomy is indicated whenever a mucinous ovarian tumor is removed.

4. **B,** Page 958. Ovarian neoplasms are formed from tissues that constitute the normal ovary. These include the epithelial lining (which is the most common source of tumors), germ cells, sex cord cells, and stroma. Very rarely, tumors arise from lymphatics, blood vessels, or nerves within the ovary. Occasionally, carcinoma originating in other organs metastasizes to the ovary.

5. **E,** Pages 958, 988. Sertoli-Leydig cell tumors are the male homologue of granulosa theca cell tumors. They are very rare and may produce androgens that cause virilization in young women. Most behave as low-grade malignancies, with 5-year survival rates of 70% to 90%. Survival rates are higher when the tumor is better differentiated. Polyembryomas and dysgerminomas are both rare malignancies of germ cell origin. Mucinous tumors are derived from the epithelium of the ovary, and a fibroma arises from nonfunctioning stroma.

6. **D,** Page 962. The ovary decreases in size in the postmenopausal years and should be no larger than 1.5 cm in greatest diameter. At this age, no physiologic enlargement should occur. Direct visualization by surgery is indicated if the mass is greater than 5 cm in diameter. Recent studies suggest that a simple cystic mass less than 5 cm in size in postmenopausal patients can be managed with follow-up. Ultrasonography aids in determining whether there are solid areas or papillae, both indications for surgical intervention.

7. **B,** Page 962. The addition of CA-125 may aid in the management of postmenopausal women with adnexal masses. Levels above the normal of 35 U/mL indicate a higher likelihood of malignancy. Such levels are also associated with benign conditions such as endometriosis, but using this serum assay in conjunction with ultrasound imaging appears to help determine when surgical intervention is appropriate in the postmenopausal patient.

8. **E,** Page 989. Krukenberg tumors of the ovary contain mucin-producing signet-ring cells and are usually metastatic from the gastrointestinal tract (most commonly) or the breast. In this case, with a known mucin-secreting tumor of the breast, bilateral ovarian metastases are most likely. Dysgerminomas may occur in older adults but are more common in young women; they are also rarely bilateral. Fibromas and Brenner tumors are also rarely bilateral, and clear cell carcinomas are relatively rare malignant ovarian epithelial tumors. In this case, it would be extremely unwise to dismiss the ovaries, which are described as enlarged, as being normal.

9. **E,** Pages 171–173, 959, 965. In a reproductive-aged woman who is not taking birth control pills or other ovarian suppressive treatment, the development of physiologic ovarian cysts is common and requires only observation for a short time. Most physiologic ovarian cysts resolve within one cycle. However, because birth control pills containing more than 35 µg of ethinyl estradiol are likely to suppress physiologic ovarian cysts, any cyst that occurs while such oral contraceptives are being taken is much more likely to be a neoplasm. In this patient, the 8-cm size also arouses concern. Therefore, such patients should be evaluated surgically. CT or ultrasonography cannot reliably distinguish between physiologic and neoplastic lesions, although identification of anything other than a unilocular cyst would increase the need for surgical exploration.

10. **C,** Page 958; Table 31–3 in Stenchever. Epithelial tumors are the most common neoplasms of the ovary, and serous tumors are the most common epithelial tumors. Like most ovarian neoplasms, serous tumors can be either benign or malignant. Malignant serous tumors have the worst prognosis of all the epithelial tumors. They are bilateral in 33% to 66% of cases.

11. **C,** Pages 974–975. Alkeran (melphalan) causes bone marrow depression within 2 weeks. Alkylating agents also have the long-term side effect of increasing the risk of leukemia. This risk may range from 2% to as high as 10% within 8 years of therapy. It is therefore important to give such agents only if the benefits of their use are significant. Chemotherapy with paclitaxel, carboplatin, or cisplatin is the more usual chemotherapy at this time. Platinum-based chemotherapy may increase the risk of leukemia also, but such therapy still has a positive risk/benefit ratio. Stomatitis commonly occurs as an acute side effect of antimetabolites. Pulmonary fibrosis occurs with bleomycin use, and cardiac toxicity occurs with doxorubicin use. Renal damage is a significant concern with cisplatin.

12. **E,** Page 986. Sex cord–stromal tumors account for about 6% of all ovarian neoplasms. Some of these produce hormones. This woman has signs of an estrogen effect without taking any replacement hormones or medications. Such symptoms together with a firm adnexal mass make the possibility of a granulosa or theca cell tumor highly likely. Inhibin may serve as a tumor marker for some granulosa cell tumors. These tumors behave as low-grade carcinomas and are primarily treated surgically. A total abdominal hysterectomy and bilateral salpingo-oophorectomy should be performed in a patient of this age with such a tumor.

13. **E,** Pages 969, 970. Primary peritoneal carcinoma is associated with the BRCA-1 and BRCA-2 gene mutations. It can occur even though the ovaries have been removed. Therefore, patients cannot be promised that they will never get ovarian type of cancer even if they undergo oophorectomy. However, the risk is decreased.

14. **B,** Page 978. Physiologic cysts are the most common cause of ovarian enlargement but they are not neoplasms. Of the neoplasms, epithelial tumors are the most common (approximately 65%) and germ cell–derived tumors are the second most common (approximately 20% to 25%). The most frequent germ cell tumor is the benign cystic teratoma, which, as its name implies, is benign and can be treated by simple removal. Only 2% to 3% of germ cell tumors are malignant. These include some very rare tumors, such as the polyembryoma, embryonal carcinoma, endodermal sinus tumors, and the relatively more common dysgerminoma.

15. **E,** Pages 983–984. Insofar as patients with dysgerminoma are young, preservation of the childbearing function is desirable, if possible. The tumor can spread within the peritoneal cavity and to retroperitoneal nodes, a more likely occurrence with larger dysgerminomas. If the tumor is confined to one ovary, a unilateral salpingo-oophorectomy should be performed and the abdomen thoroughly explored to determine the presence of intraperitoneal and retroperitoneal spread. Pelvic and paraaortic nodes should be sampled and any enlarged nodes excised. Markers, such as α-fetoprotein, should be obtained to rule out any other germ cell tumor types. If frozen section indicates pure dysgerminoma and there is no evidence of spread outside the primary tumor, only a unilateral salpingo-oophorectomy is indicated. The 5-year survival rate exceeds 90%. Approximately 20% of cases recur, but they can be treated by chemotherapy, radiotherapy, or additional surgery. These tumors are extremely radiosensitive, but the tumors are also very sensitive to chemotherapeutic agents, and multiagent chemotherapy has fewer side effects.

16. **A,** Page 966. In the 24-year-old patient described, if the frozen section obtained at the time of laparotomy for a suspected ovarian tumor cannot confirm the diagnosis of malignancy, the procedure should be terminated after removal of the ovarian tumor alone. A second procedure can subsequently be performed if malignancy is confirmed after detailed evaluation of the permanent sections. This is preferable to performing an unnecessary hysterectomy or other procedure in a patient who otherwise might desire to preserve her childbearing potential.

17–19. 17, **E**; 18, **A**; 19, **B**; Pages 960, 961, 964; Figures 31–2, 31–3, 31–6 in Stenchever. Serous cystadenomas, mucinous cystadenomas, endometrioid carcinomas, clear cell carcinomas, and Brenner cell tumors are the five cell types that constitute the epithelial tumors of the ovary. They may form tumors that are either benign or malignant. Serous tumors are the most common neoplasm and are the most common of the malignancies. Their lining epithelium resembles tubal epithelium. Mucinous tumors resemble endocervical mucinous cells, and endometrioid tumors resemble the endometrium. The Brenner cell tumor has islands of cells that resemble the Walthard cell nests of the ovary or the transitional epithelium of the bladder. Ovarian stroma is found between these islands of epithelial cells. The Brenner cell tumor is rare and almost always benign. Clear cell tumors are found in the endometrium, the ovary, and vagina. They have clear cells, show a hobnail pattern, and are very malignant.

20–23. 20, **A**; 21, **B**; 22, **D**; 23, **C**; Pages 980, 983, 987, 989; Figures 31–17, 31–20, 31–22, 31–24 in Stenchever. Benign mature cystic teratomas (dermoids) contain cells derived from all germ layers. They can occur at any time, but they are most common during the reproductive years. There is histologic differentiation into different adult tissues. Cystic teratomas may even contain functional glands such as thyroid (struma ovarii). The histologic picture shown is that of benign adult tissue. The rare malignant variants usually are associated with differentiation of the squamous components. The ovarian dysgerminoma consists of multiple germ cells with a stroma infiltrated by lymphocytes. It is analogous to the seminoma in the male. Dysgerminomas are most common in women younger than 30 and are bilateral in about 10% of cases. The Krukenberg tumor contains mucin-filled signet-ring malignant cells. They are metastatic to the ovary, usually from the gastrointestinal tract or the breast. Therefore, if one is found in the ovary, the primary lesion should be carefully sought. Granulosa cell tumors are made up of granulosa cells from the specialized stroma of the ovary. They contain some fibroblasts and theca cells in varying proportions. The histopathologic section shown also contains Call-Exner bodies. These are eosinophilic bodies surrounded by granulosa cells. Call-Exner bodies are also found in normal follicles. Granulosa cell tumors are rare, but they are mentioned infrequently because they can secrete hormones (primarily estrogen) and cause premature puberty and postmenopausal bleeding. Granulosa cell tumors behave like low-grade malignancies and have a greater than 90% 10-year survival rate.

24. **E**, Page 957; Table 31–1 in Stenchever. Despite numerous epidemiologic investigations, a clear-cut cause of ovarian cancer has not been defined. The only listed proven risk factor is the BRCA-2 gene mutation. BRCA-1 mutation is also a proven risk factor, and increasing number of years of ovulation may be involved. The use of oral contraceptives decreases the risk by about 40%. Breast-feeding and pregnancy also are protective. Tubal ligation and, to a lesser extent, hysterectomy with ovarian preservation also lower the risk of ovarian cancer. It has been suggested that ovulation-inducing drugs such as clomiphene (Clomid) increase the risk of ovarian cancer, as noted by Whittemore and colleagues. In a more recent study, Rossing and coworkers reported an increase in risk from a population-based study that suggested that the risk was associated with prolonged use of clomiphene inasmuch as no association was noted with less than 1 year of use. The results of the study were significant but involved wide (95%) confidence limits; only 11 cancer cases occurred in the clomiphene group among 3837 women studied in the infertility clinic.

25. **D**, Page 957. Lynch and associates have reported on families with these hereditary ovarian cancers. They noted that these cancers tend to occur at a younger age than among the general population. It appears that germline mutations of the BRCA-1 tumor suppressor gene on chromosome 17q are responsible for a large proportion of these hereditary cancers. The degree to which such genetic changes are predictive of cancer development in the general population is not known, but the potential of future genetic identification of such changes would allow the definition of the population at increased risk who are in need of increased surveillance.

26. **A**, Pages 962–963. CA-125 was described by Bast and colleagues in the 1980s. It is expressed by approximately 80% of ovarian epithelial carcinomas but less frequently by the mucinous tumors in this group. The marker is elevated in endometrial and tubal carcinoma, in addition to ovarian carcinoma and in other malignancies, including those originating in the lung, breast, and pancreas. CA-125 is also elevated in many nonmalignant conditions such as inflammatory disease, endometriosis, and pregnancy. A level of greater than 35 U/mL generally is considered elevated.

27. **D**, Pages 835, 975. Debulking is important to increase the effect of chemotherapy and survival. Platinum-based agents, such as cisplatin or carboplatin, and paclitaxel constitute the most common first-line chemotherapy. Other combinations are being evaluated for their efficacy.

28. **A** and **C**, Page 957. Women who ovulate less frequently, either because they took birth control pills or were often pregnant, appear to be less prone to ovarian carcinoma. Tubal ligation is also protective. Factors that increase the risk of ovarian carcinoma are living in an industrialized country and eating a diet high in animal fat. Eating vegetable fiber may reduce the risk. Familial factors are also important, such as the increased risk due to BRCA gene mutations.

29. **A, B, C** and **D**, Pages 966, 971, 973, 974. When operation for suspected ovarian carcinoma is performed, a vertical incision should be used. Peritoneal washings or ascitic fluid should be sent for cytologic study. A total abdominal hysterectomy and bilateral salpingo-oophorectomy plus omentectomy should be performed, as should biopsy of peritoneal surfaces and sampling of periaortic nodes to verify the stage. An attempt should be made to reduce the tumor to the smallest residual mass. The patient's response to postoperative therapy is improved if residual masses are less than 2 cm in diameter. As mucinous can result in pseudomyxoma peritonei, and this can also be caused by appendical mucinous cells, the appendix should be removed when any mucinous ovarian tumor is found. It is not necessary to remove the gallbladder.

30. **A, B, C,** and **D,** Page 968. The higher the stage and grade of the ovarian tumor, the poorer the prognosis. Cell type is also important, with undifferentiated and serous tumors having the worst prognosis. The amount of residual tumor after maximum removal is a factor in prognosis. The greater the amount of residual tumor, the less well the patient responds to chemotherapy. The age of the patient at the time of operation is not a prognostic indicator.

31. **A** and **D**, Pages 746, 966. The preoperative workup of a patient with suspected ovarian malignancy should always include a thorough history and physical examination and informed consent. A chest radiograph is only cost-effective if there are symptoms. An EKG is also nonrewarding if the patient is younger than 60 unless there are symptoms. Routine blood work and routine urinalysis are indicated. CT of the abdomen to look for retroperitoneal node involvement or liver metastases may also be indicated, but these studies are not very accurate. A barium enema is important to rule out bowel carcinoma and to establish a baseline of bowel integrity in the event of future radiation treatment, but usually a colonoscopy is better for this purpose. Colonoscopy is definitely superior if there is gastrointestinal bleeding. Cystoscopy need only be done if bladder involvement is suspected.

32. **A, B, C,** and **E,** Pages 966, 971. Conservative therapy for borderline tumors, which by definition must be grade 0, with preservation of childbearing function may be carried out by performing unilateral oophorectomy under the following conditions: (1) the tumor is confirmed to be stage IA, (2) a histologic sampling of the tumor confirms that it is grade 0 (borderline), (3) the contralateral ovary appears normal, (4) the biopsy specimens of omentum and peritoneum are negative, and (5) peritoneal cytologic test results are negative. Retroperitoneal nodes are not routinely sampled.

33. **B** and **D**, Page 957. About 90% of ovarian cancers are not hereditary (or familial) and develop sporadically. Hereditary ovarian cancers are rare, occur in only a few families, are mostly epithelial cancers, and are usually lethal. The term *familial ovarian cancer* denotes an inherited trait that predisposes to ovarian cancer development. Early literature studies suggested an increase from about 1.5% to 5% in the lifetime risk of ovarian cancer with one first-degree relative affected; with two or more first-degree relatives affected, the risk approaches 7%. The use of prophylactic oophorectomy in patients whose mothers had ovarian cancer has been controversial. It may be appropriate in members of families with known BRCA gene mutations as soon as childbearing has been completed. Women from such families tend to experience ovarian cancer at an earlier age than women without BRCA gene mutations.

CHAPTER 32

Neoplastic Diseases of the Vulva

1. One of the primary histologic differences between vulvar intraepithelial neoplasia and vulvar squamous hyperplasia is

   A. the degree of nuclear enlargement
   B. the thickness of the surface hyperkeratosis
   C. the depth of rete ridges
   D. the presence of perinuclear halo
   E. an intraepithelial inflammatory cell infiltrate

2. The chromosome distribution of vulvar intraepithelial neoplasia grade III (carcinoma in situ) is most likely to be

   A. haploid
   B. diploid
   C. triploid
   D. aneuploid
   E. mosaic

3. A 52-year-old woman comes to your office with a 6-month history of vulvar pruritus. Examination reveals diffuse, whitish, plaquelike areas extending from the perineal body along the lower half on the left labium majus. There is obvious excoriation around these lesions. Vulvar biopsy reveals histologic findings shown in Figure 32–1. Treatment of this patient should be

   A. wide local excision
   B. laser vaporization
   C. topical testosterone propionate
   D. topical fluorinated corticosteroids
   E. topical 5-fluorouracil

4. Taken as a whole, progression of all grades of vulvar intraepithelial neoplasia (VIN) to invasive carcinoma is estimated to be

   A. 6%
   B. 12%
   C. 19%
   D. 24%
   E. 30%

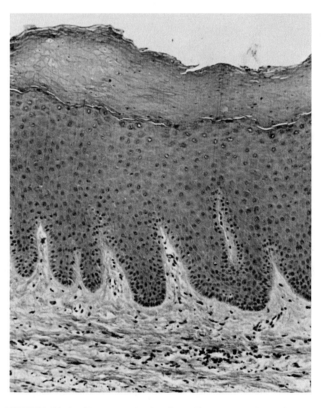

FIGURE 32–1 (From Friedrich EG, Wilkinson EJ: The vulva. In Blaustein A, ed: Pathology of the Female Genital Tract, 2nd ed. New York, Springer-Verlag, 1982.)

5. The most common human papillomavirus (HPV) subtypes found in benign vulvar warts are

   A. 6 and 11
   B. 16 and 18
   C. 31 and 33
   D. 35 and 37
   E. 40 and 41

6. In a 42-year-old patient with VIN-III (carcinoma in situ) involving the lower half of the left labium majus (approximately one quarter of the vulvar circumference), the best treatment is

   A. total vulvectomy
   B. total subcutaneous vulvectomy
   C. wide local excision of the involved area
   D. cryocautery with liquid nitrogen
   E. topical 5-fluorouracil cream

7. The main lymphatic drainage for a unilateral malignant lesion of the vulva occurring in the anterior third of the vulva is

   A. through the ipsilateral inguinal-femoral nodes
   B. through the contralateral inguinal-femoral nodes
   C. directly into the ipsilateral deep pelvic nodes
   D. directly into the contralateral deep pelvic nodes

8. The curve in Figure 32–2 that most likely illustrates the survival of a stage II vulvar epidermoid carcinoma is

   A. line *A*
   B. line *B*
   C. line *C*
   D. line *D*

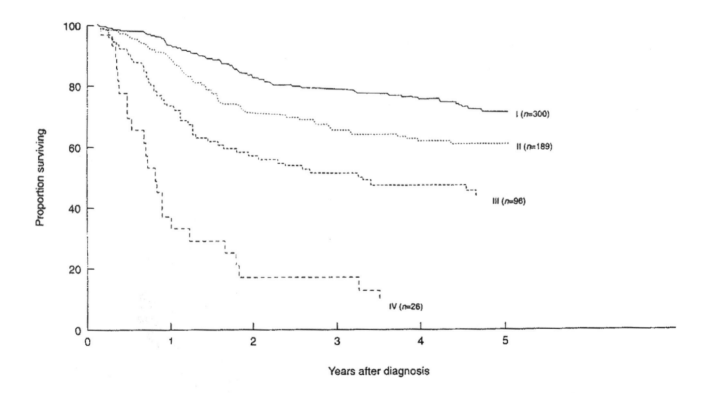

Strata	Patients (*n*)	Mean age (years)	Overall survival at					Hazards ratio[a] (95% confidence intervals)
			1 year	2 years	3 years	4 years	5 years	
I	300	64.7	92.3%	82.3%	78.7%	75.7%	71.4%	Reference
II	189	67.4	86.5%	71.0%	65.8%	62.2%	61.3%	1.94 (1.36–2.75)
III	96	69.4	72.0%	57.2%	51.3%	47.5%	43.8%	3.84 (2.55–5.78)
IV	26	72.8	33.3%	16.7%	16.7%	8.3%	8.3%	12.2 (7.08–21.2)

FIGURE 32–2 Carcinoma of the vulva: Patients treated in 1990–92. Survival by FIGO stage (epidermoid invasive cancer only) *n* = 611. (From Pecorelli S, Creasman WT, Pettersson F, et al: FIGO annual report on the results of treatment in gynaecological cancer, Epidemiol Biostat, 23, 1998.)

9. Microinvasive carcinoma of the vulva may be defined as

   A. contained within the basement membrane
   B. extending within 1 mm beyond the basement membrane
   C. extending within 3 mm beyond the basement membrane
   D. extending within 5 mm beyond the basement membrane
   E. stage IA

10. The optimal therapy for a 78-year-old patient who has diabetes mellitus, severe atherosclerotic heart disease, and stage III squamous cell carcinoma of the left labium majus is

    A. radical left hemivulvectomy with regional lymph node irradiation
    B. radical total vulvectomy with regional lymph node irradiation
    C. radiation therapy of the primary lesion alone
    D. combination radiotherapy and chemotherapy using intravenous 5-fluorouracil
    E. systemic chemotherapy alone using intravenous 5-fluorouracil

11. A 68-year-old patient has had a wide local excision (2-cm margins) for what is interpreted to be a Clark's level II superficial spreading melanoma of the vulva. The expected 5-year survival rate is

    A. 10%
    B. 25%
    C. 50%
    D. 75%
    E. 100%

12. A "sore" is noted on the left side of the clitoris. The biopsy diagnosis is squamous cell carcinoma with penetration to 5 mm and capillary space and lymphatic involvement. With the 1994 FIGO recommendations, it is determined that this is a stage I lesion. The optimal treatment would be

    A. radical vulvectomy with bilateral inguinal-femoral node dissection
    B. radical vulvectomy with left inguinal-femoral node dissection
    C. radical vulvectomy alone
    D. laser excision of the visible lesion
    E. radiation therapy of the visible lesion

13. During a lymphadenectomy of the inguinal-femoral nodes performed as part of the therapy for a 1994 FIGO stage II carcinoma of the vulva, the surgeon recognizes that several of the nodes contain tumor. Therapy now should include

    A. ipsilateral deep pelvic lymphadenectomy
    B. bilateral deep pelvic lymphadenectomy
    C. radiotherapy to ipsilateral deep pelvic nodes
    D. radiotherapy to bilateral deep pelvic nodes
    E. triple-agent chemotherapy

14. A 28-year-old woman has biopsy-proven carcinoma in situ of a 2×3-cm acuminate lesion on the posterior fourchette. The best treatment for this patient is

    A. total vulvectomy
    B. "skinning" vulvectomy
    C. topical 5-fluorouracil
    D. multiple trichloroacetic acid applications
    E. wide local excision

15. A 62-year-old woman has a lesion on the left labium majus and undergoes biopsy. The lesion is a stage IA carcinoma of the vulva based on International Society for the Study of Vulvar Disease (ISSVD) criteria. Treatment should consist of

    A. wide local excision
    B. topical 5-fluorouracil
    C. simple vulvectomy
    D. radical vulvectomy
    E. primary radiation therapy

16. A 72-year-old woman has a 9-month history of progressive vulvar pruritus. Examination of the vulva reveals diffuse erythema with excoriations and a 1.5-cm slightly raised lesion of the posterior left labium majus. The next step in her management should be

    A. excision of the raised lesion
    B. podophyllin applied to the raised lesion
    C. prescription of topical corticosteroid cream
    D. office laser vaporization of the raised lesion
    E. office cryocautery of the raised lesion

17. A 71-year-old woman comes to your office with a "swelling" in her vagina that has been present for the past 4 months. Pelvic examination is unremarkable, except for a 4×4-cm, slightly tender, moderately firm mass in the inferior medial portion of the right labium majus. The overlying skin appears normal for a woman in this age group. Your next step would be

A. vulvar colposcopy (vulvoscopy)
B. application of toluidine blue followed by acetic acid
C. to incise and drain
D. to perform biopsy on the mass
E. to ablate the mass with laser

18. Biopsy of a 9-cm condylomatous mass on the left labium majus of a 48-year-old woman reveals a verrucous carcinoma. This tumor is best managed by

A. laser ablation
B. wide local excision
C. radical vulvectomy
D. radical vulvectomy with ipsilateral inguinal-femoral lymphadenectomy
E. radical vulvectomy with bilateral inguinal-femoral lymphadenectomy

19. A 71-year-old woman with a 2-year history of progressive vulvar itching comes in for treatment. The vulva has a homogeneous "onion skin" appearance. A vulvar biopsy specimen obtained as part of your evaluation is shown in Figure 32–3. The correct diagnosis is

A. squamous hyperplasia
B. vulvar intraepithelial neoplasia (VIN) II
C. Paget disease
D. carcinoma in situ
E. lichen sclerosus

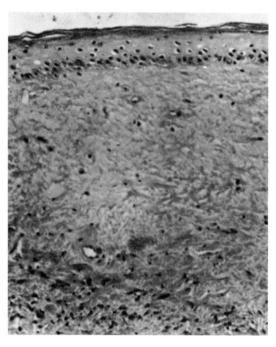

FIGURE 32–3 (From Friedrich RG, Wilkinson EJ: The vulva. In Blaustein A, ed: Pathology of the Female Genital Tract, 2nd ed. New York, Springer-Verlag, 1982.)

20. The next step in your management of the patient in Question 19 should be

A. oral conjugated estrogens
B. topical estrogen cream
C. vulvar colposcopy
D. simple vulvectomy
E. topical testosterone cream

DIRECTIONS:

for Questions 21–22: For each numbered item, select the one heading most closely associated with it. Each lettered heading may be used once, more than once, or not at all.

21–22. Match Figures 32–4 and 32–5 with the most likely diagnosis.

A. Paget disease
B. lichen sclerosus
C. verrucous carcinoma
D. squamous hyperplasia
E. melanoma

21. Figure 32–4

22. Figure 32–5

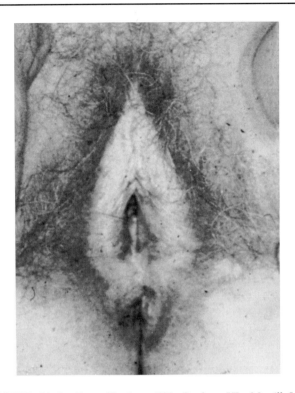

FIGURE 32–4 (From Kaufman RH, Gardner HL, Merrill JA: Diseases of the vulva and vagina. In Romney SL, et al, eds: Gynecology and Obstetrics. New York, McGraw-Hill, 1980.)

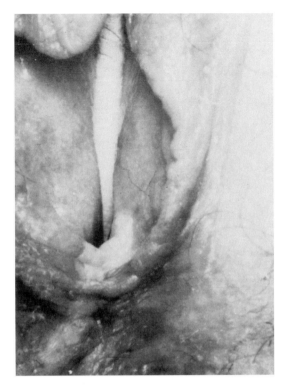

FIGURE 32–5 (From Kaufman RH, Gardner HL, Merrill JA: Diseases of the vulva and vagina. In Romney SL, et al, eds: Gynecology and Obstetrics. New York, McGraw-Hill, 1980.)

DIRECTIONS:

for Questions 23–30: Select the one best answer or completion.

23. A 68-year-old woman has just had surgery for stage IB carcinoma of the vulva. She has positive inguinal femoral nodes. Factors important in determining her chance of long-term survival include all the following *except*

   A. number of metastatic nodes
   B. size of metastatic nodes
   C. proximity of metastatic nodes to the primary tumor
   D. total nodal volume

24. A 72-year-old woman has an 18-month history of progressive pruritus. The vulvar skin has a diffuse, reddened eczematoid apperance. The vulvar biopsy specimen is reproduced in Figure 32–6. This patient should undergo all the following tests or treatments *except*

   A. stool test for blood
   B. mammography
   C. total vulvectomy
   D. chest radiography (posteroanterior and lateral)

25. In a 52-year-old woman excisional biopsy of a 3-mm, pigmented, ulcerated lesion is performed on the left labium minus, near the clitoral hood. Histologic diagnosis confirms malignant melanoma. The currently recommended treatment for this patient is

   A. simple excision
   B. wide local excision
   C. simple unilateral vulvectomy
   D. simple complete vulvectomy
   E. radical vulvectomy

26. A 68-year-old patient is evaluated for a 1-year history of vulvar pruritus. On physical examination, she has diffuse, patchy, hyperkeratotic white lesions scattered around the posterior two thirds of the vulva. Based on the physical examination assessment alone, the correct term applied to these lesions is

   A. leukoplakia
   B. leukoplakic vulvitus
   C. vulvar atypia
   D. hyperplastic dystrophy

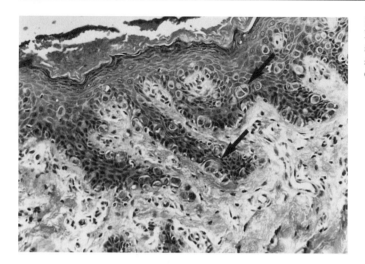

FIGURE 32–6 Vulvar epidermis with Paget's disease. Malignant cells *(arrows)* are seen infiltrating epidermis and spreading along dermal-epidermal junction. (Hematoxylin-eosin stain ×160.) (Courtesy Dr. Anthony Montag, The University of Chicago.)

27. In assessing suspected vulvar atypia, solutions that can be used to highlight abnormal areas include

   A. Lugol's solution
   B. toluidine blue
   C. acetic acid
   D. Monsel's solution
   E. Burow's solution

28. Which of the following is a true statement regarding the likelihood that VIN will progress to invasive carcinoma?

   A. The progression of VIN to invasive carcinoma is common.
   B. The risk of progression of VIN to invasive cancer is higher in older patients.
   C. The risk of invasion is higher in those with a flat appearance.
   D. Lesions that contain HPV DNA are less likely to progress to invasive carcinoma.

29. What is the latency period between lichen sclerosus and squamous cell carcinoma for the small proportion of patients in which there appears to be a potential for malignant progression?

   A. 2 years
   B. 4 years
   C. 8 years
   D. 16 years

30. Paget disease of the vulva is associated with which of the following cancers?

   A. gastrointestinal (GI) tract
   B. lung
   C. brain
   D. skin
   E. liver

ANSWERS

1. **A,** Page 1061. Nomenclature for describing vulvar disease process has changed. Currently, non-malignant vulvar disease is classified as VIN; lichen sclerosus (which has not changed); squamous hyperplasia (not otherwise specified), which was previously referred to as hyperplastic dystrophy; and miscellaneous diagnoses, including dermatoses and Paget disease. The main difference between simple squamous hyperplasia and VIN is the degree of nuclear enlargement. VIN of the vulva almost always contains nuclei that have a fourfold of greater difference in size, whereas differences in the size of nuclei in condyloma or nonneoplastic epithelia are threefold or less. Depth or confluence of the rete ridges, degree of hyperkeratosis, inflammatory cell infiltrate, and perinuclear halo do not relate to the degree of atypia. Abnormal mitoses are usually observed in vulvar intraepithelial neoplasia.

2. **D,** Page 1006. Nuclear characteristics of carcinoma in situ of the vulva are similar to those of the cervix. In many lesions, there are multinucleated cells, abnormal mitoses, increased cell density, and an increase in the nuclear/cytoplasmic ratio. Studies of the chromosome distribution of these lesions have indicated that they are aneuploid as measured by DNA analysis.

3. **D,** Page 1006; Figure 32–1 (in Stenchever), from Friedrich EG, Wilkinson EJ: The vulva. In Blaustein A, ed: Pathology of the Female Genital

Tract, New York, Springer-Verlag, 1982. Areas of squamous hyperplasia are frequently whitish lesions that appear thickened in focal or multifocal areas rather than the diffuse "onion skin" appearance of lichen sclerosus. Biopsy is necessary to establish the diagnosis. The histologic appearance shown in Figure 32–1 is characteristic. It includes benign hyperplastic dystrophy, hyperkeratosis, acanthosis, and mild inflammation. In addition to local measures to diminish irritation, topical fluorinated corticosteroids are helpful in controlling the itching. Frequently used preparations are 0.025% or 0.1% triamcinolone acetonide (Aristocort, Kenalog), fluocinolone acetonide (Synalar), or betamethasone valerate (Valisone). These agents are usually applied twice daily to control the itching, which is relieved in 1 or 2 weeks. Since prolonged use of these relatively strong topical corticosteroids may be associated with vulvar atrophy, long-term control of symptoms may be affected by intermittent use of 1% hydrocortisone.

4. **A**, Page 1006. Progression of VIN to invasive carcinoma is rare; it has been estimated to occur in about 6% of all cases. A comparable proportion of VIN spontaneously regresses. Although VIN is being diagnosed more commonly in younger women, the risk of progression to invasive cancer is higher for those who are older and those who are immunosuppressed.

5. **A**, Page 1007. The potential role of HPV has begun to be extensively studied in cases of VIN. HPV vulvar infection is widespread and is associated histologically with koilocytosis and intraepithelial neoplasia in some patients. Currently, HPV types 6 and 11 are generally recognized as found more frequently in benign vulvar warts, whereas HPV types, 16, 18, 31, 33, and 35 are more frequently associated with intraepithelial neoplasia and even invasive carcinoma.

6. **C**, Page 1008. Management of VIN is particularly complicated and requires long-term follow-up. Many lesions are multifocal, with involvement of widely separated areas. Lesions of intraepithelial neoplasia tend to be posterior, predominantly in the perianal or lower labial areas. Types of therapy have changed in the last few years. In the past, simple vulvectomy was widely used. This was later replaced by a "skinning vulvectomy." Both of these operations are disfiguring and probably unnecessary unless the entire vulva is covered with lesions. Wide local excision of the affected area can be used for approximately 70% of patients not experiencing a recurrence. This is comparable to either a total or a "skinning vulvectomy." If topical ablation is to be used, laser vaporization is preferable to liquid nitrogen cryotherapy. Although topical 5-fluorouracil

cream has been used, it is associated with particularly bothersome complications over a prolonged time. Therefore it is generally not prescribed.

7. **A**, Page 1001; Figure 32–13 in Stenchever. Tumors in the anterior third or middle of either labium tend to drain initially into the ipsilateral inguinal-femoral nodes, whereas perineal or clitoral tumors may spread into either the right or the left side. Although there has been concern in the past that tumors in the clitoral-urethral area would spread directly to the deep pelvic nodes, current evidence indicates that this rarely, if ever, occurs.

8. **B**, Pages 1011–1012. The prognosis of vulvar carcinoma is related to the stage of the disease, lesion size, and presence of regional nodes. Worldwide actuarial 5-year survival rates are: stage I, 71.4%; stage II, 61.3%; stage III, 43.8%; and stage IV, 8.3%.

9. **E**, Page 1012. The term *microinvasive carcinoma of the vulva* has no uniformly accepted definition. Part of the confusion is due to different points from which the depth of invasion is measured—that is, from the surface of the tumor or from the basement membrane. The International Society for the Study of Vulvar Disease (ISSVD) has recommended that the term *microinvasion* be dropped and the designation *stage IA* be used for tumors less than 2 cm in diameter with depth of invasion less than 1 mm from the dermal stromal junction (basement membrane).

10. **D**, Pages 1017–1018. Combined use of chemotherapy and radiation has been introduced as a new and apparently effective means of treating recurrent and occasionally large primary vulvar carcinomas, particularly in patients who are not good operative candidates. The patient illustrated in this case, who has atherosclerotic heart disease and diabetes, might be such a candidate. This type of combined chemotherapy and radiation therapy is being used more widely in the treatment of squamous cell carcinomas of the lower genital tract and is described further in Chapter 29 of Stenchever.

11. **E**, Pages 1017–1018. The prognosis for vular melanoma has improved in part because most of these carcinomas are of the superficial spreading variety (good prognosis) rather than the nodular variety (poor prognosis). Although firm recommendations from available data are not possible, a reasonable approach is to excise a melanoma with a 2-cm margin without node dissection for tumors that are less than 2 mm thick. Long-term results for lesions that corresponds to Clark level I or II suggest 5-year survival rates in the vicinity of 100%.

12. **A**, Pages 1013–1015. Effective therapy for stage I or stage II and some early stage III vulvar

carcinomas can be accomplished with a radical vulvectomy and bilateral inguinal-femoral node dissection. Previous recommendations suggested that, because of the patterns of lymphatic drainage, it is important with all invasive vulvar carcinomas to perform bilateral groin dissection. In view of recent evidence that suggests that deep pelvic nodes are virtually never involved unless the inguinal nodes are also involved, most oncologists now remove only the inguinal-femoral nodes at the time of primary operation. Likewise, unless the lesion is central, such as clitoral, most oncologists perform only an ipsilateral dissection. Laser excision or primary radiation is unacceptable treatment. A deep pelvic node dissection can be done if, in the frozen or permanent section of histologic specimen, the inguinal-femoral nodes are found to be involved with tumor.

13. **D,** Page 1015. A recent national cooperative randomized study suggested that radiation therapy to the deep pelvic nodes is superior to operative therapy when it is known that the inguinal-femoral nodes contain tumor. This report indicated improved survival associated with less morbidity for patients who received radiation of 4500 to 5000 rad. Although chemotherapy may be used for disseminated disease as a palliative measure, no chemotherapeutic regimen has been successful in treatment of this disease.

14. **E,** Page 1008. Wide local excision is the best treatment for a patient with an isolated lesion of the posterior fourchette that proves to be carcinoma in situ. In the past, simple vulvectomy was widely practiced to treat carcinoma in situ of the vulva, but this disfiguring operation is now infrequently used and has been shown to be unnecessary. This is particularly true in younger women. "Skinning" vulvectomy followed by split-thickness vulvar skin grafting has been advocated. In this case, with a small lesion such a procedure would constitute more treatment than is necessary. 5-Fluorouracil cream has also been used to treat carcinoma in situ of the vulva. This treatment is successful in approximately 75% of cases. However, this treatment causes severe vulvar edema and pain over a prolonged time and usually is not prescribed for isolated lesions. Applications of concentrated trichloroacetic acid are used to treat condyloma acuminatum when this condition is *not* associated with severe VIN. This treatment is unacceptable for cases of true carcinoma in situ.

15. **A,** Pages 1012–1013. For stage IA lesions, as defined by the ISSVD, therapy may be less extensive than is usually employed for invasive vulvar carcinoma. Based on currently available evidence, treatment for these lesions is controversial.

Protocols are being developed to evaluate the best therapy. It appears that most patients with stage IA carcinoma of the vulva would no longer be treated with a modified radical or radical vulvectomy. The lymph node dissection is omitted or deferred, depending on the final pathologic evaluation of the primary tumor. A wide local excision appears to be adequate therapy.

16. **A,** Page 1013. A typical invasive vulvar carcinoma usually appears as a slightly raised or polyploid mass. The patient frequently complains of a "sore" that has not healed. Prolonged vulvar pruritus is frequently associated with this disease. Delay in diagnosis is common because many older patients fail to seek prompt medical attention, and often, when they do, a biopsy is not initially performed. In patients with this presentation, it is mandatory that an office biopsy be performed immediately and certainly before treatment is initiated. If possible, wide local excision should be done because this approach may be adequate treatment. Topical treatment with corticosteroids or podophyllin is contraindicated before a tissue diagnosis is made. Both laser vaporization and office cryocautery of lesions such as these are also contraindicated until a specific diagnosis is made.

17. **D,** Page 1017. Bartholin gland carcinoma is an adenocarcinoma that accounts for 1% to 2% of vulvar cancers. An enlargement of the Bartholin gland in a postmenopausal woman should raise suspicion for this malignancy. Since this complaint is rarely associated with acute inflammation in a postmenopausal woman, all such masses appearing in this age group should undergo biopsy. Empiric treatment with laser or topical agents is not warranted unless indicated by the biopsy results. Examination with a magnifying device such as a colposcope would not be useful in this patient because the lesion is below the epithelium. For the same reason, the use of toluidine blue or any other adjunct designed for epithelial diagnosis would not be indicated. (See Question 27 for further discussion of the limitations of toluidine blue as a diagnostic tool.) Simple incision and drainage are not appropriate unless representative samples of tissue are first submitted for pathologic examination. These tumors are treated similarly to primary squamous cell carcinoma of the vulva. Radical vulvectomy with bilateral inguinal-femoral lymphadenectomy is the treatment of choice.

18. **B,** Page 1017. Verrucous carcinoma is a rare tumor that may attain considerable size but is generally indolent. Wide local excision is usually effective therapy. Radical vulvectomy alone or with ipsilateral or bilateral inguinal lymphadenectomy is not necessary. Laser ablation is insufficient to

remove the deeper tissues. Radiation therapy is ineffective, can worsen the prognosis, and therefore is contraindicated.

19. **E,** Pages 1000–1001. The changes shown in this photomicrograph are typical for lichen sclerosus. Usually the epithelium becomes markedly thinner with the loss or blunting of the rete ridges. The superficial portion of the dermis is hyalinized, whereas the deep portion contains a lymphocytic infiltrate. This is not a premalignant condition, but it tends to be multifocal and usually recurs.

20. **E,** Page 1006. The next step in managing lichen sclerosus is topical testosterone cream. The efficacy of testosterone is excellent. It is important to remember that estrogen does not significantly effect changes in vulvar skin, although it promotes maturation and thickening of the vaginal epithelium. Vulvar colposcopy (vulvoscopy) is difficult and nonessential since the vulva has a homogeneous appearance. If colposcopy is readily available and will not add significantly to the cost of care, its use cannot be criticized. Simple vulvectomy is unnecessary because the condition is benign. As an alternative to 2% testosterone proprionate in petrolatum, clobetasol proprionate 0.05% twice daily has also been used with success in patients with lichen sclerosus.

21–22. 21, **B;** 22, **D;** Page 1005; Figures 32–8 and 32–9 in Stenchever. (From Kaufman RH, Gardner HL, Merrill JA: Diseases of the vulva and vagina. In Romney SL, et al, eds: *Gynecology and Obstetrics,* New York, McGraw-Hill, 1980.) A clinical diagnosis must not replace a histologic diagnosis. Lesions of the vulva should undergo biopsy. Figure 32–4 depicts tissue of the labia minora and perineum that has a white, brittle "cigarette paper" appearance. Figure 32–5 depicts squamous hyperplasia, formerly called hyperplastic dystrophy. Note the sharply demarcated, raised white area at the lower tip of the white pointer. These lesions usually appear thickened, and the process tends to be focal or multifocal rather than diffuse. A biopsy is necessary to establish the diagnosis.

23. **C,** Page 1016. Survival of patients with vulvar carcinoma is directly related to the presence of metastatic disease in regional lymph nodes. After radical vulvectomy and bilateral node dissection, there is about a 95% 5-year survival rate for patients with negative regional lymph nodes. As the number of metastatic nodes increases, the 5-year survival rate diminishes progressively. There is also a direct correlation between survival and metastatic nodal size. Lesions associated with higher nodal tumor volume are generally related to earlier recurrence and decreased survival rates.

24. **D,** Page 1008. This is a patient with Paget disease, which is a condition of the vulva generally occurring in postmenopausal women with a long history of vulvar pruritus. It is frequently associated with other invasive carcinomas, including squamous carcinoma of the vulva or cervix, adenocarcinoma of the sweat glands of the vulva, or Bartholin gland carcinoma. Cases of adenocarcinoma of the gastrointestinal tract accompanying Paget disease also have been reported. Thus, once a diagnosis of Paget disease of the vulva is made, it is important to rule out the presence of malignancy at other sites, including the breast. If no primary malignancy is uncovered, a total vulvectomy is usually performed. It is important to remove the full thickness of the skin to the subcutaneous fat to be certain that all the skin adnexal structures are excised because they may have a subclinical malignancy. Since the disease may recur, resulting in multiple surgical procedures, some experts have advocated less extensive initial therapy. Women who have been treated for Paget disease of the vulva should have, as part of routine follow-up, an annual examination of the breast, cytologic evaluation of the cervix and vulva, and screening for gastrointestinal disease (at least by testing for occult blood in the stool). A chest radiograph is not a good general screening tool, and this patient is not at increased risk for pulmonary disease by virtue of her Paget disease. Therefore, there is no indication to perform chest radiography.

25. **B,** Pages 1017–1018; Figure 32–7. Melanoma is the most common non-squamous-cell malignancy of the vulva, accounting for about 5% of primary cancers of this area. The diagnosis may be established by excisional biopsy. For many years, the treatment was provided by radical vulvectomy and bilateral inguinal-femoral lymphadenectomy. The currently recommended treatment is wide local excision only.

26. **C,** Page 1000. In the past a number of ambiguous terms have been used to describe gross lesions of the vulva. Terms such as *leukoplakia, hyperplastic dystrophy,* and *leukoplakic vulvitis* have been discarded because they imply, without biopsy confirmation, both precancerous lesions and inflammation. Under the new classification scheme used by the International Society for the Study of Vulvar Diseases and adopted by the International Society for Gynecologic Pathology, these gross lesions should be called *vulvar atypia,* with biopsy confirmation needed to make the final diagnosis. The histologic architecture of these lesions defines whether or not surgical or medical therapy should be offered.

27. **C,** Pages 1002–1003. Certain diagnostic aids may be useful in the initial evaluation of a patient with suspected vulvar atypia in preparation for

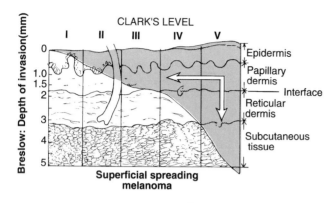

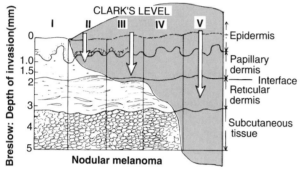

FIGURE 32–7 Level of invasion for superficial spreading melanoma and nodular melanoma. (From Podratz KC, Caffey TA, Symmonds RE, et al: Gynecol Oncol 16:153, 1983.)

biopsy. As a cytoplasmic stain, Lugol's solution is not particularly helpful because of the numerous false-positive areas and the fact that it does not penetrate the hyperkeratosis associated with many of these disorders. Toluidine blue, which is a nuclear stain, may assist in delineating vulvar atypia, since the superficial keratin layers of the vulva do not normally contain nuclei. It should be remembered, however, that ulcerations and fissures in the skin also retain this dye. Because of the lack of specificity of toluidine-blue staining, this technique has generally been discarded. Monsel's solution (ferrous subsulfate)

and Burow's solution (aluminium acetate) are not used for diagnosis. Monsel's solution is useful in achieving hemostasis in minor office procedures, whereas Burow's solution is a useful adjunct to the treatment of vulvar itching. Acetic acid is used in patients who have suspected vulvar atypia in preparation for colposcopic (vulvoscopic) examination of the vulva. The magnification of the colposcope is practical in following patients with VIN. With this instrument, directed biopsy is performed. The colposcope is not used for routine vulvar examination. It is primarily used for patients who are being evaluated or followed up for vulvar atypia or intraepithelial neoplasia.

28. **B,** Page 1006. Progression of VIN to invasive carcinoma is rare. It has been estimated to occur in approximately 6% of all cases. Moreover, a comparable proportion of VIN cases spontaneously regress. The risk of progression to invasive cancer is higher for those who are older and those who are immunosuppressed. Furthermore the risk of invasion is higher in women who have raised lesions with irregular surface patterns or lesions that contain HPV DNA. Thus, patients who are older and those with irregular raised lesions have the greatest risk of unrecognized invasive cancer.

29. **B,** Page 1001. In the past, patients with lichen sclerosus were thought not to be at increased risk for vulvar carcinoma. It is now thought that there is a small premalignant potential of lichen sclerosus. The risk appears to be 4.5% that a patient with lichen sclerosus will experience squamous cell carcinoma of the vulva, with an average of 4 years of latency between symptomatic lichen sclerosus and cancer.

30. **A,** Page 1002. Paget disease in the vulva histologically resembles Paget disease of the breast. Paget cells are large pale cells that often occur in nests and infiltrate up through the epithelium. There is an increased association of Paget disease of the vulva with invasive GI and breast cancers.

CHAPTER
33

Neoplastic Diseases of the Vagina

DIRECTIONS:

for Questions 1–32: Select the one best answer or completion.

1. **Recurrences of squamous cell carcinoma of the vagina are most likely to occur as**

   A. local recurrences
   B. bone metastases
   C. liver metastases
   D. lung metastases
   E. brain metastases

2. **Of the following treatment modalities, the most frequently used in the treatment of squamous cell carcinoma of the vagina is**

   A. laser ablation
   B. wide local excision
   C. radical surgery
   D. radiation therapy
   E. chemotherapy

3. **Premalignant disease of the vagina is primarily identified with**

   A. screening colposcopy
   B. cytologic screening
   C. vaginal washings
   D. targeted biopsies in high-risk populations

4. **A "field defect" in gynecology denotes**

   A. a blind spot in the visual field as a result of metastatic genital cancer
   B. the propensity of the squamous epithelium of the lower genital tract to undergo premalignant change
   C. herniation of fatty tissue through the inguinal canal
   D. adenosis of the vagina as a result of in utero exposure to diethylstilbestrol
   E. an area not affected by radiation therapy

5. **A stage II vaginal cancer indicates that**

   A. there is ureteric involvement
   B. the lesion extends to the pelvic wall
   C. the lesion is limited to the vaginal wall
   D. the lesion involves subvaginal tissue but does not extend to the pelvic wall
   E. the lesion involves the rectal mucosa

6. **An 80-year-old woman who is in good health has a routine gynecologic examination. She had a total abdominal hysterectomy at age 45 for benign disease. The Pap smear is reported as showing severe atrophy with inflammatory changes and a few atypical cells. The appropriate management is to**

   A. prescribe topical 5-fluorouracil
   B. repeat the Pap smear in 1 year
   C. prescribe a course of estrogen followed by a repeat Pap smear in 3 months
   D. perform colposcopy
   E. perform a vaginectomy

7. **A patient with primary squamous cell carcinoma of the vagina is found to have hydronephrosis. The tumor seems to be filling the pelvis, but the bladder and rectum appear to be free of disease. The remainder of her evaluation does not reveal distant disease. The appropriate stage to be assigned to this patient is**

   A. 0
   B. I
   C. II
   D. III
   E. IV

8. A 60-year-old gravida 6 has recently experienced vaginal bleeding. Until this event she was healthy and was not receiving any medications. On examination a fungating, ulcerative lesion is found on the left lateral wall of the vagina near the fornix. The next step in her medical care is to

    A. perform a Pap smear
    B. look at the lesion with a colposcope
    C. perform a biopsy of the lesion
    D. perform vaginectomy
    E. order radiation therapy

9. A 41-year-old patient underwent a total abdominal hysterectomy for moderate dysplasia of the cervix and uterine myomata. This patient should be advised that she

    A. does not need to have vaginal cytology
    B. needs a Pap smear every 4 to 5 years
    C. needs a Pap smear every 2 to 3 years
    D. needs a Pap smear annually
    E. should be followed with yearly colposcopic examinations

10. In vaginal carcinoma in situ (VAIN-3), abnormal cells

    A. are confined to the outer one third of the epithelium
    B. are confined to the inner two thirds of the epithelium
    C. are throughout the entire thickness of the epithelium
    D. have invaded the basement membrane
    E. have invaded subepithelial tissues

11. A 2-year-old is seen after passing a "grapelike" structure from the vagina. Otherwise the child is asymptomatic. One should

    A. obtain vaginal secretions for culture and sensitivity
    B. admit the child for observation in the hospital
    C. empirically treat the child with penicillin
    D. warn the parents about the problem of children inserting foreign objects into the vagina
    E. perform vaginoscopy with the patient under anesthesia

12. A 40-year-old patient, at 5 years after vaginal hysterectomy for carcinoma in situ of the cervix, is found to have diffuse multicentric vaginal intraepithelial neoplasia (VAIN). The most appropriate treatment is

    A. surgical excision
    B. laser ablation
    C. 5-fluorouracil cream
    D. radiation therapy
    E. systemic chemotherapy

13. Which of the following is appropriate therapy for vaginal intraepithelial neoplasia?

    A. radical hysterectomy
    B. vaginectomy
    C. radiation therapy
    D. local excision

14. All of the following are appropriate therapy for stage II clear cell adenocarcinoma of the vagina *except*

    A. radical hysterectomy
    B. vaginectomy
    C. pelvic lymphadenectomy
    D. diverting colostomy

15. Which of the following is the most common therapy for stage III squamous cell carcinoma of the vagina?

    A. partial vaginectomy
    B. total vaginectomy
    C. radiation therapy
    D. 5-FU

16. Clear cell carcinoma of the vagina is associated with what histologic finding?

    A. hobnail cells
    B. Call-Exner bodies
    C. signet-ring cells
    D. giant cells

17. What is the appropriate treatment for pseudosarcoma botryoides?

    A. 5-FU
    B. local excision
    C. vaginectomy
    D. radiation

18. Which of the following is a risk factor for the development of vaginal intraepithelial neoplasia?

    A. diethylstilbestrol (DES) exposure in utero
    B. infection with papillomavirus
    C. bacterial vaginosis
    D. mother with VAIN

19. Which of the vaginal cancers is typically associated with adults?

    A. endodermal sinus tumor
    B. sarcoma botryoides
    C. clear cell adenocarcinoma
    D. squamous cell carcinoma

20. **All the following are similarities between CIN and VAIN** *except*

    A. detected by Pap smear
    B. herpesvirus is risk factor
    C. requires radiation therapy
    D. characterized by abnormal maturation of epithelium

21. **Which tumor is the most likely to metastasize to the vagina?**

    A. endometrium
    B. ovary
    C. rectosigmoid
    D. thyroid

22. **Which of the following statements correctly characterizes malignant melanoma of the vagina?**

    A. affects younger patients
    B. invades superficially
    C. responsive to chemotherapy
    D. recurs frequently

23. **The diagnosis of sarcoma botryoides has been established in a 2-year-old. Management of this patient should include**

    A. chemotherapy
    B. operation
    C. radiation therapy
    D. all the above

24. **An early symptom commonly associated with vaginal cancer is**

    A. urinary frequency
    B. pelvic pain
    C. abnormal vaginal bleeding
    D. tenesmus

25. **The presence of an abnormal vaginal epithelium can be detected through**

    A. Lugol's stain
    B. colposcopy
    C. vaginal cytology
    D. all the above

26. **All the following are appropriate therapies for VAIN** *except*

    A. cryotherapy
    B. laser ablation
    C. 5-fluorouracil cream
    D. radiation therapy

27. **All the following are appropriate modalities used in the treatment of carcinoma in situ of the vagina** *except*

    A. radiation therapy
    B. laser ablation
    C. 5-fluorouracil cream
    D. local excision

28. **The interpretation of routine Pap smears is adversely affected by**

    A. vaginal infection
    B. menopausal changes
    C. menstruation
    D. all the above

29. **Factors affecting the prognosis of patients with clear cell adenocarcinoma of the vagina embody the**

    A. age of the patient
    B. size of the tumor
    C. depth of invasion
    D. all the above

30. **The usual treatment of a patient with a malignant melanoma of the vagina is**

    A. radiation
    B. chemotherapy
    C. hormonal treatment
    D. surgery

31. **alpha-Fetoprotein is secreted by**

    A. an endodermal sinus tumor of the vagina
    B. a vaginal squamous cell carcinoma
    C. sarcoma botryoides
    D. all the above

32. **Laser therapy is an appropriate therapy for**

    A. VAIN
    B. melanoma of the vagina
    C. clear cell adenocarcinoma
    D. endodermal sinus tumor
    E. pseudosarcoma botryoides

ANSWERS

1. **A,** Page 1031. Initially squamous cell carcinoma of the vagina recurs locally, just as squamous cell carcinomas of the cervix and vulva do. Although distant metastases occur, most patients initially have local recurrences. Since an effective chemotherapy program for recurrent vaginal carcinoma has not been developed, in patients who have only localized recurrence an exenterative procedure should be considered if the tumor was initially treated with radiation.

2. **D,** Page 1030. In recent years radiation therapy has been the most frequent mode of treatment for squamous cell carcinoma of the vagina. External radiation therapy with megavoltage equipment is used initially to shrink the tumor. This is then followed by a local cesium or radium implant placed interstitially with needles or by intracavitary radiation using a tandem similar to the delivery systems used for cervical carcinoma.

3. **B,** Page 1027. Since premalignant disease of the vagina is generally asymptomatic, detection is primarily a function of cytologic screening. Most frequently these findings occur in patients who have undergone previous treatment for cervical intraepithelial disease. A colposcopically directed biopsy is usually required in order to obtain histologic identification.

4. **B,** Page 1027. A "field defect" describes the propensity of squamous epithelium of the lower genital tract (cervix, vagina, and vulva) to undergo premalignant changes. The epithelium of the lower genital tract is derived from a common embryonic origin. Since these structures are subjected to similar environmental stimulants (e.g., human papillomavirus and herpes simplex virus type II), similar premalignant changes might be anticipated. Areas of such neoplastic changes need not be contiguous; in fact, they may arise in multiple sites throughout the genital tract. The recognition of field defect phenomenon is important because patients with cervical intraepithelial neoplasia are more likely to also develop vaginal intraepithelial neoplasia and vulvar intraepithelial neoplasia.

5. **D,** Page 1028, Table 33–1. The staging of vaginal cancer according to FIGO is done after clinical evaluation, which includes examination with the patient under anesthesia, cystoscopy, sigmoidoscopy, and imaging studies (i.e., intravenous pyelogram, barium enema). Stage II involves the subvaginal tissue but does not extend to the pelvic wall.

6. **C,** Page 1027. An abnormal Pap smear requires further evaluation. Since an estrogen-deficient state may adversely affect the interpretation of a

TABLE 33–1

International Federation of Gynecology and Obstetrics (FIGO) Staging Classification for Vaginal Cancer

Stage	Characteristics
0	Carcinoma in situ
I	Carcinoma limited to vaginal wall
II	Carcinoma involves subvaginal tissue but has not extended to pelvic wall
III	Carcinoma extends to pelvic wall
IV	Carcinoma extends beyond true pelvis or involves mucosa of bladder or rectum (bullous edema as such does not assign a patient to stage IV)

Pap smear, it should be repeated after the patient is given estrogen replacement therapy. Colposcopic evaluation of the atrophic vaginal epithelium may be difficult because of the chronic inflammatory changes. If the repeat Pap smear after estrogen replacement therapy is abnormal, colposcopic evaluation and biopsies will be necessary at that time. A vaginectomy performed without a histologic diagnosis may constitute either overtreatment or undertreatment.

7. **D,** Page 1028; Table 33–1. The lesion extends into the pelvis and obstructs a ureter, indicating that the lesion has extended to the pelvic wall. The appropriate stage to be assigned according to the FIGO classification is stage III.

8. **C,** Page 1029. A large fungating, ulcerative lesion in this age group is likely to be a neoplasm. A biopsy of this or any significant lesion is a rapid and accurate way of making a definitive diagnosis; it should be performed at the initial visit. Treatment should not be undertaken until a diagnosis is made. This diagnosis must be based on a biopsy—not on Pap smear or colposcopy results.

9. **D,** Page 1027. If the concept of a field defect is considered, this patient with premalignant changes of the cervix is more likely to develop premalignant changes of the vagina. If left undetected, this may later progress to invasive cancer. A patient who has had moderate cervical dysplasia is at an increased risk of developing a vaginal or vulvar malignancy. As a screening tool, vaginal cytology (rather than colposcopy) remains most cost-effective.

10. **C,** Pages 1023, 1025; Figure 33–1. Vaginal carcinoma in situ (VAIN-3) denotes an intraepithelial neoplasm that has not invaded the basement

FIGURE 33–1 (From Stenchever MA, Droegemueller W, Herbst AL, Mishell DR Jr: Comprehensive Gynecology, 4th ed: St Louis, Mosby, 2001.)

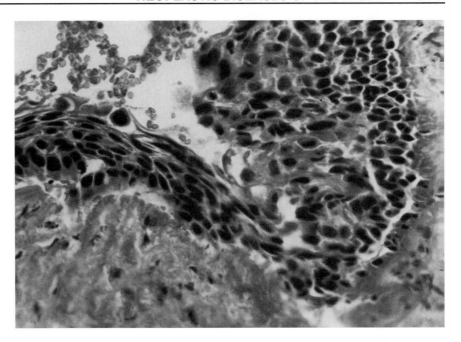

membrane or does not involve the subepithelial tissues, but in which dysplastic cells extend throughout the entire epithelial layer.

11. **E,** Page 1031. Although children sometimes insert foreign bodies into the vagina, passing a "grapelike" structure by a 2-year-old strongly suggests the presence of sarcoma botryoides. Since the prognosis of the child is directly related to the rapidity with which the diagnosis is established, vaginoscopy should be performed with the patient under anesthesia and biopsy should be done on all suspicious lesions as soon as possible.

12. **C,** Page 1028. Fluorouracil cream is most appropriate for diffuse, multicentric lesions, whereas surgical excision is reserved for apical lesions, commonly found after hysterectomy. Laser ablation is generally used for discrete lesions.

13. **D,** Page 1028. As is true for cervical intraepithelial neoplasia, the abnormal vaginal epithelium must be completely eradicated. Small lesions, particularly those at the vaginal apex in patients who have undergone hysterectomy, usually are excised.

14. **D,** Page 1032. In general, operation is the primary treatment modality because of the young age of the patients. For stage I and early stage II tumors, radical hysterectomy with partial or complete vaginectomy, pelvic lymphadenectomy, and replacement of the vagina with split-thickness skin grafts has been the most common approach. In most cases ovarian function is preserved. In addition, efforts have been made to preserve fertility in patients who have small tumors of the vagina by the use of local irradiation of the primary tumor and immediate adjacent tissues to spare the ovaries. Since metastases to regional pelvic nodes can occur even with small stage I tumors, retroperitoneal lymph node dissections are usually performed before local therapy.

15. **C,** Page 1031. Radiation therapy has been the most common mode of treatment. External radiation therapy with megavoltage equipment is initially used to shrink the tumor. This is then followed by a local cesium or radium implant placed interstitially with needles or by intracavitary radiation using a tandem or ovoids, similar to the delivery systems used for cervical carcinoma (particularly in the case of a tumor in the upper third of the vagina if the cervix is present). The treatment is individualized, depending on tumor size and stage. Some therapists have advocated using only local sources of radiation if the primary carcinoma is small (less than 2 cm) and accessible to needle implantation. For large lesions the dosage of the external component of radiation therapy is increased, with a concomitant reduction in the local vaginal component of treatment of the primary tumor.

16. **A,** Page 1033; Figure 33–5 in Stenchever. The characteristic of the tubulocystic pattern of clear cell adenocarcinoma is hobnail cells extruding into the lumina of tubular structures. Clear cell adenocarcinoma also may have other patterns, such as solid or papillary.

17. **B,** Page 1035. A rare benign vaginal polyp that resembles sarcoma botryoides is found in the vagina of infants or pregnant women. Although large atypical cells may be present microscopically, strap cells are absent. Grossly these polyps do not have the grapelike appearance of sarcoma botryoides. They are called pseudosarcoma botryoides. Treatment by local excision is effective.

TABLE 33–2
Common Primary Vaginal Cancers

Tumor Type	Predominant Age (Years)	Clinical Correlations
Endodermal sinus tumor (adenocarcinoma)	<2	Extremely rare; alpha-fetoprotein secretion; often fatal; multimodality therapy
Sarcoma botryoides	<8	Aggressive malignancy; multimodality therapy
Clear cell adenocarcinoma	>14	Associated with intrauterine exposure to DES
Melanoma	>50	Very rare; poor survival
Squamous cell carcinoma	>50	Most common primary vaginal cancer

18. **B,** Page 1027. As with the cervix, predisposing factors associated with these changes may include venereal diseases, herpesvirus type II infection, and human papillomavirus infection. Additional risk factors include prior radiation therapy of the genital tract, immunosuppressive therapy in transplant patients, and chemotherapy in patients undergoing treatment for malignant disease.

19. **D,** Page 1027. As shown in Table 33–2, both squamous cell carcinoma and melanoma occur in older patients.

20. **C,** Pages 1023–1025; Figure 33–1, *A.* VAIN is the abbreviation used to describe intraepithelial neoplasms of the vagina, whereas CIN is used to describe cervical intraepithelial neoplasms. Both conditions are a result of a faulty maturation process in the surface epithelium. Risk factors include previous venereal disease, herpesvirus type II infection, human papillomavirus infection, and sexual activity at an early age with multiple sexual partners. Both lesions result in the exfoliation of abnormal cells into the vagina, which can be detected through a routine Pap smear collected from the cervix and the posterior vaginal pool. Both lesions are treated surgically. Although VAIN is most often in the upper one third of the vagina, it is commonly multifocal, requiring examination of the vagina in its entirety.

21. **A,** Page 1027. Most vaginal malignancies are metastatic, primarily from the cervix and the endometrium. Less commonly, ovarian and rectosigmoid carcinomas, as well as choriocarcinoma, metastasize to the vagina. The most common histologic type of primary vaginal cancer is squamous cell carcinoma, but numerous other types of carcinomas, as well as primary sarcomas, occur.

22. **D,** Page 1034. A malignant melanoma of the vagina is a rare neoplasm with only about 100 cases reported to date. It affects older women (mean age 60). The lesion invades deeply into the subvaginal tissue, and recurs frequently. Pigmented lesions of the lower genital tract are more likely than pigmented lesions elsewhere in the body to undergo malignant transformation. If there is any question regarding a pigmented lesion, it should be excised and submitted for histologic evaluation.

23. **D,** Page 1035. Although exenterative procedures were performed in the past in the treatment of children with embryonal rhabdomyosarcoma (sarcoma botryoides), effective control with less radical operation appears to have been achieved with a multimodality approach consisting of chemotherapy (vincristine, actinomycin D, and cyclophosphamide) usually combined with operation. Radiation therapy has also been used. Such a combined approach appears to result in effective treatment with less mutilating surgery.

24. **C,** Page 1029. The most common symptoms of vaginal cancer are abnormal vaginal bleeding and vaginal discharge. Urinary frequency is sometimes noted in patients with a large anterior lesion, whereas tenesmus is noted in patients with a large posterior lesion. These symptoms appear only when the lesions are large, and therefore they occur late in the course of disease. Similarly, pain is usually a symptom of an advanced tumor that has invaded into the deep tissues.

25. **D,** Page 1027. The presence of dysplastic vaginal epithelium is most frequently detected initially on Pap smear. The abnormal area can be delineated by colposcopy or Lugol's stain. It should undergo biopsy for histologic evaluation.

26. **D,** Page 1028. The premalignant changes of vaginal intraepithelial neoplasia (VAIN) are localized to that epithelial layer alone. Ablation of the epithelium results in eradication of the disease. Cryotherapy, laser ablation, 5-fluorouracil cream application, and surgical excision of small lesions are all acceptable methods of treating these lesions.

27. **A,** Page 1028. Although both vaginectomy and radiation therapy would ablate carcinoma in situ of the vagina, this approach would be considered overtreatment. The lesion is limited to the epithelial area, and thus removal of the epithelial layer either with laser therapy or the application of 5-fluorouracil cream is sufficient. In either instance, follow-up is required to ensure elimination of all abnormal areas. Like all patients with lower genital tract malignancies, the patient is at a higher risk of developing similar neoplasms along the lower genital tract. Therefore close gynecologic surveillance is necessary for the remainder of the patient's life.

28. **D,** Page 1027. Inflammatory changes and estrogen deficiency affect the appearance of the exfoliating cells and thus make interpretation of cytologic smears more difficult. It is recommended that an infection be treated and cleared and that patients with severe atrophic changes be given hormonal replacement treatment. The cytologic smears should be repeated after completion of therapy. Menstrual blood creates technical difficulties by obscuring the sample.

29. **D,** Page 1032. Factors favorable in the survival of patients with clear cell adenocarcinoma of the vagina include:
    1. low stage
    2. older age
    3. tubulocystic pattern
    4. small tumor diameter
    5. reduced depth of invasion
    6. no lymph node involvement
    7. positive DES history

30. **D,** Page 1034. Treatment of patients with malignant melanoma of the vagina consists of radical operation with wide excision of the vagina and uterus and dissection of the retroperitoneal nodes (pelvic and inguinal). Lower vaginal lesions require treatment similar to that of vulvar carcinoma, whereas upper vaginal lesions require treatment similar to that of cervical carcinoma. Adjunctive radiation therapy and chemotherapy also have been used. Despite all this, the 5-year survival is dismal. Local recurrence is common and the disease is usually fatal.

31. **A,** Page 1034. An endodermal sinus tumor (adenocarcinoma) is a rare vaginal tumor. It affects very young girls, usually less than 2 years old. The tumor is aggressive and has an unfavorable prognosis because the tumor is usually fatal. It produces α-fetoprotein, which can be detected in the serum and can serve as a tumor marker.

32. **A,** Page 1023. Laser (Light Amplification by Stimulated Emission of Radiation) is an energized source of light that can be used to vaporize tissue and to treat intraepithelial neoplasia.

Malignant Disease of the Fallopian Tube

for Questions 1–27: Select the one best answer or completion.

1. The least common primary female genital tract malignancy originates in the

    A. ovary
    B. fallopian tube
    C. uterus
    D. vagina
    E. vulva

2. What is the most frequent presenting symptom in cancer of the fallopian tube?

    A. pain
    B. weight loss
    C. anorexia
    D. bloating
    E. abnormal bleeding or discharge

3. The diagnosis of primary tubal carcinoma is most commonly made by

    A. history
    B. physical examination
    C. ultrasound examination
    D. computed tomography (CT)
    E. surgical exploration

4. A 62-year-old patient has persistent uterine bleeding despite two dilatation and curettage (D&C) procedures and two trials on conjugated equine estrogens–progestin therapy. No endometrial pathologic condition has been found, and the pelvic examination is unremarkable. The next step should be

    A. vaginal hysterectomy
    B. abdominal hysterectomy
    C. laparoscopy/laparotomy
    D. irradiation of the pelvis
    E. hysteroscopy/laser ablation of the endometrium

5. A 57-year-old patient complains of vaginal bleeding; a profuse, intermittent watery discharge; and lower abdominal pain. On pelvic examination, a 5-cm right adnexal mass is palpated. These findings are most typical of

    A. a functional ovarian cyst
    B. ovarian carcinoma
    C. endometrial carcinoma
    D. a fallopian tube carcinoma
    E. a leiomyosarcoma

6. The percentage of patients with fallopian tube carcinoma in whom cytologic testing of the vagina yields positive results is

    A. <1%
    B. 2%–5%
    C. 10%–10%
    D. 50%–60%
    E. >70%

7. At the time of exploratory laparotomy for a right adnexal mass in a 60-year-old patient, a dilated right fallopian tube is discovered. When opened, it is filled with tumor. No other tumors are noted, but the peritoneal fluid is found to be positive for malignant cells. The "unofficial stage" of the tubal carcinoma is

    A. IA
    B. IB
    C. IC
    D. II
    E. III

8. The most frequent site of metastatic spread of tubal carcinoma is

   A. liver
   B. lung
   C. bone
   D. peritoneum
   E. retroperitoneal nodes

9. At the time of exploratory laparotomy, a 30-year-old gravida 1, para 1, is found to have a primary tubal carcinoma confined to the right tube. The appropriate operation is

   A. right salpingectomy
   B. right salpingo-oophorectomy
   C. bilateral salpingectomy
   D. bilateral salpingo-oophorectomy
   E. total abdominal hysterectomy with bilateral salpingo-oophorectomy

10. In performing an exploratory laparotomy for a suspected tubal carcinoma, the first step on entering the abdominal cavity should be

   A. ligation of the distal and proximal ends of the affected tube
   B. palpation of the liver
   C. palpation of the paraaortic nodes
   D. obtaining a peritoneal cytologic specimen
   E. palpation of the omentum

11. Recent data suggest that prognosis is worsened if the level of what assay is elevated?

   A. αFT
   B. human chorionic gonadotropin (hCG)
   C. carcinoembryonic antigen (CEA)
   D. thyroid-stimulating hormone (TSH)
   E. CA-125

12. The family of a patient with tubal carcinoma confined to the tube (stage I) asks about the prognosis. It would be accurate to inform them that 5-year survival rate is

   A. <5%
   B. 10%–20%
   C. 30%–40%
   D. 50%–60%
   E. 70%–80%

13. In a postmenopausal woman, the classic symptoms suggestive of tubal carcinoma are included in the triad of

   A. pain, watery discharge, anorexia
   B. bleeding, watery discharge, adnexal mass
   C. bleeding, pain, adnexal mass
   D. anorexia, watery discharge, bleeding
   E. anorexia, pain, adnexal mass

14. Adenocarcinoma of the fallopian tube occurs most commonly in patients who are

   A. 40–49 years old
   B. 50–59 years old
   C. 60–69 years old
   D. 70–79 years old
   E. 80–89 years old

15. Which of the following should be performed at the time of laparotomy for removal of tubal carcinoma?

   A. paraaortic node sampling
   B. peritoneal washings
   C. omentectomy
   D. all the above

16. For what stage(s) of tubal carcinoma is pelvic irradiation recommended after surgery?

   A. I
   B. II
   C. III
   D. IV

17. Which of the following is the most common histologic type of primary tubal carcinoma?

   A. papillary-alveolar
   B. endometrioid
   C. serous
   D. clear cell

18. The criteria used to diagnose primary tubal carcinoma include the following

   A. The tumor is primarily within the lumen of the tube.
   B. The mucosa of the tube is involved with the tumor.
   C. A transition can be demonstrated between the malignant and the nonmalignant tubal epithelium.
   D. All the above.

19. Which statement accurately describes the staging of tubal carcinoma?

   A. It was officially adopted by FIGO in 1986.
   B. It is based on clinical findings.
   C. It is based on the system used for primary ovarian carcinoma.
   D. It accounts for the grade of tumor.

20. **A 52-year-old patient is found to have a stage IA carcinoma of the fallopian tube. Proper therapy should include**

    A. total abdominal hysterectomy, bilateral salpingo-oophorectomy, paraaortic node biopsy, omentectomy
    B. intraperitoneal ^{32}P
    C. cyclophosphamide (Cytoxan) and megestrol acetate (Megace)
    D. all the above

21. **A 58-year-old asymptomatic patient is seen for a routine office visit. A Pap smear is performed. It is reported as "cells consistent with adenocarcinoma." The differential diagnosis should include adenocarcinoma of the**

    A. endometrium
    B. ovary
    C. fallopian tube
    D. all the above

22. **A 48-year-old patient undergoes surgery for a left adnexal mass. While exploring the pelvis, you note a tumor of the left fallopian tube. If you suspect metastatic cancer to the tube, you should pay particular attention to the**

    A. ovaries
    B. intestines
    C. uterus
    D. all the above

23. **Abnormal uterine bleeding is the most common complaint associated with malignancies of all the following *except***

    A. cervix
    B. fallopian tube
    C. ovary
    D. uterus

24. **The term *hydrops tubae profluens* is associated with**

    A. vaginal discharge
    B. a disappearing pelvic mass
    C. pelvic pain
    D. all the above

25. **Peritoneal implants of tubal carcinoma of 2-cm size are used to define what FIGO stage?**

    A. I
    B. II
    C. III
    D. IV

26. **Which of the following is a suggested predisposing factor for tubal carcinoma?**

    A. pelvic infection
    B. multiparity
    C. family history of the condition
    D. all the above

27. **Figure 34–1 is a high-powered microscopic view of a section through a tumor of the fallopian tube. It is a**

    A. papillary adenocarcinoma
    B. medullary adenocarcinoma
    C. carcinosarcoma
    D. mixed mesodermal tumor
    E. choriocarcinoma

ANSWERS

1. **B,** Page 1039. Fallopian tube carcinoma accounts for approximately 0.3% to 1.1% of gynecologic malignancies. Up to 90% are metastatic from other sites, usually the ovary or the uterus. Metastatic fallopian tumors are 10 times more common than primary tumors.

2. **E,** Page 1040. In none of the malignancies of the female genital tract does pain represent the most common presenting symptom. In the case of tubal carcinoma, pain may occur, but it is a less common presenting symptom than abnormal or excessive vaginal bleeding or discharge.

3. **E,** Pages 1040, 1041. Although tubal carcinoma may appear with excessive bleeding or discharge, and although an adnexal mass is occasionally found, history and physical examination do not usually lead to the correct diagnosis. Similarly, imaging studies are not pathognomonic. The diagnosis is most frequently made after operative exploration for other diagnoses.

4. **C,** Page 1040. In a patient with postmenopausal uterine bleeding for whom two D&Cs fail to reveal the cause of bleeding, the possibility of tubal carcinoma must be considered. Laparoscopy can aid in establishing this diagnosis. Hysterectomy would not necessarily address the possibility of an adnexal pathologic condition, although an abdominal approach would allow thorough inspection

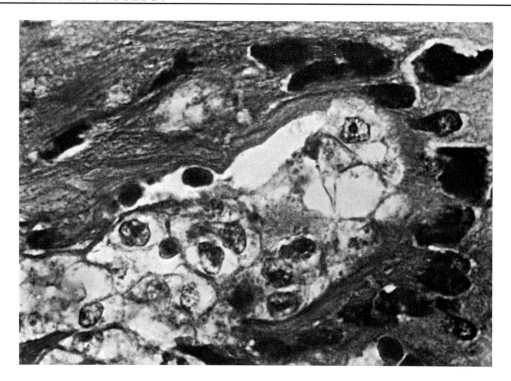

FIGURE 34–1

of tubes and ovaries. Irradiation of the pelvis for bleeding of unknown cause is inappropriate. Hysteroscopy with laser ablation of the endometrium would not rule out an adnexal cause for the bleeding.

5. **D,** Page 1040. The triad of bleeding, watery discharge, and adnexal mass (hydrops tubae profluens) in a postmenopausal woman is considered highly suggestive of tubal carcinoma. These findings, however, only rarely occur together. The diagnosis is usually made postoperatively because the physician's index of suspicion is usually low. An adnexal mass in a postmenopausal patient must not be considered functional. The diagnosis of ovarian carcinoma is less likely because of the watery vaginal discharge. Postmenopausal bleeding should be considered endometrial carcinoma until proven otherwise, but the watery discharge and an adnexal mass suggest a different primary process. Leiomyosarcoma would appear as a uterine mass rather than an adnexal mass and without the watery discharge.

6. **C,** Page 1040. (Benedet JL, White GW, Fairey RN, Boyes DA: Adenocarcinoma of the fallopian tube. Obstet Gynecol 50:654, 1977: Hirai Y, Kaku S, Teshima H, et al: Clinical study of primary carcinoma of the fallopian tube: experience with 15 cases. Gynecol Oncol 34:20, 1989.) Only 10% of the patients with tubal carcinoma in the series by Benedet have positive vaginal cytologic findings, whereas Hirai and coworkers have reported positive preoperative cytology in 6 of 15 cases (40%).

Therefore, the Pap smear is not a reliable screening tool, and a negative smear does not rule out the possibility of tubal carcinoma.

7. **C,** Page 1043; Table 34–1. FIGO staging places a tumor confined to one tube with positive washings at stage IC. If the washings had been negative, the stage would be IA. If the tumor is confined to both tubes with negative washings, the stage would be IB.

8. **D,** Page 1041. The peritoneum is the most common site of metastatic spread of tubal carcinoma. Retroperitoneal nodes are also a common site. Hepatic and lung metastases are less common and denote stage IV disease.

9. **E,** Page 1041. Although the patient described is young (30 years old) and of low gravidity and parity, the appropriate operation is total abdominal hysterectomy with bilateral salpingo-oophorectomy. If no intraperitoneal spread is apparent, paraaortic node biopsy should be performed. An omentectomy should also be done with an attempt to remove all from disease.

10. **D,** Page 1041. In carrying out operative staging for presumed tubal or ovarian cancer, the first surgical procedure performed once in the peritoneal cavity should be peritoneal cytologic testing. It is done by lavage using 200 to 300 mL of normal saline mixed with 5000 units of heparin. If any other manipulations are carried out before obtaining appropriate cytologic samples, one runs the risk of shedding tumor cells into the peritoneal cavity, thus altering the staging evaluation.

11. **E,** Page 1041. Hefler and associates found that CA-125 levels were prognostic, with elevated levels associated with a worse prognosis.

12. **E,** Page 1043. The overall 5-year survival rate for all stages of tubal carcinoma combined is 38%. Patients with disease confined to the tube have the best prognosis, expecting a 70% to 80% 5-year survival rate.

13. **B,** Page 1040. The classic description of tubal carcinoma is the triad of abnormal uterine bleeding, adnexal mass, and watery discharge in a postmenopausal woman. Pain is reported but less frequently. Anorexia is not typically associated with tubal carcinoma.

14. **B,** Page 1040; Figure 34–2. The average age of women with adenocarcinoma of the fallopian tube is 54.9 years. The decade in which most cases occur is 50 to 59 years.

15. **D,** Page 1041. The diagnosis of primary tubal carcinoma is most frequently made at the time of operative exploration. Once the diagnosis is established, frequently by frozen section, a thorough operative staging procedure is carried out, including a total abdominal hysterectomy and bilateral salpingo-oophorectomy. Peritoneal cytologic testing is performed. If there is no evidence of intraperitoneal spread, a paraaortic node sampling should be performed to rule out extrapelvic spread. This is particularly important in cases of large or poorly differentiated tumors, in view of the fact that these carcinomas often metastasize to the paraaortic nodes. An omentectomy should also be performed.

16. **B,** Page 1047. Operation by TAH-BSO is adequate for stages IA and IB. For stage IC, either ^{32}P or adjuvant chemotherapy with platinum-containing regimens is appropriate. For stages II and III, chemotherapy would be chosen by most therapists after operation, although some centers might advocate whole abdominal radiation with a pelvic boost for stage II disease. Chemotherapy would be most likely used for stage IV disease.

17. **C,** Page 1041. A serous histologic pattern resembling ovarian carcinoma is most common, but endometrioid, clear cell, and other rare patterns have been reported.

18. **D,** Page 1040. Hu CY, Taymor ML, Hertig AT: Primary carcinoma of the fallopian tube. Am J Obstet Gynecol 59:58, 1950. The criteria used in the diagnosis of primary tubal carcinoma were suggested by Hu and associates. They include:
    1. The primary tumor is grossly within the lumen of the tube.
    2. The mucosa of the tube is involved with the tumor, which displays a papillary or medullary pattern.
    3. A transition can be demonstrated between the malignant and the nonmalignant tubal epithelium if the tubal wall is involved to a great extent.

19. **C,** Page 1041. A staging system for primary tubal carcinoma was officially adopted by FIGO in 1991. It resembles staging for ovarian cancer. The suggested staging system is accomplished at the time of operation. The histologic grade is used in determining the staging of endometrial, not tubal, adenocarcinoma.

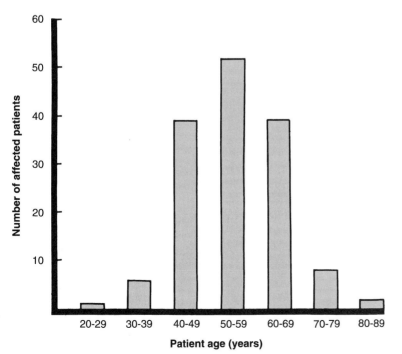

FIGURE 34–2 Histogram illustrating age distribution of patients with tubal carcinomas.
(From Podezaski D, Herbst AL: Cancer of the vagina and fallopian tube. In Knapp RC, Berkowitz RS, ed: Gynecologic Oncology, New York, Macmillan, 1983.)

20. **A,** Page 1041. Therapy for stage IA tubal carcinoma confined to the lumen with negative cytologic findings usually consists of a primary operation only (total abdominal hysterectomy bilateral salpingo-oophorectomy, paraaortic node biopsy, and omentectomy). If peritoneal cytology is positive, intraperitoneal ^{32}P or whole abdominal radiation is also used. Chemotherapy is reserved for widespread intraperitoneal disease or recurrent metastatic carcinoma.

21. **D,** Page 1040. Vaginal cytologic findings have been reported to be positive in 10% to 40% of fallopian tube carcinomas. Ruling out endometrial carcinoma must be the primary consideration; however, the diagnoses of tubal carcinoma, as well as endocervical or ovarian carcinoma, should be considered in patients with vaginal cytologic findings positive for adenocarcinoma in whom endometrial carcinoma has been excluded.

22. **D,** Page 1039. Since 90% of tubal cancers are metastatic, it behooves the clinician to know the likely primary sites (ie, ovary, uterus, or intestines).

23. **C,** Page 1040. Abnormal or excessive vaginal bleeding is the most commonly associated sign of cancers of the uterus, fallopian tubes, and cervix. Cervical cancer is classically associated with contact bleeding (postcoital or postdouche). Ovarian cancer tends to present as vague swelling of the abdomen caused by ascites, unless the ovarian neoplasm is the relatively rare granulosa cell tumor.

24. **D,** Page 1040. Hydrops tubae profluens, sometimes associated with tubal carcinoma, refers to a symptom complex of abnormal vaginal discharge and pelvic pain associated with a pelvic mass. This mass may disappear after the discharge is noted. This symptom complex is presumably explained by blockage of the distal part of the tube, peristalsis of the tube resulting in vaginal discharge, and disappearance of the mass as the dilated tube is emptied.

25. **C,** Page 1043. Among the definitions for stage III tubal carcinoma are:
    (a) Tumor involving one or both tubes with histologically confirmed implants of abdominal peritoneal surfaces, none exceeding 2 cm in diameter. Lymph nodes are negative.
    (b) Abdominal implants greater than 2 cm in diameter or positive retroperitoneal or inguinal nodes, or both.

26. **A,** Page 1039. Baekelandt and coworkers noted a history of infertility, low parity, and pelvic infection as possible predisposing factors. In a recent molecular genetic study, abnormalities of p53 and c-*erbB*-2 protooncogenes were observed similar to those noted in ovarian carcinoma, suggesting a possible similar biologic behavior between fallopian tube and ovarian carcinoma.

27. **E,** Page 1041. The photomicrograph depicted in Figure 34–1 is a high-power view of a choriocarcinoma. Central pale cytotrophoblasts are surrounded by syncytiotrophoblasts. These tumors tend to be hemorrhagic and necrotic. No villi are visible. Choriocarcinoma of the tube is thought to result from trophoblastic disease associated with ectopic pregnancy.

CHAPTER 35

Gestational Trophoblastic Disease

DIRECTIONS:

Select the one best answer or completion.

1. A 37-year-old gravida 5, para 4, is referred with a confirmed diagnosis of a hydatidiform mole. This was not a planned pregnancy; the patient thought that she had completed her childbearing. During the evaluation of this patient, it is noted that the uterus is greater than expected by dates and that she has bilateral ovarian cysts approximately 10 cm in diameter. Which of the following is the best therapy?

    A. sharp curettage
    B. chemotherapy
    C. hysterotomy
    D. hysterectomy
    E. hysterectomy with bilateral oophorectomy

2. Which is the most common site of metastasis for gestational trophoblastic tumor (GTT)?

    A. brain
    B. lung
    C. liver
    D. ovary
    E. vagina

3. A 30-year-old gravida 3, para 2, delivered a normal 3000-g male infant. On the first postpartum day, she had a bilateral tubal ligation. She experienced excessive bleeding 3½ weeks postpartum. A dilatation and curretage (D&C) was performed 4 weeks postpartum. The tissue is pictured in Figure 35–1. What does it show?

    A. a hydatidiform mole
    B. a partial mole
    C. a choriocarcinoma
    D. evidence or retained secundines
    E. a normal finding

4. A 22-year-old gravida 2, para 1, delivered a 3600-g female infant by cesarean section. Bleeding could not be controlled, and a hysterectomy was performed. The tissue is pictured in Figure 35–2. What is shown?

    A. a hydatidiform mole
    B. a partial mole
    C. a choriocarcinoma
    D. evidence of retained secundines
    E. a normal finding

5. Choriocarcinoma is most likely to develop after a(n)

    A. normal pregnancy
    B. partial mole
    C. hydatidiform mole
    D. ectopic pregnancy
    E. incomplete abortion

6. The risk of developing a hydatidiform mole is highest if pregnancy occurs in women who are

    A. younger than 20
    B. 20 to 29
    C. 30 to 39
    D. 40 to 49
    E. older than 50

7. A 20-year-old gravida 1, para 0, is seen at 21 weeks of pregnancy by menstrual dates. The uterus is the size of a 25-week gestation. Having made the diagnosis of a hydatidiform mole, you would

    A. start oxytocin immediately
    B. evacuate by hysterotomy
    C. give prophylactic chemotherapy
    D. perform a suction curettage
    E. perform a hysterectomy

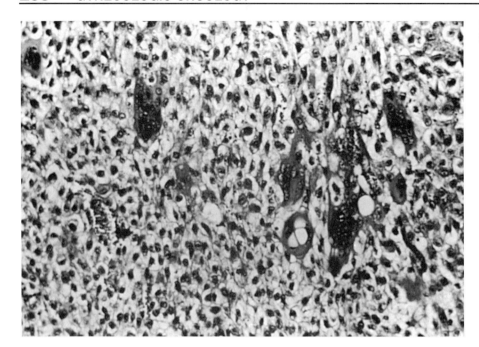

FIGURE 35–1 (Courtesy of Robert C. Maier, MD, Medical College of Georgia.)

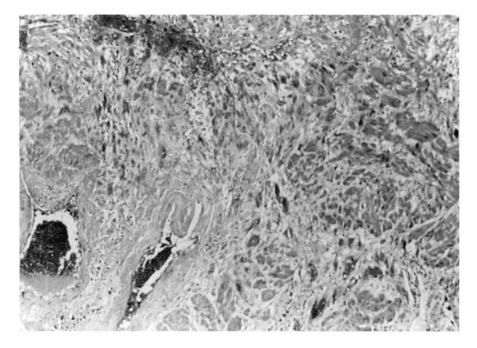

FIGURE 35–2 (Courtesy of Robert C. Maier, MD, Medical College of Georgia.)

8. Signs and symptoms of a complete hydatidiform mole include all the following *except*

   A. abdominal pain
   B. ovarian enlargement
   C. hyperemesis gravidarum
   D. fetal heart tones
   E. uterus small for dates

9. Which of the following patterns of blood types is associated with a higher risk of choriocarcinoma?

   A. wife, A; husband, A
   B. wife, A; husband, O
   C. wife, B; husband, A
   D. wife, AB; husband, O
   E. The couple's blood type has not been shown to be a risk factor.

10. Factors associated with high-risk metastatic gestational trophoblastic disease include all the following *except*

    A. pretreatment serum β human chorionic gonadotropin (β-hCG) greater than 40,000 mIU/mL
    B. duration of disease greater than 4 months
    C. previous chemotherapy failure
    D. liver metastasis
    E. vaginal metastasis

11. Which of the following is associated with some normal and some swollen villi plus fetal, cord, or amniotic membrane elements associated with polyploidy?

    A. androgenesis
    B. partial mole
    C. complete mole
    D. gestational trophoblastic tumor
    E. placental-site trophoblastic tumor

12. Which of the following is associated with a placental abnormality involving swollen placental villi and trophoblastic hyperplasia with loss of fetal blood vessels?

    A. androgenesis
    B. partial mole
    C. complete mole
    D. gestational trophoblastic tumor
    E. placental-site trophoblastic tumor

13. All the following are typical for a partial mole *except*

    A. hyperplasia of the syncytiotrophoblast
    B. hyperplasia of the cytotrophoblast
    C. both maternal and paternal origin
    D. nuclear DNA is completely paternal, and mitochondrial DNA is maternal

14. Etoposide (VP-16) is typically reserved for high-risk and drug-resistant cases of metastatic GTT because of subsequent

    A. nausea and vomiting
    B. alopecia
    C. secondary malignancies
    D. stomatitis
    E. neuritis

15. Each of four patients has had a hydatidiform mole evacuated from her uterus. After consulting the graph in Figure 35–3, indicate which patient should be treated for gestational trophoblastic tumor.

    A. patient 1
    B. patient 2
    C. patient 3
    D. patient 4

16. All the patients whose β-hCG is depicted in Figure 35–3 are in their late 20s, are multigravidas, and had their last menstrual period 14 weeks ago. Their uteri are consistent with a 14-week pregnancy, and their ovaries are not palpable. If you assume that all additional relevant studies are normal, management of the patient(s) with gestational trophoblastic neoplasia identified in Question 15 should include all the following *except*

    A. a chest radiograph
    B. single-agent chemotherapy
    C. a sensitive test specific for β-hCG every 2 weeks for 1 year
    D. contraception for 1 year

17. Malignant sequelae associated with a hydatidiform mole appear to be more common when the signs and symptoms include

    A. hyperemesis gravidarum
    B. a uterus normal for dates
    C. ovarian enlargement
    D. vaginal bleeding

18. A 32-year-old gravida 5, para 4, is now 20 weeks pregnant according to her menstrual dates. The uterus is felt to be the size of a 16-week gestation. Ultrasonography results in a series of views as depicted in Figure 35–4. The β-hCG is markedly elevated for 20 weeks. In discussing the possible outcomes, you should tell this patient that

    A. the fetus has a life expectancy of less than 1 month
    B. she will not need to have serial β-hCG levels obtained postpartum
    C. there is a 20% risk of malignant sequelae
    D. there is evidence that her disease has spread to the ovary

19. It is established that persons who are likely to experience a hydatidiform mole include all the following *except*

    A. a history of a prior hydatidiform mole
    B. a history of recurrent abortions
    C. poor nutrition
    D. age over 40 years

20. Approximately what proportion of cases of gestational trophoblastic tumors occurs after molar pregnancy?

    A. 10%
    B. 25%
    C. 50%
    D. 75%
    E. 90%

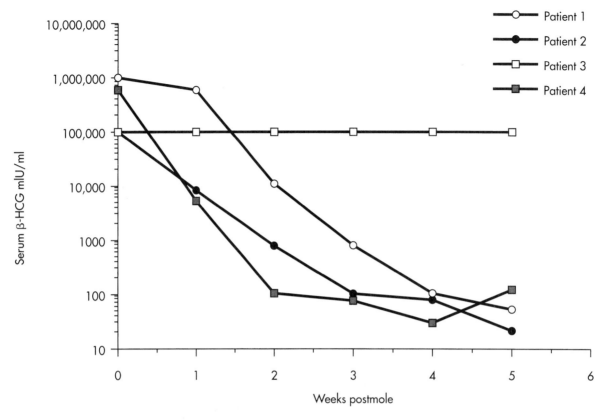

FIGURE 35–3

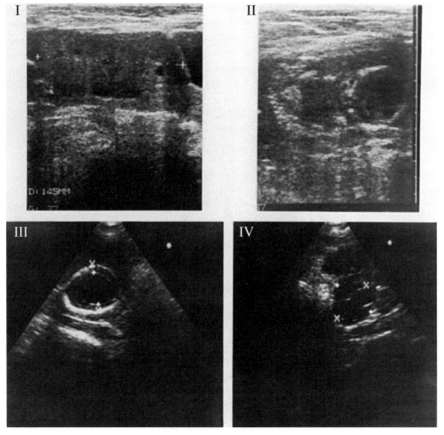

FIGURE 35–4

21. Which test is currently used to establish the diagnosis of a complete or partial mole?

    A. arteriogram
    B. computed tomography (CT)
    C. ultrasound imaging
    D. magnetic resonance imaging (MRI)

22. A patient's uterus is symmetrically large for dates. The referring physician ordered a β-hCG measurement. The result is charted on the laboratory report shown in Figure 35–5. An abdominal ultrasound study is requested and is shown in Figure 35–6. Based on this information, the most likely diagnosis is

    A. twins
    B. a complete mole
    C. incorrect dates
    D. theca-lutein cyst
    E. normal early intrauterine gestation

23. A 29-year-old multigravid patient has just delivered a full-term infant after an uncomplicated pregnancy. Of significance in her history is a previous molar pregnancy, for which she was treated. Which of the following tests is appropriate at this time?

    A. hCG level
    B. CT of pelvis
    C. pelvic ultrasonography
    D. chest radiography
    E. liver function tests

24. In the staging of GTT, stage III is defined by evidence of metastases to what organ?

    A. brain
    B. liver
    C. lung
    D. vagina
    E. bladder

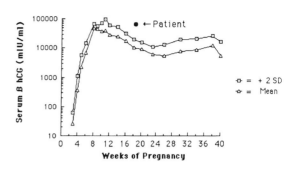

FIGURE 35–5

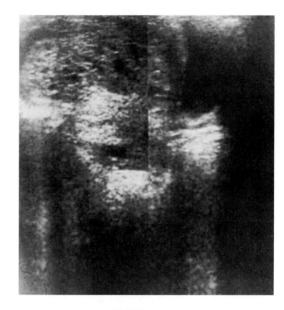

FIGURE 35–6

25. A 30-year-old woman delivered a full-term infant 2 months ago but has persistent vaginal bleeding for which she has undergone D&C. The pathology report shows trophoblastic tissue. What should be the clinician's primary concern?

    A. hydatidiform mole
    B. invasive mole
    C. partial mole
    D. choriocarcinoma
    E. misinterpretation by the pathologist

ANSWERS

1. **D,** Page 1054. If the patient has completed childbearing, hysterectomy should strongly be considered if the patient is older and has an enlarged uterus or theca-lutein cysts. The ovarian lutein cysts regress after termination of the pregnancy, and oophorectomy should not be performed unless there is other ovarian pathology or there is an acute episode such as rupture. Older patients or those with risk factors for ovarian carcinoma may wish to consider elective removal.

2. **B,** Page 1056. The most frequent site of metastatic GTT is the lungs (80% to 90% of cases), and less frequently the liver, brain, ovary, and vagina. However, metastatic disease can occur at any site. Given the diagnosis of GTT, a careful survey for metastatic disease should be initiated using CT examination of the brain and the abdomen. Tests of renal and liver chemistries should also be performed in addition to a hematologic profile.

3. **C,** Page 1051. The photomicrograph depicted in Figure 35–1 is high-power view of a choriocarcinoma. Both pale cytotrophoblasts and syncytiotrophoblasts can be seen. These tumors tend to be hemorrhagic and necrotic. No villi are visible. With a complete or partial hydatidiform mole, the villi are edematous and lack fetal blood cells. One would expect to see villi rather than hemorrhage or necrosis with retained secundines. Choriocarcinoma may develop after a normal pregnancy. Trophoblastic tissue regresses within 2 to 3 weeks after normal delivery. The finding of trophoblastic cells in the uterus more than 3 weeks after delivery should lead one to consider the possibility of choriocarcinoma. This scenario is indeed rare since the incidence of choriocarcinoma following a normal term pregnancy is 1 in 40,000 in the United States.

4. **D,** Page 1051. This photomicrograph depicts decidua and syncytiotrophoblasts within the myometrium. One should remember that trophoblasts invade the myometrium in a normal pregnancy. This is *not* indicative of gestational trophoblastic neoplasia. In all probability, this patient will have no further difficulties. She does not require β-hCG monitoring.

5. **C,** Page 1052. Although most choriocarcinomas occur after complete molar pregnancies, occurrences have been reported after incomplete moles and rare choriocarcinomas have developed after a normal pregnancy (1 per 40,000 term pregnancies). The disease also follows incomplete abortion and ectopic pregnancy.

6. **E,** Page 1052; Table 35–1 in Stenchever. The risk of developing a hydatidiform mole in women who are pregnant is lowest in the 25- to 29-year age bracket. If the risk assigned to this group is 1, the risk in a woman younger than 20 is 1.53 and in women older than 50 is 80.76, this being the highest risk group. Since not many women who are 50 years old become pregnant, numerically few hydatidiform moles occur in this age group.

7. **D,** Page 1054. Intravenous oxytocic agents are used during the evacuation and immediately postoperatively to aid in uterine contraction and to help reduce blood loss. However, it is not advisable to use oxytocic drugs before evacuation of the molar pregnancy because of the risk of disseminating abnormal trophoblastic cells. Suction curettage has proved to be safe and effective even with a larger uterus. After evacuation by suction curettage is complete, a gentle, sharp curettage should be performed to ensure completion of the procedure. There is no need for hysterotomy. Prophylactic chemotherapy has not gained widespread acceptance because giving chemotherapy at the time of evacuation of the mole exposes the patient to toxic and dangerous drugs, and 80% of patients with a complete mole do not require further treatment. Since this patient is 20 years old and a gravida 1, it should be assumed that she has not completed childbearing. Therefore, she is not a candidate for a hysterectomy.

8. **D,** Page 1052. Signs and symptoms associated with a hydatidiform mole include abnormal bleeding in early pregnancy, lower abdominal pain, preeclampsia before 24 weeks of gestation, hyperemesis gravidarum, a uterus large for dates, a uterus small for dates, enlargement of the ovaries, absent fetal heart tones and fetal parts, expulsion of swollen villi, and rarely hyperthyroidism. With an incomplete, not a complete, hydatidiform mole, a fetus is usually present.

9. **B,** Page 1052. No differential in the risk for hydatidiform mole for ABO blood groups has been demonstrated. However, studies have shown that women with type A blood who are married to men with type O and vice versa are at higher risk for choriocarcinoma compared with matings of other blood groups.

10. **E,** Page 1057. Each of these factors is considered to be a marker for high-risk metastatic gestational trophoblastic disease except for vaginal metastases, which are generally excluded from the diagnosis.

11–12. 11, **B;** 12, **C;** Page 1049. A hydatidiform mole is a placental abnormality involving swollen placental villi and trophoblastic hyperplasia with loss of fetal blood vessels. There are two types, partial and complete. A partial mole is a molar pregnancy with some normal and some swollen villi plus some fetal, cord, or amniotic membrane elements associated with polyploidy. A complete mole is the most common type of gestational trophoblastic disease (GTD), occurring in the United States in 0.75 per 1000 pregnancies.

13. **B,** Page 1049. The three morphologic characteristics of a complete mole are (1) a mass of distended villi that appears as large grapelike dilations, (2) a loss of fetal blood vessels in the villi, and (3) hyperplasia of the syncytiotrophoblast and cytotrophoblast. With a partial mole, in addition to the presence of a fetus, there is hyperplasia of the syncytiotrophoblast only. In a complete mole, only paternal chromosomes are believed to be present; there are 46 chromosomes and they are nearly always 46,XX, although a few moles with 46,XY karyotype have been reported. This is the result of a process known as androgenesis, which is the impregnation of an inactive egg by a paternal haploid sperm that duplicates its chromosomes to provide a diploid complement (see Figure 35–2). The nuclear genome is entirely paternal, whereas the mitochondrial genome

is maternal as usual. This anomaly is due to a fertilization error occurring at the time of maternal meiosis II.

Incomplete or partial moles are triploid and have 69 chromosomes of both maternal and paternal origin (see Figure 34–3 in Mishell). The most common mechanism for the origin of a partial mole is a haploid egg being fertilized by two sperm, resulting in three sets of chromosomes. In all instances, mitochondrial DNA is maternal. Not all triploidic concepti demonstrate molar degeneration since duplication of paternal DNA plays some unknown role. Consequently, a 69,XXY fetus in which two of three haploid sets are maternal (eg, maternal meiotic I error) would have a normal placenta. The ultimate severity of the triploidic phenotype depends on this imprinting mechanism.

14. **C,** Page 1058. As described in Chapter 26 of Stenchever, etoposide (VP-16) is usually reserved for high-risk and drug-resistant cases because secondary malignancies have been reported following its use.

15. **C,** Pages 1001–1002. Usually, there is a gradual decline of β-hCG evacuation of a hydatidiform mole, reaching a normal range of 3 to 5 mIU/mL by the 14th week after evacuation. An abnormal regression curve may be noted after evacuation of a mole, as shown in patient 3, and in such instances the patient requires therapy for a gestational trophoblastic tumor. A rise in titer or a plateau in titer (failure to decrease over a 3-week interval) indicates the presence of postmolar trophoblastic neoplasia. Although patient 4 may eventually require further therapy, additional evaluation is indicated before this decision is reached.

16. **C,** Page 1001. Management of a patient with a hydatidiform mole includes the following:
    a. A chest radiograph initially; repeated if results are abnormal or if the β-hCG plateaus or rises
    b. Contraception for 1 year
    c. A pelvic examination every 2 weeks until normal, then every 3 months
    d. Weekly serum determinations of β-hCG until normal for two values, then monthly for 1 year
    In this question, the option was to monitor β-hCG every 2 weeks, not weekly. Single-agent therapy is sufficient because, with the information given, it appears that patient 3 has nonmetastatic disease. Before chemotherapy is initiated, however, a CT of the brain and the liver should be obtained as well as a pelvic ultrasonography; renal and liver studies, and a hematologic profile.

17. **C,** Pages 1001–1002. Although hyperemesis gravidarum and vaginal spotting are more common in patients with molar pregnancies, there is no predictive value for malignancy associated with their presence. Malignant sequelae following a hydatidiform mole appear to be more common among women with an enlarged uterus. Enlargement of the ovaries is associated with a higher frequency of future malignant sequelae (approximately 50%), as compared with less than 15% for those without ovarian enlargement.

18. **A,** Pages 1049, 1054. The ultrasound view depicted in Figure 35–4 reveals placental tissue suggestive of a hydatidiform mole (I), oligohydramnios (II), hydrocephaly (III), and a cystic structure (IV), which in this patient is a theca-lutein cyst. This is a case of a partial mole associated with an abnormal fetus. Survival of such an infant beyond the early neonatal period has not been reported. Partial moles are rarely associated with the subsequent development of malignant trophoblastic disease. In spite of this fact, patients with partial moles need the same follow-up as those with complete moles, including serial β-hCG determinations.

19. **C,** Page 1051. A history of prior hydatidiform mole increases the risk of a subsequent mole by 20 to 40 times. Recurrent spontaneous abortion is also a risk factor, as is advanced maternal age. The increased frequency of moles in lower socioeconomic groups and in underdeveloped areas has led to the suggestion that poor nutrition is a factor in the development of the disease. The evidence is conflicting, and a dietary cause is not supported by current data.

20. **C,** Page 1056. GTT develops after approximately 20% of complete hydatidiform moles. Conversely, about one half the cases of GTT arise after molar pregnancy, whereas one fourth occur after normal pregnancy and one fourth after abortion or ectopic pregnancy.

21. **C,** Page 1053. The most valuable aid in the diagnosis of a hydatidiform mole is ultrasonography. Other diagnostic tests, such as amniograms and arteriograms, were previously used. CT and MRI may be useful in the evaluation of possible metastatic disease, but these methods are not necessary to establish an initial diagnosis.

22. **B,** Page 1053. Levels of β-hCG can appear elevated in a twin pregnancy. This patient's value would fall into an acceptable range if she were really 12 weeks, not 18 weeks. Patients with a complete mole usually have an elevated β-hCG. A single β-hCG measurement is often not diagnostic, especially if the level is not elevated. In 30% to 50% of cases, the uterus is large for dates. Patients with an incomplete mole tend to have lower levels of β-hCG. The ultrasound study shown in Figure 35–6 is typical of that seen in molar pregnancy, effectively eliminating these other possibilities. Theca-lutein cysts are not uncommonly found in patients with molar pregnancies, but their ultrasonographic appearance is very different.

23. **A,** Page 1059. If pregnancy occurs after GTD, it is important to perform ultrasonography early in the gestation to identify a gestational sac in the uterus as well as document fetal heart tones. After delivery, hCG levels should be obtained to rule out any recurrences of GTD. The placenta should be examined histopathologically also.

24. **C,** Page 1047. The stages of GTT include I (confined to uterus); II (metastases to pelvis and vagina); III (metastases to lung); and IV (distant metastases, eg, liver and brain).

25. **D,** Page 1050. After delivery, trophoblastic tissue typically regresses after 2 to 3 weeks. The processes that lead to this normal regression are unknown. The finding of trophoblastic tissue in the uterus more than 3 weeks after delivery should raise the possibility of choriocarcinoma.

PART FIVE

Reproductive Endocrinology and Infertility

Primary and Secondary Dysmenorrhea and Premenstrual Syndrome

for Questions 1–33: Select the one best answer or completion.

1. A 36-year-old gravida 3, para 3, who underwent a tubal ligation 8 years ago is undergoing treatment for premenstrual syndrome (PMS). She has responded well to ovarian suppression with danazol. No other previous therapy has been beneficial, and she now seeks a more permanent solution. She should be offered

   A. hysterectomy
   B. hysterectomy with bilateral oophorectomy
   C. endometrial ablation
   D. dilatation and curettage (D&C)
   E. presacral neurectomy

2. A 32-year-old woman has been arrested and charged with the murder of her husband. In her defense, she has entered a plea of temporary insanity by virtue of PMS. You have been subpoenaed to testify. On the witness stand, the prosecuting attorney asks you to define "premenstrual syndrome." Your testimony should indicate that the symptoms of PMS

   A. occur no more than 14 days before menstruation
   B. occur no more than 5 days before menstruation
   C. occur in a severe form in more than 10% of patients
   D. are sometimes absent immediately after menstruation
   E. are primarily emotional, not physical

3. The woman's defense attorney (Question 2) has entered into evidence a graph of the defendant's "symptoms" over the past 2 months. You are asked to review the defendant's exhibit A (Figure 36–1). Based on this graph, you might reasonably testify that the accused

   A. has PMS
   B. is manic-depressive
   C. was insane at the time of the murder
   D. has severe dysmenorrhea
   E. none of the above

4. A 20-year-old nulligravida complains of severe lower abdominal cramping pain, nausea, vomiting, and diarrhea, which occur approximately 8 hours after the onset of menstruation and last for 1 to 2 days. The patient's periods take place regularly every 26 to 28 days and last 5 days. The woman is not sexually active, uses no birth control, and normally takes Extra Strength Tylenol (acetaminophen) with little relief. Her physical examination, including the pelvic examination, is unremarkable. The cause of these symptoms is most likely

   A. adenomyosis
   B. endometriosis
   C. cervical stenosis
   D. excess prostaglandin
   E. leiomyomata

EXHIBIT A

Severity of symptoms that defendant associates with PMS

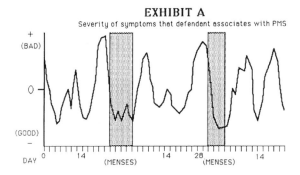

FIGURE 36–1

5. **Which of the following may be an effective alternative to nonsteroidal anti-inflammatory drugs (NSAIDs) as treatment for primary dysmenorrhea?**

   A. oral contraceptives
   B. analgesics
   C. transcutaneous nerve stimulation
   D. all the above

6. **Functional bowel disorder occurs in approximately what percentage of women with dysmenorrhea?**

   A. 20%
   B. 40%
   C. 60%
   D. 80%

7. **Which of the following has been linked to the cause of PMS?**

   A. serotonin
   B. endorphins
   C. progesterone
   D. all the above

8. **PMS is diagnosed by using**

   A. serum progesterone
   B. serum follicle-stimulating hormone (FSH)
   C. thyroid function tests
   D. symptom diary

9. **Which treatment for PMS is associated with neuropathy?**

   A. magnesium
   B. vitamin B$_6$ (pyridoxine)
   C. diuretics
   D. progesterone

10. **Which of the following is demonstrated by patients who complain of premenstrual bloating?**

    A. change of abdominal girth
    B. change of weight
    C. altered perception of body size
    D. all the above

11. **Which of the following is characteristic of primary dysmenorrhea?**

    A. likely to have a familial pattern
    B. probable diagnosis for menstrual discomfort in a 42-year-old multipara
    C. associated with throbbing abdominal pain and a sense of pelvic heaviness
    D. all the above

12. **All the following are characteristic of primary dysmenorrhea except**

    A. likely to improve with analgesics of mild to moderate strength
    B. generally associated with a normal pelvic examination result
    C. symptoms start 3 to 4 days before menses
    D. major cause of school absences

13. **Which of the following progesterone treatments has been used to treat PMS?**

    A. vaginal progesterone suppository
    B. oral medroxyprogesterone acetate
    C. oral micronized progesterone
    D. all the above

14. **The likely basis on which estradiol patches with oral norethindrone works for PMS is**

    A. normalization of estrogen level
    B. normalization of progesterone level
    C. suppression of ovulation
    D. modulation of serotonin

15. **Which of the following describes the current status of psychotherapy in the management of PMS?**

    A. preferred as adjunctive therapy
    B. no role
    C. best used after operative castration
    D. best primary therapy for young patients

16. **Which of the following NSAIDs is in the same chemical family as aspirin?**

    A. ibuprofen
    B. fenamates
    C. naproxen
    D. ketoprofen

17. **A 19-year-old nulligravid college student requests contraception. Her only significant history is that of dysmenorrhea for 6 years. Her physical examination result is normal. Recommended contraceptive choices for her should include all the following except**

    A. oral contraceptives
    B. a diaphragm
    C. a copper-containing intrauterine device (IUD)
    D. Depo-Provera

18. Of the following, which is the most likely cause of PMS?

    A. prolactin excess
    B. hypothyroidism
    C. serotonin deficiency
    D. testosterone deficiency

19. A 17-year-old nulligravida requests treatment of her primary dysmenorrhea. Contraindications to the use of NSAIDs in this patient include

    A. aspirin-sensitive asthma
    B. a history of diarrhea with menstruation
    C. premenstrual irritability and bloating
    D. diabetes mellitus

20. Which of the following would be useful in making the diagnosis of PMS?

    A. clinical trial of 200 mg/day of vitamin B_6
    B. serum estrogen level test
    C. diary of symptoms over 2 to 3 months
    D. history of cyclic depressive symptoms

21. A 32-year-old desires treatment for PMS. She has previously taken bromocriptine and asks about taking it again. She should be told that it

    A. is appropriate when breast tenderness is the major symptom
    B. causes a greater improvement in mood than does placebo treatment
    C. reduces the elevated level of prolactin found in patients with PMS
    D. is most beneficial if taken all month

22. Prostaglandin F_{2a} has been implicated as a possible cause of primary dysmenorrhea because

    A. it is found in higher amounts in women with dysmenorrhea
    B. it is capable of stimulating the smooth muscle of the uterus
    C. inhibition of its production through the use of NSAIDs results in the relief of symptoms
    D. all the above

23. The role of progesterone in the treatment of PMS is based on

    A. the observation that PMS symptoms are absent during pregnancy
    B. well-controlled studies
    C. the reduced levels of progesterone in patients with PMS
    D. the elevated progesterone levels in women who are asymptomatic

24. Appropriate initial therapy for premenstrual symptoms in a 29-year-old gravida 3, para 2, ab 1, female who has had her "tubes tied" includes

    A. reassurance
    B. a balanced diet
    C. vitamin B_6 100 mg PO twice a day
    D. all the above

25. In a 19-year-old nulligravida with the clinical diagnosis of primary dysmenorrhea, appropriate therapy consists of two tablets at the onset of pain and then one tablet three times a day PRN of

    A. Anaprox 275 mg
    B. Ponstel 250 mg
    C. Motrin 800 mg
    D. all the above

26. A 30-year-old patient is referred for cyclic fluid retention as a primary focus of PMS. She should be told that fluid retention has been implicated in PMS because the symptom complex is associated with

    A. an increase in total body weight
    B. an increase in abdominal girth
    C. a perception of swelling
    D. all the above

27. A 36-year-old gravida 3, para 3, who owns a health food store asks your opinion about using vitamin B_6 in a dosage of 650 mg twice a day for the treatment of PMS. You can respond that this regimen

    A. has no apparent effect on estrogen metabolism
    B. is potentially dangerous
    C. has not been proved effective
    D. all the above

28. A 34-year-old gravida 1, para 1, who is using an IUD for contraception complains of heavy, crampy periods since the birth of her child 1 year ago. She had experienced menstrual pain during most of her periods before her pregnancy. This discomfort had responded to therapy with ibuprofen (Motrin). Her current discomfort is somewhat worse than it was previously. She has tried an over-the-counter ibuprofen medication without success. This patient's physical examination, including pelvic examination, is normal and her IUD string is visible. Possible diagnoses include all the following except

    A. primary dysmenorrhea
    B. secondary dysmenorrhea
    C. PMS
    D. endometriosis

29. **In an effort to help the patient in Question 28, you might reasonably recommend**

    A. an oral contraceptive agent
    B. an NSAID
    C. removal of the IUD
    D. all the above

30. **A 16-year-old has disabling primary dysmenorrhea. Her history is otherwise negative, and her physical examination results are normal. Initial therapeutic options include**

    A. oral contraceptives
    B. prostaglandin synthetase inhibitors (NSAIDs)
    C. analgesics
    D. all the above

31. **Factors that affect the severity of PMS symptoms include**

    A. age
    B. number of children
    C. evidence of clinical depression
    D. all the above

32. **A 38-year-old gravida 4, para 4, has a 2-year history of emotional lability, irritability, and difficulty with fellow workers. She admits to episodes of inexplicable crying and feels that sometimes people are "out to get her." She has not sought help for this but thinks that it may be PMS. In addition to PMS, a differential diagnosis for this patient should include**

    A. anxiety
    B. depression
    C. psychosis
    D. all the above

33. **A 32-year-old gravida 1, para 1, has a 4-year history of increasing dysmenorrhea. She reports that she had had minor cramping as a teenager that was easily controlled by over-the-counter medications. She got pregnant without difficulty at age 27 but required a cesarean section because of a breech presentation. After the delivery of her child, she was treated for a recurrent low-grade squamous intraepithelial lesion (LGSIL) with cryo-cautery of the cervix. Over the past 4 years, she has noted increasing pain with her menses, prolonged bleeding (increased from 4 to 7 days), and significantly decreased flow. Although each of the following is plausible, which is the most likely cause of the secondary amenorrhea?**

    A. cervical stenosis
    B. chronic endometritis
    C. endometriosis
    D. pelvic congestion
    E. pedunculated submucosal myoma

ANSWERS

1. **B,** Pages 1074–1075. As reported recently, some patients who respond to ovarian-suppression doses of medication may be candidates for hysterectomy and bilateral salpingo-oophorectomy as the definitive treatment for PMS. Removing the uterus alone will not alter the symptoms because it only eliminates the source of bleeding and not the source of other premenstrual symptoms. Endometrial ablation would also only reduce or eliminate menstrual bleeding while not addressing the symptoms. D&C and presacral neurectomy have no role in the treatment of PMS. Hysterectomy with bilateral oophorectomy should be used only in the unusual case in which other therapies have failed and in a patient who clearly responds to ovarian suppression. In addition to danazol, gonadotrophin-releasing hormone (GnRH) agonists have been used to treat PMS successfully. Patients who undergo surgical castration can be given estrogen replacement therapy without symptoms recurring.

2. **A,** Page 1070. Probably the best working definition of PMS is one that restricts the recurrence of significant distressing emotional and physical symptoms to no more than 14 days before menses. These symptoms must recur episodically and predictably and do not need to occur every month, although they usually do so. In addition, the symptoms must spontaneously and completely disappear with, or soon after, the onset of menstrual flow. Although PMS is thought to affect

anywhere from 5% to 95% of women, only about 2% to 3% have severe symptoms.

3. **E,** Pages 1070–1071. The pattern of symptoms illustrated in Figure 36–1 is typical of patients who have complaints that become linked or entrained with the recurrent rhythm of the period, not true PMS. Note that there is no true symptom-free period following each menstrual flow. Menstrual pain has not been mentioned, which does not support the diagnosis of dysmenorrhea. As a gynecologist, you are not in a position to diagnose what that disorder is or to make legal assessments regarding the patient's guilt or accountability.

4. **D,** Pages 1065–1066. Primary dysmenorrhea is caused by an excess of prostaglandin F_{2a}. This prostaglandin excess also is responsible for the presence of nausea, vomiting, and diarrhea, which do not occur with adenomyosis or cervical stenosis. The pain associated with endometriosis generally precedes the onset of menstrual flow and improves after the flow is established.

5. **D,** Pages 1066–1067. Although NSAIDs are the standard therapy for primary dysmenorrhea, other approaches are possible. Oral contraceptives relieve the symptoms of primary dysmenorrhea in about 90% of patients. Analgesics may be necessary in treating patients with primary dysmenorrhea, but they should be used as backup drugs when the desired therapeutic effect is not achieved with NSAIDs or oral contraceptives. Recently, Kaplan and colleagues reported on the use of transcutaneous electrical nerve stimulation (TENS) for two menstrual cycles in 61 Israeli women with primary dysmenorrhea. Thirty percent reported marked pain relief; 60%, moderate relief; and 10%, no change in symptoms. These authors suggested that this method could be considered primary therapy or for use in conjunction with pharmacologic therapy.

6. **C,** Page 1070. In a study by Crowell and associates, dysmenorrhea was diagnosed in 19.8% of 383 women. Functional bowel disorder, defined as abdominal pain with altered bowel function, occurred in 61% of the women with dysmenorrhea but in only 20% of the others. Although neuroticism was diagnosed significantly more often in patients with functional bowel disorder, with or without dysmenorrhea, bowel symptoms were significantly correlated with dysmenorrhea even after controlling for the effects of neuroticism. Prostaglandin levels in vaginal fluid were elevated in patients with dysmenorrhea but did not consistently differentiate the diagnostic groups. These authors concluded that there was a strong covariance of menstrual and bowel symptoms, along with an overlap in their diagnosis, suggesting a common physiologic basis.

7. **D,** Pages 1071–1072. In 1981, Reid and Yen reviewed the literature on PMD and concluded that it was a multifactorial psychoendocrine disorder. Recent studies indicate that alterations in serotoninergic neuronal mechanisms in the central nervous system may have major involvement. The fact that ovulation (and therefore progesterone) production is important in this syndrome has been known for some time, but studies of the relationship of progesterone in the circulation and the severity of the symptoms have not been fruitful. In fact, some have demonstrated an increased level of progesterone in the circulation in women with PMS, whereas others have shown a decrease or no change at all. Chuong and coworkers recently demonstrated that β-endorphin levels throughout the periovulatory phase were lower in patients with PMS than in controls.

8. **D,** Page 1072. No laboratory tests are available to confirm the diagnosis of PMS. Although it has been reported that many patients with PMS suffer thyroid hypofunction, a recent study demonstrated that there was no significant thyroid disease in 44 carefully studied patients with PMS who were compared with 15 normal controls. The diagnosis of PMS is made by symptom diary and elimination of other diagnoses.

9. **B,** Pages 1072–1073. Vitamin B_6 deficiency in patients with PMS has been suggested because this vitamin is a coenzyme in the biosynthesis of dopamine and serotonin, and the possibility that this agent may be involved in the etiologic complex of PMS has been raised. Higher doses of pyridoxine should be administered with caution since neuropathy occurred in several patients treated with as little as 100 to 200 mg daily. Such symptoms as sensory deficit, paresthesia, numbness, ataxia, and muscle weakness may occur. The physician therefore should review the patient's diet and initially suggest a high-protein, well-balanced diet. Supplemental vitamins may be used, and the physician may elect to suggest that the patient use a vitamin B_6 (pyridoxine) supplement (50 mg/day).

10. **C,** Page 1073. Although many patients do report a feeling of fluid retention during the luteal phase, this effect has been difficult to demonstrate. Perceived swelling of the body is difficult to prove unless actual careful weight analysis is done. The symptoms of bloatedness are most noticeable during the premenstrual phase of the cycle. Despite elevated scores for bloatedness, there is no increase in body weight or measured body-dimension changes during this period. The patient does perceive an increase in body size, and a discrepancy between the perceived body size and the actual body size is noted.

11–12. 11, **A**; 12, **C**; Pages 1066–1068. The best therapy for secondary dysmenorrhea is ultimately directed toward the cause, but both primary and secondary dysmenorrhea may be treated successfully with analgesics. The distinction between primary and secondary is most often based on normal pelvic examination results associated with primary dysmenorrhea. The peak age of incidence for primary and secondary dysmenorrhea is very different. Primary dysmenorrhea is much more likely in younger women. Thus, it accounts for a significant number of school absences. In older women, secondary dysmenorrhea is more apt to be the correct diagnosis, even though primary dysmenorrhea is still possible. Although causes of secondary dysmenorrhea such as myomata may have a familial pattern, it is primary dysmenorrhea that is most closely associated with a familial tendency. The symptoms of pelvic heaviness and throbbing pain are more common with secondary dysmenorrhea. The pain of primary dysmenorrhea is usually described as sharp or "laborlike." In neither primary nor secondary dysmenorrhea do the symptoms start appreciably before the onset of menstrual flow.

13. **D**, Pages 1073–1074. Although Dalton advocates the use of naturally occurring progesterone, the fact that progesterone receptors respond to both synthetic progestins and progesterone implies that any reasonable progestational agent would be appropriate. However, in all double-blind studies to date, progesterone has not been shown to be effective. In the rare patient in whom progesterone is to be tried, a regimen of 10 to 20 mg/day of medroxyprogesterone acetate (Provera) or 50 to 100 mg twice a day of progesterone vaginal suppositories can be tried. Oral micronized progesterone has also been described as treatment for PMS.

14. **C**, Page 1074. Some relief of symptoms was noted in a double-blind, placebo-controlled, crossover study using estradiol patches (200 mg every 3 days) and norethindrone (5 mg on days 19 to 26 of each cycle) when compared with placebo by Watson and colleagues. The authors realized that they were suppressing ovulation and that this may have been the mechanism for symptom relief.

15. **A**, Page 1074. Studies in the 1950s showed that 50% of patients improved with psychotherapy alone. However, this change is similar to the response rate of many placebo therapies. If patients have obvious psychiatric problems as detected by history, psychotherapy certainly should be added. Psychotherapy is less effective as a primary therapy.

16. **B**, Pages 1066–1067. Although the pathogenesis of dysmenorrhea is still unknown, the fact that there is a close association between an elevated prostaglandin F_{2a} level in the secretory endometrium and the symptoms of dysmenorrhea has led to the theory that prostaglandin F_{2a} is associated with the pathogenesis of dysmenorrhea. NSAIDs are prostaglandin synthetase inhibitors and have been demonstrated to alleviate these symptoms. These substances are nonsteroidal and anti-inflammatory. They have been used as analgesics for a number of conditions, including arthritis, and generally are divided into two chemical groups—the arylcarboxylic acids, which include acetylsalicylic acid (aspirin) and fenamates, and the arylalkanoic acids, including the arylpropionic acids (ibuprofen, naproxen, and ketoprofen) and the indoleacetic acids (indomethacin).

17. **C**, Pages 1066–1067. Because primary dysmenorrhea is associated with ovulatory cycles, suppression of ovulation with oral contraceptives or Depo-Provera often provides at least some relief. A diaphragm would be an acceptable barrier form of contraception if the patient were sufficiently motivated to use it correctly. Her dysmenorrhea would then need to be treated with an NSAID. Although some studies indicate no effect of IUD use on the incidence of dysmenorrhea, many authors think that IUDs may contribute to menstrual pain and classify the device as a cause of secondary dysmenorrhea. Progesterone-containing IUDs are less likely to be associated with dysmenorrhea. The patient in this question, however, is a nulligravida. Therefore, the potential adverse effect on fertility must be weighed, and the IUD should be avoided.

18. **C**, Page 1071. Although many possible causes for PMS have been advanced over the years, all remain unproven. Currently, the best that can be said is that PMS is a multifactorial psychoendocrine disorder. There is growing evidence that serotonin and endorphins may have a central role in PMS.

19. **A**, Pages 1066–1067. Aspirin-sensitive asthma, inflammatory bowel disease, and gastric ulcer are contraindications for most NSAIDs. Although there is an incidence of 3% to 10% of diarrhea with the use of NSAIDs, many studies have indicated that these drugs reduce the incidence of period-related diarrhea. PMS is not a contraindication to these drugs; indeed, patients may respond favorably to their use. Diabetes is also not a contraindication to the use of NSAIDs.

20. **C**, Page 1072. The most useful tool for making the diagnosis of PMS is a diary of symptoms. There is no evidence that changes in estrogen levels aid the diagnosis. Since the value of vitamin B_6 therapy is debatable, any response noted would be nondiagnostic because of the possibility of a

placebo effect. A history of depressive symptoms is helpful, but a prospective calendar more accurately documents the cyclic nature of these symptoms.

21. **A,** Page 1074. Studies have been unable to demonstrate an abnormal level of prolactin in women with PMS. In controlled studies of bromocriptine use in the treatment of PMS, only breast tenderness responded and only in doses above 5 mg/day.

22. **D,** Pages 1066–1067. Prostaglandin F_{2a} has been found in levels of 5 to 10 times the usual amount in women with primary dysmenorrhea. Prostaglandin F_{2a} is a potent stimulator of smooth muscle, both in the uterus and in the gastrointestinal tract. In the uterus, this action may be responsible for intrauterine pressures in excess of 400 mm Hg. (During contractions of the uterus during menstruation, the uterine pressure is 60 to 80 mm Hg.) In the gastrointestinal tract, the increased motility caused by the stimulatory effects of prostaglandin F_{2a} may account for the frequent observation of nausea, vomiting, and diarrhea in patients with primary dysmenorrhea. Although the success of NSAID therapy supports the role of prostaglandins in primary dysmenorrhea, it does not by itself conclusively establish a cause-and-effect relationship.

23. **A,** Pages 1073–1074. The use of progesterone therapy in the treatment of PMS has been most vocally championed by Katharina Dalton of England. She observed that PMS symptoms were absent in her own pregnancy and in her patients during pregnancy. This has led to the use of progesterone in uncontrolled open trials of more than 30,000 patients worldwide. Despite this experience, no controlled blind study has confirmed the superiority of progesterone over placebo. No study of any kind has confirmed any consistent alteration of progesterone levels.

24. **D,** Pages 1072–1073. Although no double-blind trials have proved this, reassurance, a good diet, and an exercise program are always appropriate. Exercise may help induce endogenous endorphin production. A substantial number of patients benefit from just undergoing the process of investigation and the identification of a diagnostic condition. Supplementation with small doses of vitamin B_6, which is a coenzyme in the production of serotonin, is probably reasonable therapy in almost any patient with PMS.

25. **D,** Pages 1066–1067; Table 36–2. Anaprox (naproxen sodium), Ponstel (mefenamic acid), and Motrin (ibuprofen) are all approved for the treatment of dysmenorrhea and are appropriate in the absence of contraindications. Because of evidence of receptor site activity by the fenamates (Ponstel and Meclomen), these agents may confer some

theoretical advantage. In practice, this may be reflected in a slightly faster onset of action. For most patients, however, these differences are probably of little consequence.

26. **C,** Page 1073. Controlled studies have been unable to demonstrate any changes in abdominal measurements or in total body weight, even in patients who complain of swelling and bloating. These patients do think that they are bloated and swollen during the period of symptoms.

27. **D,** Pages 1072–1073. The rationale for using vitamin B_6 as therapy for PMS comes from the fact that it is a coenzyme in the production of serotonin in the brain. Because reduced levels of serotonin have been found in patients with depression, some authors have postulated that replacing vitamin B_6 may favorably affect the emotional symptoms of PMS. Vitamin B_6 therapy for PMS has not been adequately studied to make any case for efficacy. Although some patients may experience improvement, there are no blind studies to suggest a response greater than what occurs with placebo. Peripheral nerve damage has been reported in dosages above 200 mg/day. Dosages in the magnitude suggested for this patient should not be used.

28. **C,** Pages 1065–1070. Although the most likely diagnosis for this patient is dysmenorrhea secondary to the presence of an IUD, continuing primary dysmenorrhea is still a possibility. The patient's history is not typical of PMS. The history does suggest that this patient may have had primary dysmenorrhea before her pregnancy. Studies reported by Dawood indicate that pregnancy and delivery do not relieve dysmenorrhea. As many as 20% of women with dysmenorrhea experience a return of symptoms with the resumption of ovulation. The lack of response of the patient's symptoms to over-the-counter strengths of ibuprofen most likely reflects inadequate dosage rather than a non–prostaglandin-mediated cause. The patient's history is compatible with early endometriosis, but there is no documentation (via laparoscopy or biopsy).

29. **D,** Pages 1065–1066. When IUD use was more common, IUDs were a not uncommon cause of secondary, although iatrogenic, dysmenorrhea. It has been postulated that the increased prostaglandins related to IUD use not only may have been partially responsible for the contraceptive effect but also may have been the cause of the accompanying menstrual pain. This association is supported by studies that indicate moderate success in treating these women with therapeutic doses of prostaglandin inhibitors. To attempt to differentiate between secondary dysmenorrhea associated with this patient's IUD and primary

dysmenorrhea, it may be necessary to advise the removal of the IUD. If this is done, an alternative contraceptive should be provided. Sterilization would not be appropriate because it does not address the complaint of dysmenorrhea. Oral contraceptives might be the most logical option.

30. **D,** Page 1067. Oral contraceptives relieve the symptoms of primary dysmenorrhea in 90% of patients. This may be due to a modulating effect on the hypothalamus or a reduction in the amount of endometrium. Prostaglandin synthetase inhibitors are a logical alternative. Analgesics can be used as backup drugs if the other two options are ineffective. Narcotics must be avoided.

31. **D,** Pages 1071–1072. It is known that environmental stressors do affect the severity of the symptoms of PMS. In one study, 34% of symptom severity was attributable to PMS in the patient's mother, a low level of exercise, a younger age, and a larger number of children. In another study, patients with PMS were shown to have episodes of "luteal phase depression" when compared with controls, but it was noted that these episodes were different from those suffered by patients with "endogenous depression."

32. **D,** Page 1071. PMS must be differentiated from other psychiatric disorders, such as depression, anxiety reactions, and psychosis. A critical point in making the diagnosis of PMS is that PMS symptoms occur only during the luteal phase. A prospective symptom diary over several months will help to identify this pattern. Although continuous use of psychoactive drugs, such as tricyclics and lithium, has not yielded good relief of PMS symptoms, alprazolam or fluoxetine hydrochloride given on days 20 through 28 of the cycle has significantly relieved the severity of premenstrual nervous tension, mood swings, irritability, anxiety, depression, fatigue, forgetfulness, crying, cravings for sweets, abdominal bloating, cramps, and headaches. Fluoxetine hydrochloride should not be given to patients with bipolar depression. Alprazolam and fluoxetine seem to hold promise for relieving PMS symptoms when properly used, and they appear to be required in small doses only.

33. **A,** Page 1068. This patient has a typical history for cervical stenosis—history of a cervical procedure, scant menstrual flow, and secondary dysmenorrhea. The treatment for this patient will consist of cervical dilatation. Although endometriosis may have been caused by the stenosis, the primary problem is the stenosis. Chronic endometritis causes secondary dysmenorrhea, but the menstrual flow should be increased and other symptoms of dyspareunia or abnormal discharge is likely present. Pelvic congestion is a diagnosis of exclusion. A submucosal pedunculated myoma is a possible cause with a ball-valve type of action. However, given the history, attempts at cervical dilation constitute the first step, followed perhaps by hysteroscopy to rule out a polyp or myoma.

Abnormal Uterine Bleeding

for Questions 1–18: Select the one best answer or completion.

1. **A woman complaining of menorrhagia has flow lasting a total of 10 days. Most of her menstrual blood loss most likely occurs**

   A. within the first 3 days of menstruation
   B. during the 4th, 5th, and 6th days of menstruation
   C. during the last 3 days of menstruation
   D. at a different time each month

2. **A 38-year-old gravida 3, para 3, has a history of progressive menorrhagia over the past 8 months. This has never happened previously. The patient weighs 170 pounds and is 5 feet 2 inches tall. She has no rash, but her skin is dry. An office endometrial aspirate at her initial visit 1 month ago revealed proliferative endometrium. Her hemoglobin was 10.8 g. The systemic disease most likely to be associated with these findings is**

   A. systemic lupus erythematosus (SLE)
   B. idiopathic thrombocytopenic purpura (ITP)
   C. von Willebrand disease
   D. hypothyroidism
   E. diabetes mellitus

3. **The mechanisms that normally stop menstrual blood loss include all the following except**

   A. localized vasoconstriction
   B. formation of a platelet plug
   C. vascular fibrin deposition
   D. fibrinolysis
   E. myometrial contraction

4. **Anovulatory patients have heavier bleeding than ovulatory patients because anovulatory patients appear to have a deficiency in**

   A. prostaglandin F_{2a}
   B. prostaglandin E_2
   C. thromboxane
   D. prostacyclin
   E. arachidonic acid

5. **A 28-year-old gravida 1, para 1, with menorrhagia over the past 6 months had an endometrium sample taken on day 22 of her cycle. The report states "secretory endometrial fragments." Since the biopsy, her menstrual flow has been heavier and longer. A workup for other potential causes of this bleeding is unrevealing. The next step in her management should be**

   A. a repeat office endometrial aspiration
   B. dilatation and curettage (D&C)
   C. vaginal probe ultrasonography
   D. hysteroscopy
   E. a midluteal progesterone level test

6. **In treating patients with severe menorrhagia secondary to anovulation, a theoretical advantage of high-dose conjugated equine estrogens over a high-dose combination oral contraceptive is that estrogen alone**

   A. promotes rapid endometrial growth
   B. increases spiral artery recoil
   C. increases platelet aggregation
   D. promotes synthesis of prostaglandin F_{2a}
   E. can be given intravenously

7. A 13-year-old virgin complains of a 3-month history of menometrorrhagia. The rectal abdominal examination result is normal. Office urine pregnancy test results are negative. The hemoglobin and hematocrit are 9.8 g and 29%, respectively. The treatment of choice for this patient is

   A. combination oral contraceptives
   B. cyclic progestin therapy for 10 days every month
   C. D&C
   D. outpatient hysteroscopy
   E. daily high-dose conjugated oral estrogen

8. An 18-year-old gives a 2-month history of intermittent, irregular bleeding. Her last normal menstrual period was 3 months ago. Before that, her cycle was regular at 28 days. Pelvic examination results are normal. The next step in management should be

   A. endometrial aspiration
   B. pelvic ultrasound imaging
   C. a pregnancy test
   D. laparoscopy
   E. hysteroscopy

9. A 45-year-old gravida 3, para 3, who has had menorrhagia for 6 months underwent a hysteroscopy and D&C 4 weeks ago. The uterus size was normal. The cavity was smooth and without polyps, and the pathologist reported that the endometrium was secretory. The patient smokes 10 cigarettes per day. The preferred management is

   A. a levonorgestrel-releasing intrauterine device (IUD)
   B. continuous medroxyprogesterone acetate
   C. continuous conjugated estrogens
   D. cyclic danazol
   E. combination oral contraceptives

10. An 18-year-old has had one extremely heavy period for which she was prescribed conjugated estrogens, 10 mg in divided doses. Her pregnancy test result is negative. The patient denies sexual activity. Assuming that the bleeding is markedly diminished within 24 hours, the next step in the treatment of this patient should be

    A. conjugated estrogens, 10 mg/day in divided doses plus medroxyprogesterone acetate, 10 mg/day for 2 weeks
    B. conjugated estrogens, 20 mg/day in divided doses for 2 weeks
    C. a cycle of oral contraceptives containing 30 to 35 mg of ethinyl estradiol
    D. vitamin E for 30 days
    E. office endometrial aspiration

11. The mean volume of blood lost during normal menstruation is

    A. 15 mL
    B. 35 mL
    C. 55 mL
    D. 75 mL
    E. 95 mL

12. A 38-year-old gravida 2, para 1, ab 1, states that she has had heavy vaginal bleeding for 9 days. Her pulse is 110, blood pressure is 80/60, and pelvic examination is normal. A titer for β human chorionic gonadotropin (β-hCG) is negative, hemoglobin is 10 g, and hematocrit is 30%. The most efficacious treatment is

    A. parenteral high-dose conjugated estrogens for 10 days
    B. D&C
    C. medroxyprogesterone acetate, 20 mg/day for 10 days
    D. danazol, 400 mg/day for 10 days
    E. oral contraceptive tablets, four tablets per day for 10 days

13. A 14-year-old comes to the emergency department with a 3-day history of excessive menstrual flow. Her hemoglobin is 8.2 g, and her hematocrit is 23%. The pregnancy test result is negative. The blood pressure is 80/40, and the pulse is 120. The most likely diagnosis is

    A. von Willebrand disease
    B. prothrombin deficiency
    C. leukemia
    D. anovulation
    E. endometrial polyp

14. A 28-year-old woman has been about 7 days late for her period three or four times per year for the past 2 years. The flow eventually starts with spotting. A β-hCG titer is negative at the time of her office visit. An endometrial biopsy done on the fourth day of her "late flow" reveals mixed proliferative and secretory endometrium. These findings indicate

    A. an inadequate corpus luteum
    B. anovulation
    C. repetitive subclinical abortions
    D. a chronic ectopic pregnancy
    E. a persistent corpus luteum (Halban syndrome)

15. A 41-year-old, 5-feet 4-inch, 135-pound gravida 2, para 2, woman has a 4-month history of irregular menstruation. She has very heavy flow every 60 to 120 days. A β-hCG titer is negative. The pelvic examination result is normal. The next step in management should be

    A. office hysteroscopy
    B. office endometrial aspiration
    C. serum clotting studies
    D. hysterosalpingogram
    E. pelvic ultrasound imaging

16. After successful treatment of an acute episode of anovulatory bleeding in a 13-year-old, long-term treatment is best accomplished by

    A. D&C
    B. cyclic oral contraceptives
    C. cyclic conjugated estrogens
    D. cyclic medroxyprogesterone acetate
    E. cyclic danazol

17. A 42-year-old woman with class III valvular heart disease has a history of progressive menorrhagia over the past 8 months. Previous attempts to decrease the bleeding with medroxy-progesterone acetate have failed. An endometrial aspiration is reported to be proliferative endometrium without inflammation. The hemoglobin is 10.8 g. At this point you would

    A. start cyclic oral contraceptives
    B. start nonsteroidal anti-inflammatory drugs (NSAIDs)
    C. start antibiotic therapy
    D. perform an endometrial ablation procedure
    E. perform D&C

18. The rationale for the therapeutic use of conjugated estrogens for the immediate treatment of dysfunctional uterine bleeding is based on the fact that it

    A. stabilizes endogenous serum clotting factors
    B. causes a decrease in platelet adhesiveness
    C. causes decidualization of the endometrium
    D. leads to rapid proliferation of the endometrium
    E. is followed by a uniform endometrial slough on withdrawal

DIRECTIONS:

for Questions 19–21: For each numbered item, select the one heading most closely associated with it. Each lettered heading may be used once, more than once, or not at all.

19–21. Appropriate therapeutic agent

    (A) danazol
    (B) ergot alkaloid
    (C) tranexamic acid (AMCA)
    (D) medroxyprogesterone acetate

19. Which is an inhibitor of fibrinolysis and is associated with a 60% reduction in menstrual blood loss in patients with menorrhagia?

20. Which is an inhibitor and does not reduce menstrual blood loss in patients treated for menorrhagia?

21. Which is an inhibitor and enhances activity of 17-α-dehydrogenase to favor conversion of estradiol to estrone?

DIRECTIONS:

for Questions 22–31: Select the one best answer or completion.

22. In assessing the quantity of blood loss during menstruation, the most reliable feature obtained by history is the

    A. number of days of flow
    B. number of sanitary pads used
    C. patient's description of passage of blood clots
    D. patient's quantification as "heavy"

23. The histologic appearance of the endometrium of a patient who is anovulatory is likely to show all the following except

    A. an eosinophilic infiltrate
    B. areas of necrosis of the endometrium
    C. lack of spiraling arterioles
    D. proliferation of the endometrium

24. Complications that are more commonly associated with endometrial ablation than with hysterectomy include all the following except

    A. fluid overload
    B. hematometra
    C. infection
    D. thermal damage
    E. uterine perforation

25. A 35-year-old gravida 2, para 2, with a negative workup is having persistent menorrhagia despite medical management. An endometrial ablation is elected as the treatment approach. Which of the following techniques does not require pretreatment?

    A. laser ablation
    B. roller-ball thermal ablation
    C. thermal balloon ablation
    D. none of the above; they all require pretreatment

26. The following are all pharmacologic actions of NSAIDs used in treating menorrhagia except

    A. blocking formation of prostacyclin
    B. inhibition of fibrinolysis
    C. interference in the conversion of arachidonic acid to prostaglandin
    D. inhibition of platelet aggregation

27. The hematologic profile of a group of women who lose more than 80 mL of blood each menstrual cycle would typically include all the following except

    A. increased bleeding time
    B. lower mean corpuscular volume
    C. lower mean hemoglobin level
    D. lower mean hematocrit level
    E. reduced serum iron levels

28. Medroxyprogesterone acetate has all the following actions except that it

    A. activates 17-hydroxysteroid dehydrogenase
    B. does not alter high-density lipoprotein, low-density lipoprotein (HDL/LDL) levels as much as the 19-nortestosterones
    C. inhibits replenishment of estrogen receptors in the cell
    D. reduces vascularity in the basalis layer of the endometrium

29. Therapeutic agents that are efficacious in reducing mean menstrual blood loss include all the following except

    A. cyclic synthetic progestins
    B. danazol
    C. methylergonovine maleate
    D. NSAIDs
    E. progestin-releasing IUDs

30. The advantages of "roller-ball" electrocautery ablation of the endometrium over laser ablation include the fact that the former

    A. can be done with a paracervical block
    B. involves considerably shorter operative time
    C. has fewer long-term complications
    D. hormonal "pretreatment" is not necessary
    E. is less expensive

31. A 20-year-old gravida 0 complains of "heavy menstruation," which is now in its seventh day. The pelvic examination result is normal except for the presence of clotted blood filling the posterior fornix. A β-hCG titer is negative, and an office hematocrit is 35%. The recognized standard management options include all the following except

    A. D&C
    B. high-dose conjugated estrogen therapy (10 mg/day in divided doses until bleeding stops)
    C. medroxyprogesterone acetate (10 mg/day for 10 days)
    D. oral contraceptive pill (50 mg of estrogen) four times a day until bleeding is stopped for 1 week

ANSWERS

1. **A,** Pages 1080–1081. Menorrhagia has been reported in up to 14% of healthy women participating in studies of measurement of menstrual blood loss. In women complaining of menorrhagia, just as with women who have normal menstruation, 70% of the blood is lost within the first 2 days of menstruation and 92% is passed by the end of the third day. There seems to be no relation between the number of days of menstrual bleeding and total menstrual blood loss. The majority of patients with menorrhagia did not have increased duration of flow but rather had a marked increase in the amount of menstrual flow for the first few days.

2. **D,** Page 1082. Hypothyroidism is frequently associated with menorrhagia and intermenstrual

bleeding. Thyroid-stimulating hormone (TSH) should be measured in women with menorrhagia of undetermined cause. In a study by Wilansky and Greisman, 15 of 67 women had early hypothyroidism, which was detected by an abnormal thyrotropin-releasing hormone (TRH) stimulation test. After treatment, the TSH levels in the affected women returned to normal and the menorrhagia disappeared within 3 to 6 months. Although this study awaits corroboration, hypothyroidism should be kept in mind in patients with otherwise unexplained menorrhagia. The history given in this question is not typical for diabetes mellitus, SLE, ITP, and von Willebrand disease.

3. **E,** Page 1083. The mechanism for hemostasis in reaction to vascular injury is similar in the endometrium to that in other injured tissues of the body. There are five basic actions, including (1) localized vasoconstriction, (2) platelet adhesion, (3) formation of the platelet plug, (4) reinforcement of the platelet plug with fibrin, and (5) removal of the coagulated material by fibrinolysis. This process is slightly altered in the endometrial vessels compared with vessel damage elsewhere in that the hemostatic plugs in the endometrium are smaller, have a different morphologic pattern, and persist for a shorter time than those in other tissues.

4. **A,** Page 1083. Smith and colleagues found that the levels of prostaglandin F_{2a} were lower in women with anovulatory abnormal uterine bleeding with a persistently proliferative endometrium than were the levels in women with a normal secretory endometrium. Prostaglandin F_{2a} is known to promote vasoconstriction in the spiral arterioles of the endometrium. It has been shown that prostaglandin F_{2a} binds to receptors in the spiral arteries in the late secretory phase to cause vasoconstriction and presumably to help control menstrual flow. Prostaglandin E_2 is a vasodilator. Thromboxane promotes platelet aggregation, whereas prostacyclin inhibits this process. Arachidonic acid is the precursor for both prostaglandin F_{2a} and prostaglandin E_2.

5. **D,** Page 1084. In patients who are ovulating and have menorrhagia, it is important to rule out a uterine lesion, such as an endometrial polyp, submucous myoma, or carcinoma. Although a number of tests, including vaginal probe ultrasonography, might reveal the source of the problem, many authors prefer hysteroscopy, which can be performed in the office with the patient under local anesthesia. It has been estimated that a D&C misses the diagnosis in 10% to 25% of patients. Gimpelson and Rappold found that hysteroscopy permitted accurate diagnosis in 60 of 342 patients in whom the diagnosis was not made

by D&C. March has reported that one fourth of patients with a presumptive diagnosis of dysfunctional bleeding were found to have a uterine lesion at the time of hysteroscopy.

6. **A,** Page 1085. To control an acute bleeding episode, after organic causes have been ruled out, the use of oral conjugated estrogens in very high doses (10 mg in four divided doses) is a therapeutic regimen that many authors consider to be clinically useful. Although high-dose combination oral contraceptives have been found to be effective, some studies suggest that this approach is not as efficacious as high doses of conjugated estrogens alone. The difference might be due to the fact that the combined use of estrogen and progestin does not afford as rapid an endometrial growth as estrogen alone. The progestin decreases the synthesis of estrogen receptors and increases estradiol dehydrogenase in the endometrial cell, inhibiting the growth-promoting action of estrogen. Other mechanisms, such as estrogen's effect on spiral artery recoil, platelet function, or prostaglandin synthesis, seem to be unrelated. A great deal of controversy surrounds the issue of what constitutes the best treatment. As evidenced by the ear, nose, and throat literature, estrogen may have a direct effect on blood vessels. Authors who prefer a combination of estrogen and progestin point out that the progestin in a combination oral contraceptive acts more slowly and thus does not initially counter the effects of estrogen on endometrial growth.

7. **B,** Pages 1085–1086. This question ignores the possibility of a blood dyscrasia, which should always be considered, especially in a teenager. Adolescent anovulatory patients represent an ideal model for the use of progestins in the treatment of dysfunctional uterine bleeding. Since these patients exhibit immaturity of the hypothalamic pituitary axis, this treatment is preferred over oral contraceptives because the therapy does not prolong hypothalamic pituitary inhibition and may, according to the older literature, delay the maturation of this axis. In the young virginal patient with these findings, D&C and hysteroscopy are not necessary. Treating the patient with estrogen alone will not help because her problem is primarily that of unopposed estrogen secretion.

8. **C,** Page 1082. The most common causes of vaginal bleeding during the reproductive age are accidents of pregnancy such as a threatened, incomplete, or missed abortion or an ectopic pregnancy. This warrants a sensitive β-hCG test, either by serum or urine, as part of the immediate diagnostic evaluation. Endometrial aspiration and hysteroscopy are contraindicated in this patient until

pregnancy is ruled out. After the results of the pregnancy test are available, one might perform pelvic ultrasonography or laparoscopy in this patient with a normal pelvic examination result if there is concern about a pregnancy abnormality.

9. **A,** Page 1086. After hysteroscopy and D&C are used to evaluate acute bleeding in a woman in her late reproductive years, further therapy is indicated if the histologic findings show secretory endometrium. This can be accomplished by using cyclic medroxyprogesterone acetate to effect orderly withdrawal bleeding each month. Continuous medroxyprogesterone acetate is associated with degrees of endometrial atrophy due to hypothalamic-pituitary-ovarian suppression from which the patient is likely to bleed again. Both cyclic and continuous conjugated estrogens are contraindicated since they cause excessive endometrial proliferation, which may cause further irregular, heavy bleeding. Cyclic danazol is not indicated and is less cost-effective in controlling bleeding. The use of a norgestrel-containing IUD as a treatment for menorrhagia causes, on average, an 80% reduction in menstrual blood loss within 3 months. Since this woman is 45 and thus is in a perimenopausal age group, she should be treated even though the endometrium is secretory. At this time, it is possible that she is not ovulating each month. Oral contraceptives are a less safe choice in this patient.

10. **A,** Page 1085. When high-dose conjugated estrogen therapy has been successful in reducing the amount of uterine bleeding within the first 24 hours, immediate progestin support of the endometrium is also required. Therefore, conjugated estrogen therapy is continued at the same dosage and a progestin, usually medroxyprogesterone acetate, 10 mg/day, is added. Both hormones are continued for 2 weeks, after which treatment is stopped to allow withdrawal bleeding. Doubling the conjugated estrogen dose for 2 weeks is likely to cause abnormal hyperplasia of the endometrium and more bleeding. Initiation of oral contraceptives at this point is another option in this patient, but there is no compelling reason to switch to another regimen, especially since she is not sexually active. This regimen is a combination estrogen-progestin oral contraceptive three or four times a day for one pack. Vitamin E has not been scientifically proved to be of benefit. Since this patient has responded to high-dose conjugated estrogen therapy, office endometrial aspiration is unnecessary at this point. If the patient had not responded to the above outlined therapy, endometrial sampling would be indicated.

11. **C,** Page 1080. There are two reliable objective methods that can be used to quantify menstrual blood loss. One involves radioisotope tagging of a patient's red blood cells; the other is photometric measurement to quantify the amount of hematin collected on sanitary napkins. With these techniques, recent studies have found that the mean amount of menstrual blood loss in healthy women (women with normal hemoglobin, hematocrit, and plasma iron) is about 55 mL, which is up from earlier studies done in the 1960s and 1970s.

12. **B,** Pages 1088–1089. D&C should be used to stop the acute bleeding episode in patients over the age of 35 since the incidence of anatomic problems and pathologic findings is increased in this age group. D&C can be both diagnostic and therapeutic. D&C is the quickest way to stop acute bleeding. It is indicated in patients with severe menorrhagia who may be hypovolemic. It should be remembered that, although D&C is effective for the treatment of acute bleeding, long-term cures are unusual because the underlying pathophysiologic condition is unchanged.

13. **D,** Page 1081. Certain systemic diseases, especially disorders of blood coagulation such as von Willebrand disease and prothrombin deficiency, may often first appear as abnormal uterine bleeding. Other disorders that produce platelet deficiencies, such as leukemia, occasionally are initially noted in this fashion. Although older studies indicated a 20% incidence, a more recent study by Falcone noted that coagulation disorders are found in about 5% of adolescent females who require hospitalization for abnormal uterine bleeding. This is still frequent enough that such teens should be checked for bleeding disorders.

14. **E,** Pages 1082–1083. Certain disorders that may cause dysfunctional uterine bleeding relate to the life span of the corpus luteum. Prolonged life of the corpus luteum has been reported as a cause for abnormal bleeding similar to that presented by this patient (Halban syndrome or a persistent corpus luteum). The cause is uncertain, and the treatment is expectant. This entity must be differentiated from early pregnancy loss by obtaining a sensitive serum or urine pregnancy test. Since this disorder is associated with a normal-appearing secretory endometrium, the diagnosis is made when a biopsy obtained on the fourth day of the patient's flow is both proliferative and secretory and the β-hCG assay is negative.

15. **B,** Page 1084. In this age group, having ruled out pregnancy and with a normal pelvic examination, one must rule out malignancy even though it is unlikely. A cost-effective method is to perform an office endometrial aspiration. An endometrial biopsy is ideally obtained at the onset of the bleeding episode to help determine whether ovulation has occurred. This knowledge helps determine

therapy. Office hysteroscopy is not indicated until the endometrial histologic picture is known. A hysterosalpingogram and pelvic ultrasonogram are unnecessary at this time. Serum clotting studies are largely unrevealing in a patient in this age group with a short history of a bleeding abnormality.

16. **D,** Pages 1085–1086. Anovulatory adolescent patients present an ideal model for the use of progestins in the treatment of dysfunctional uterine bleeding. Because these teenagers are likely to have an immature hypothalamic-pituitary axis, progestin therapy for cycle days 16 to 25 is a reasonable mode of treatment to produce regular cyclic bleeding until the positive feedback system matures. By giving medication on cycle days 16 to 25 rather than calendar days this is mimics and then merges with ovulatory cycles once the system matures. Although controversial, oral contraceptives probably should not be used in these patients unless there is a need for contraception, since this therapy prolongs hypothalamic-pituitary inhibition. D&C is not indicated in this patient, whose acute bleeding episode has been controlled. Cyclic conjugated estrogens and cyclic danazol therapy are not valid choices. Danazol is expensive and carries with it the risk of undesirable side effects.

17. **D,** Pages 1090–1092. Laser photovaporization of the endometrium for treatment of menorrhagia has been advocated by some investigators. This procedure for endometrial ablation may be used as an alternative to hysterectomy in patients for whom other modalities have failed or are contraindicated. A study by Erian in the *British Journal of Obstetrics and Gynecology* (volume 101, 1994) involving 1866 patients found that with laser ablation for severe menorrhagia, 56% of patients became amenorrheic, 38% had reduced or normal menses, and 7% had no improvement. Endometrial ablation can also be accomplished with electrocautery applied through a ball-end electrode attached to a urologic resectoscope. In a study of 200 women by Paskowitz, 40% had amenorrhea and 60% reported decreased bleeding. Cyclic oral contraceptives are contraindicated in this patient. The effectiveness of NSAIDs and antifibrinolytics in patients with systemic disease is poor, but some would argue for a trial before attempting an operative procedure, such as an ablation or D&C. The latter may afford only temporary relief.

18. **D,** Page 1085. The rationale for the therapeutic use of estrogen for the immediate treatment of abnormal uterine bleed is based on the fact that, in pharmacologic doses, estrogen causes rapid growth of the endometrium. Thus, bleeding that results from most causes of dysfunctional bleeding responds to such therapy because a rapid growth of endometrial tissue occurs over the denuded and raw epithelial surface. Acute bleeding from most causes is usually controlled by this method. Appreciable changes in either systemic or local clotting factors or changes in platelet adhesiveness have not been well documented. Decidualization of the endometrium does not occur in the absence of progestin therapy. Likewise, uniform endometrial slough after estrogen withdrawal does not occur unless the estrogen treatment has been followed by adequate doses of progestins. As suggested in the answer to Question 6, there are many respected physicians who would opt to use a combination oral contraceptive.

19–21. 19, **C;** 20, **B;** 21, **D;** Pages 1087–1088. Tranexamic acid (AMCA) is one of a number of potent inhibitors of fibrinolysis and therefore has been used in the treatment of various hemorrhagic conditions including menorrhagia. It is associated with a significant (50%) reduction of blood loss in these patients. The blood loss reduction was greatest in patients who originally exhibited the greatest loss. Ergot derivatives are not recommended; they are rarely effective and have a high incidence of side effects, including nausea, vertigo, and abdominal cramps. One study demonstrated no reduction in blood loss in 82 women with menorrhagia treated with ergot alkaloid preparations. This therapy is not effective at the cellular level. It is efficacious postpartum because myometrial contractions are important in reducing blood loss. One mechanism of action of medroxyprogesterone acetate is to enhance the conversion of a potent estrogen, estradiol, to the less potent estrogen, estrone. This effectively reduces the cellular proliferation of the endometrium and reduces menstrual flow in patients with menorrhagia.

22. **C,** Pages 1080–1081. A woman's perception of menstrual blood loss correlates poorly with the actual amount lost. Determining the number of sanitary pads used is an unreliable method of gauging menstrual blood loss, except when a patient is soaking a large number of pads. Absorption varies greatly among different types of products, as does fastidiousness in changing pads. Asking the patient to estimate the amount of blood loss is also unreliable; for example, it has been shown that 40% of women with a blood loss greater than 80 mL consider their menstrual flow to be light or moderate. The patient's age alone does not correlate with menstrual blood loss unless a concomitant pelvic pathologic condition such as myomata is found. Likewise, the number

of days of flow has not correlated in patients who bleed 7 days or less. Queries about the passage of blood clots or the degree of inconvenience caused by the bleeding are most helpful in assessing the amount of blood lost during menses.

23. **A,** Pages 1082–1083. In most patients with dysfunctional uterine bleeding, ovulation fails to occur. There is continuous estradiol production without corpus luteum formation and progesterone secretion. This leads to a continually proliferating endometrium and the formation of areas of necrosis, which occur as the endometrium outgrows its blood supply. In contrast with normal menstruation, a uniform slough of the endometrium to the basalis layer does not occur and there is excessive uterine blood flow. Spiraling of the arterioles is a morphologic change noted in the presence of progesterone (ovulation). Acute inflammation or eosinophilic infiltration typically is not part of the histologic picture of the endometrium of patients with dysfunctional uterine bleeding. Chronic endometrial inflammation may contribute to irregular bleeding patterns (see Chapter 23).

24. **C,** Pages 1090–1092. Complications of hysteroscopic endometrial ablation include fluid overload, uterine hemorrhage, uterine perforation, thermal damage to adjacent organs, and hematometra. Most of these complications occur because the ablation extends too deep into the endometrium, opening up uterine vessels and "drowning" adjacent tissues with thermal injury. Guidelines for the safe and effective practice of endometrial ablation, including correct patient selection, were recently summarized by Garry after a meeting of a group of experts. These experts concluded that correct patient selection should be restricted to women with heavy prostaglandins. In addition, these agents may block the action of prostaglandins by interfering directly at their receptor sites. All NSAIDs are cyclooxygenase inhibitors and thus block the formation of both thromboxane and the prostacyclins. Thromboxane increases platelet aggregation. A number of agents are available, including mefenamic acid, meclofenamate, and naproxen sodium. These drugs are usually given for the first 3 days of menses or throughout the bleeding episode. They appear to have similar levels of effectiveness. The antifibrinolytic drugs are tranexamic acid and paraaminomethylbenzoic acid.

25. **C,** Pages 1090–1092. Both the roller-ball technique and laser ablation require preoperative medication for several weeks to cause endometrial atrophy. They also require experience with operative hysteroscopy and the use of general anesthesia. Although the time to learn the roller-ball technique is shorter than for the laser and the equipment is less expensive, the roller-ball technique is still more involved than balloon thermal ablation. Balloon thermal ablation does not require pretreatment of the endometrium, does not require hysteroscopy training, and can be performed with local anesthesia.

26. **B,** Pages 1086–1087. NSAIDs are prostaglandin synthetase inhibitors. They inhibit the biosynthesis of cyclic endoperoxides, which catalyze the conversion of arachidonic acid to prostaglandins. In addition, these agents may block the action of prostaglandins by interfering directly at their receptor sites. All NSAIDs are cyclooxygenase inhibitors and thus block the formation of both thromboxane and the prostacyclins. Thromboxane increases platelet aggregation. A number of agents are available, including mefenamic acid, meclofenamate, and naproxen sodium. These drugs are usually given for the first 3 days of menses or throughout the bleeding episode. They appear to have similar levels of effectiveness. The antifibrinolytic drugs are tranexamic acid and paraaminomethylbenzoic acid.

27. **A,** Pages 1080–1081. Using quantitative methods, Hallberg and colleagues found that persons with a monthly menstrual blood loss greater than 80 mL have significantly lower mean hemoglobin, hematocrit, and serum iron levels. Therefore, a menstrual blood loss greater than 80 mL should be regarded as hypermenorrhea. The anemia demonstrated in these patients is secondary to blood loss (decreased iron) and is only very rarely related to abnormal clotting factors or platelet aggregation abnormalities. Abnormalities of these factors may contribute to excessive blood loss in a smaller select group of patients. Prolonged bleeding time would indicate such a problem.

28. **D,** Pages 1085–1086. Medroxyprogesterone acetate, given to patients with adequate amounts of endogenous estrogen, produces regular withdrawal bleeding. When used as maintenance therapy over a longer time, medroxyprogesterone acetate is usually prescribed in a dose of 10 mg daily for 10 to 13 days each month. Progestins act as antiestrogens. They diminish the effect of estrogen on the target cells by inhibiting estrogen receptor replenishment in the cytosol and influence the activation of 17-dehydroxysteroid dehydrogenase, which converts estradiol to the less active estrone. These findings account for the antimitotic, antigrowth effect of progestins. Although other progestins have been used, medroxyprogesterone acetate does not alter serum lipids as much as the 19-nortestosterone derivatives and thus may have fewer adverse long-term effects. Natural progesterone stimulates secretory

activity, which does not occur with long-term use of medroxyprogesterone acetate. No evidence suggests that medroxyprogesterone acetate reduces endometrial vascularity.

29. **C,** Pages 1085–1088. All the listed treatments may be efficacious in reducing menstrual blood loss. Progestins not only stop endometrial growth but also support and organize the endometrium in such a way that an organized slough occurs after its withdrawal. This organized slough to the basalis layer allows a rapid cessation of bleeding. In addition, progestins stimulate arachidonic acid formation in the endometrium, increasing the prostaglandin F_{2a}/prostaglandin E ratio. The progesterone-releasing IUD has also been found to be effective in the treatment of women with ovulatory abnormal uterine bleeding. In various studies, a 60% to 80% reduction in menstrual blood loss has occurred 1 year after the introduction of a progestin-releasing IUD. Several NSAIDs have been administered during menstruation to groups of women with menorrhagia and ovulatory abnormal uterine bleeding. These drugs have reduced mean menstrual blood loss by about 20% to 50%. Danazol has been used by several investigators for the treatment of menorrhagia. Doses of 200 and 400 mg daily have been given over 12 weeks after careful pretreatment observation and evaluation. Menstrual blood loss was markedly reduced in these studies from more than 200 mL to less than 25 mL. The interval between bleeding episodes also increased. Reduction of dosage from 400 to 200 mg daily decreased the side effects but did not alter the reduction in blood loss. Ergot derivatives are not recommended for therapy because they are rarely effective and have a high incidence of side effects (nausea, vertigo, and abdominal cramps).

30. **E,** Pages 1090–1093. Both laser ablation and electrocautery of the endometrium can successfully treat patients with heavy menstrual flow. It is suggested that with both methods, patients be pretreated for approximately 1 to 2 months with a hormonal agent to effect endometrial atrophy. This increases the effectiveness of laser or cautery ablations. High-dose progestins or danazol may be used in this capacity. The long-term effects of all techniques of endometrial ablation are not yet known. The clinician should be aware that a certain percentage of patients return with continued menstrual flow and that these patients may need a second treatment with these techniques. In addition, the long-term effect on the rates of potentially serious endometrial pathologic conditions, such as endometrial carcinoma, are not known. The time needed to learn the roller-ball technique is shorter than that for laser, and the equipment is considerably less expensive.

31. **A,** Pages 1085–1086. There are several approaches to the treatment of acute "endocrinologic" uterine bleeding. Each has its advocates. In such a 20-year-old patient, acute bleeding usually can be controlled adequately by administration of oral conjugated estrogens in a dose of 10 mg/day in divided doses until the bleeding markedly slows or stops or by the use of medroxyprogesterone acetate, 10 mg/day for 10 days. According to some authors, medroxyprogesterone acetate is less effective in providing immediate relief from the bleeding. Oral contraceptive agents containing 50 mg of estrogen have been used in the immediate treatment of this problem. In this age group, it is important to rule out pregnancy. Judging from the amount of bleeding and the age of the patient, the bleeding is likely to be secondary to anovulation. Endometrial sampling is not indicated in this patient, in whom the risk of neoplastic disease is low. This procedure will not remove the underlying cause for her bleeding. D&C is not necessary unless there is a poor clinical response to estrogen therapy.

CHAPTER
38

Primary and Secondary Amenorrhea

DIRECTIONS:

for Questions 1–25: Select the one best answer or completion.

---

1. **Normal pubertal development is the result of**

   A. adrenal maturation
   B. increased sensitivity of the hypothalamic-pituitary-gonadal axis to circulating estrogen
   C. decreased rapid-eye-movement (REM) sleep
   D. maturation of the hypothalamic-pituitary-gonadal axis
   E. weight loss

2. **A 17-year-old states that she has never had a period. The examination findings are as shown in Figure 38–1. The most likely diagnosis is**

   A. pregnancy
   B. androgen insensitivity
   C. gonadal dysgenesis
   D. imperforate hymen
   E. Rokitansky-Küster-Hauser syndrome

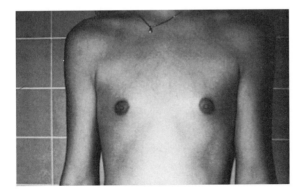

FIGURE 38–1

3. **Given the probable diagnosis in Question 2, the most useful initial diagnostic test would be a**

   A. buccal smear
   B. follicle-stimulating hormone (FSH) determination
   C. serum estrogen determination
   D. gonadotrophin-releasing hormone (GnRH) (LH-RH) stimulation test
   E. x-ray examination to determine the patient's bone age

4. **Eight months after the delivery of her second child, a patient complains that she has not had a period. The patient did not breast-feed because she could not produce milk. Pregnancy test and progestin withdrawal test results are both negative. Of the choices given, the most likely diagnosis is**

   A. Sheehan syndrome
   B. hyperprolactinemia
   C. polycystic ovarian disease
   D. androgen insensitivity
   E. Rokitansky-Küster-Hauser syndrome

5. **Anorexia nervosa is characterized by all the following except**

   A. dry skin
   B. hypotension
   C. tachycardia
   D. hypothermia
   E. constipation

6. A 14-year-old girl with normal secondary sexual development is seen in the emergency department and complains of abdominal pain. She has never menstruated. On examination, you palpate a large central abdominopelvic mass that extends to the umbilicus and feels like an enlarged uterus. Fetal heart tones are not heard. The most likely diagnosis is

A. Rokitansky-Küster-Hauser syndrome
B. androgen insensitivity
C. complete transverse vaginal septum
D. pregnancy
E. gonadal dysgenesis

7. Of the following conditions, the most common cause of secondary amenorrhea in an adolescent woman is

A. polycystic ovarian syndrome
B. eating disorder
C. hyperprolactinemia
D. Rokitansky-Küster-Hauser syndrome
E. gonadal dysgenesis

8. A 27-year-old marathon athlete asks for your advice regarding her menstrual cycles. In the past 4$\frac{1}{2}$ years, she has menstruated only once. The examination results are within normal limits. Appropriate advice would be to ask the woman to

A. reduce her physical activity to a minimum
B. increase her caloric intake and gain weight
C. take glucocorticoids daily
D. await the results of a progestin withdrawal test
E. obtain a psychiatric evaluation

9. A 17-year-old who has had regular periods (every 28 to 30 days) since she was 12 is now 2 weeks late for her period. Her medical history is negative, and the physical examination results are within normal limits. Which of the following tests is indicated?

A. serum prolactin
B. FSH
C. β human chorionic gonadotropin (β-hCG)
D. serum estradiol
E. karyotype

10. A 16-year-old tells her physician that she is 4 weeks late for her period. She is sexually active. Her medical history is negative, and the physical examination results are within normal limits. The pregnancy test result is negative. The most likely diagnosis is

A. ectopic pregnancy
B. anovulation
C. gonadal failure
D. hypothyroidism
E. anorexia nervosa

11. The appropriate therapeutic modality for an anovulatory adolescent is

A. clomiphene citrate
B. cyclic progestin withdrawal
C. menotropins (Pergonal)
D. GnRH agonist
E. conjugated estrogens (Premarin)

12. A 14-year-old high school student is referred for evaluation of primary amenorrhea. She is an excellent athlete and runs almost 5 miles daily. On examination, her breasts are Tanner stage I; her pubic hair development is graded as Tanner stage II. The remainder of the examination results are within normal limits. The first step in her evaluation should include a

A. pregnancy test
B. serum luteinizing hormone (LH) level test
C. serum FSH level test
D. karyotype
E. serum testosterone level test

13. A 27-year-old woman has had no menstrual periods for 6 months. She feels well, exercises moderately, and has no other symptoms or complaints. She does not have a history of uterine infection. Her general physical evaluation result is normal. This woman does not have withdrawal bleeding after progesterone. Her laboratory tests include a normal complete blood count, a prolactin level of 10 ng, an LH level of 15 mIU/mL, an FSH level of 10 mIU/mL, and an estradiol level of 44 pg/mL. The most likely diagnosis is

A. polycystic ovary syndrome
B. premature ovarian failure
C. hypothalamic failure
D. gonadotrophin-resistant ovary syndrome
E. hypothalamic dysfunction

14. Typically, patients with Rokitansky-Küster-Hauser syndrome are differentiated from patients with androgen insensitivity by

A. amenorrhea
B. progesterone withdrawal test results
C. the presence of a blind vagina
D. karyotype
E. breast formation

15. One would expect a patient with anorexia nervosa to have

A. low T$_4$
B. high T$_3$
C. low FSH
D. decreased cortisol
E. high blood pressure

16. **Appropriate treatment of patients with androgen insensitivity syndrome should not include**

    A. gonadectomy
    B. vaginal dilation
    C. breast augmentation
    D. replacement estrogen
    E. maintaining their female identity

17. **Asherman syndrome is not associated with**

    A. secondary amenorrhea
    B. dilatation and curettage (D&C)
    C. elevated FSH
    D. uterine infection
    E. intraperitoneal tuberculosis

18. **The somatic features of Turner syndrome include**

    A. short stature
    B. normal breast development
    C. cubitus varus
    D. arachnodactyly
    E. clubbed feet

19. **Ovarian failure is not caused by**

    A. immune disorders
    B. X chromosome deletion
    C. autosomal recessive disorders in persons with a 46,XX karyotype
    D. chemotherapy
    E. birth order

20. **In a 15-year-old with primary amenorrhea and a large uterine mass, the least plausible diagnosis listed is**

    A. Rokitansky-Küster-Hauser syndrome
    B. imperforate hymen
    C. pregnancy
    D. transverse vaginal septum
    E. cervical agenesis

21. **The most efficient procedure in establishing the diagnosis of Asherman syndrome is**

    A. hysterography
    B. hysteroscopy
    C. laparoscopy
    D. ultrasound imaging
    E. computed tomography (CT)

22. **True statements about patients with anorexia nervosa include**

    A. They lose at least 40% of their original body weight.
    B. Onset occurs after age 25.
    C. They desire to gain weight.
    D. This condition occurs in about 1 in 1000 Caucasian women.
    E. This condition occurs more frequently in African-American women than in Caucasian women.

23. **Female athletes with exercise-induced amenorrhea have which of the following?**

    A. low prolactin levels
    B. high FSH levels
    C. high α-endorphin levels
    D. low catechol estrogen levels
    E. high LH levels

24. **The most common cause of primary amenorrhea in a nonpregnant woman is**

    A. 17-hydroxylase deficiency
    B. gonadal failure
    C. late-onset congenital adrenal hyperplasia
    D. pituitary tumor
    E. absent uterus

25. **The most common pathologic cause of amenorrhea in adolescent females is**

    A. anorexia nervosa
    B. pituitary tumor
    C. absent uterus
    D. gonadal failure
    E. 17-hydroxylase deficiency

DIRECTIONS:

for Questions 26–30: Match the women with amenorrhea with the most likely cause for their condition.

(A) gonadal failure
(B) pituitary failure
(C) intrauterine synechiae
(D) hypothalamic dysfunction
(E) late-onset congenital adrenal hyperplasia

26. **An 18-year-old who is 4 feet 8 inches tall**

27. **A 20-year-old with loss of sense of smell**

28. **A 30-year-old with recent history of spontaneous abortion followed 2 weeks later by a D&C for retained products of conception**

29. A 22-year-old who is 5 feet 6 inches tall and weighs 102 pounds

30. An 18-year-old with a chromophobe adenoma

DIRECTIONS:

for Questions 31–36: Select the one best answer or completion.

31. Of the following, which is the most common etiologic origin of secondary amenorrhea not associated with pregnancy?

    A. ovarian
    B. hypothalamic
    C. pituitary
    D. uterine

32. A 22-year-old healthy woman who is a dedicated long-distance runner has become amenorrheic since increasing her daily running distance because of training for a marathon. The most practical management of this situation is to

    A. obtain a karyotype
    B. institute estrogen and progesterone replacement
    C. instruct her to stop running
    D. give cyclic clomiphene therapy
    E. give daily cortisone replacement

33. An 18-year-old amenorrheic, nonhirsute phenotypic woman with no breast development has a low FSH level and a normal prolactin level. Her uterus is small but normal. Her karyotype is 46,XX. The next step in this patient's management is

    A. gonadectomy
    B. CT of the hypothalamus-pituitary area
    C. a GnRH stimulation test
    D. measurement of testosterone levels
    E. measurement of 17-hydroxyprogesterone levels

34. Two reasons for a woman having normal female genitalia and breasts without a uterus are congenital absence of the uterus and

    A. congenital adrenal hyperplasia
    B. gonadal dysgenesis
    C. 17-hydroxylase deficiency
    D. prolactinoma
    E. androgen resistance syndrome

35. A 14-year-old girl is brought in by her mother because she has not yet experienced menses. On physical examination, she has no breast development or pubic hair. Your initial approach to the patient is to

    A. do nothing until age 16
    B. draw blood for a serum FSH level
    C. perform a pelvic examination
    D. reassure the mother that this is normal
    E. start the patient on oral contraceptive pills

36. A 21-year-old coed presents to the physician complaining of secondary amenorrhea for 3 months. Her pregnancy test result is negative. The physical examination reveals breast and pubic hair at Tanner stage IV or V. Her FSH level is 60 mIU/mL. The next step in the evaluation would be to

    A. cycle her with medroxyprogesterone
    B. perform a karyotype
    C. reassure the patient that this is common
    D. start on oral contraceptive pills
    E. use clomiphene citrate once she desires a pregnancy

ANSWERS

1. **D,** Page 1103. Before puberty, gonadotrophin levels are low because the hypothalamic-pituitary-gonadal axis is extremely sensitive to the negative feedback of the low level of circulating estrogen. As the axis matures, this sensitivity diminishes and LH shows an episodic nocturnal rise. Next, pulses of FSH and LH are noted both at night and during the day. FSH and LH stimulate the gonad to produce estrogen, which, in turn, affects secondary sexual development.

2. **C,** Pages 1104–1106. The combination of primary amenorrhea and absent breast development suggests failure of the gonads to produce estrogen. The only condition listed that is characterized by absent estrogen production is gonadal dysgenesis. In all other conditions listed, the amenorrhea is associated with adequate and appropriate breast development. The Rokitansky-Küster-Hauser syndromes characterized by an incomplete or atretic vagina and an absent, rudimentary, or bicornuate uterus. The tubes and the ovaries are

normal, and hence pubertal development is normal except for a lack of menstruation. The lower vagina usually consists of a short blind pouch. On rare occasion, a patient may have a functional endometrium and thus experience hematometra. Renal malformations (50%) and skeletal malformations (10% to 15%) are moderately common.

3. **B,** Pages 1104–1109. Although all the tests listed have a place in the workup of a patient with delayed puberty, a determination of the FSH serum concentration would be most valuable in this patient. A high FSH level confirms gonadal failure, whereas a low FSH level suggests constitutional delay or pituitary failure. A karyotype is important after the diagnosis of gonadal failure is established because some affected patients have a mosaic containing a Y chromosome. Because a karyotype contains a great deal more information, it is preferred over a buccal smear.

4. **A,** Page 1116. This postpartum patient was unable to produce milk, which is the typical presentation of a patient whose pituitary gland was destroyed during pregnancy and delivery by hemorrhage or thrombosis. This extremely rare constellation of events is called *Sheehan syndrome*. It is important to evaluate the function of the other endocrine organs, particularly the thyroid and the adrenal glands, because "multigland" hormonal replacement therapy may be indicated. Androgen insensitivity is found in a genetic male, whereas the Rokitansky-Küster-Hauser syndrome is characterized by absence of a vagina. Neither is possible in a postpartum woman. The clinical presentation is not typical of polycystic ovarian disease because withdrawal bleeding is expected in response to progestin therapy. If she had hyperprolactinemia, she would have breast-fed easily.

5. **C,** Pages 1113–1114. Patients with anorexia nervosa have bradycardia, not tachycardia. These patients may also have dry skin, hypotension, hypothermia, and constipation. If they gain weight, their pattern of LH pulses goes through the changes that usually occur in normal puberty. The ovaries do the same, with increasing follicular size and development of a dominant follicle.

6. **C,** Pages 1106–1107. The large central mass is probably an enlarged uterus. The association of primary amenorrhea, an enlarged uterus, and pain suggests an obstruction of the outflow tract and retention of menstrual flow. The patient has normal sexual development, indicating an active hypothalamic-pituitary-ovarian axis and adequate estrogen production and excluding the possibility of gonadal dysgenesis. If, in fact, the large abdominopelvic mass is a uterus, androgen insensitivity syndrome is excluded because a uterus is absent in these patients. The absence of fetal heart tones makes pregnancy unlikely. Rokitansky-Küster-Hauser syndrome with a uterus is rare and is therefore far less likely than a complete transverse vaginal septum.

7. **B,** Pages 1113–1114. Any patient with postpubertal amenorrhea should be considered to be pregnant until proven otherwise because pregnancy is the most common cause of amenorrhea in young females. Adolescents with anorexia nervosa, excessive stress, hyperprolactinemia, Rokitansky-Küster-Hauser syndrome, and gonadal dysgenesis all can have presenting symptoms of primary amenorrhea, but eating disorders are probably the most common cause of secondary amenorrhea in adolescents who are not pregnant. Polycystic ovarian syndrome may cause amenorrhea, but it usually results in irregular uterine bleeding.

8. **D,** Pages 1110–1111, 1116–1118. It is now thought that amenorrhea associated with strenuous exercise is also related to stress. Although reducing physical activity to a minimum or increasing caloric intake to gain weight may alleviate the problem, most athletes refuse to do so. Amenorrhea by itself does the patient no harm. However, it reflects a hypoestrogenic state, which makes the patient susceptible to osteoporosis. Before the initiation of estrogen replacement therapy (ERT), estrogen can be measured or a progestin withdrawal test can be done. If estrogen is greater than 40 pg/L or if the progesterone withdrawal test is positive (bleeding occurs), the patient is presumed to be producing adequate amounts of estrogen and ERT is not required. Otherwise, ERT is suggested to prevent the deleterious effects of estrogen deficiency on the bones. There is no reason to administer glucocorticoids.

9. **C,** Pages 1116–1117. The most common cause of secondary amenorrhea in young women is pregnancy. Although hyperprolactinemia, gonadal failure, and chromosome abnormalities may cause secondary amenorrhea, these are relatively rare. This patient has not met the criteria for secondary amenorrhea. However, a pregnancy test should be performed. If the result is negative, the patient can be reassured. She will most likely resume normal menstruation. If she has 6 months of amenorrhea and is not pregnant, a workup should be initiated.

10. **B,** Pages 1116–1119. Anovulation is relatively common at both ends of the reproductive age group—that is, young adolescent girls in the first 2 years after puberty and perimenopausal women. Thus, anovulation secondary to hypothalamic-pituitary dysfunction is the most likely diagnosis in this patient who has had prior periods and whose anatomic and chromosomal study results

are probably normal. If there is doubt, other laboratory tests, such as an FSH, TSH, prolactin, estrogen, and karyotyping, can be performed.

11. **B,** Pages 1116–1118. Most young female patients who suffer from chronic anovulation have unopposed estrogen production. Overgrowth of endometrium follows, and abnormal uterine bleeding occurs after a period of amenorrhea. Although the patient can be followed without treatment, progestin withdrawal would reassure the patient that there is no significant pathology as well as counteract the action of unopposed estrogen. Even though clomiphene citrate induces ovulation, and therefore can be used to treat chronic anovulation, this medication should be reserved for patients who wish to become pregnant. Birth control pills should be used if the patient is sexually active and not seeking pregnancy.

12. **C,** Pages 1108–1109, 1110–1112; Figure 38–6. Although exercise-induced amenorrhea is relatively common in this age group, this young woman has not begun her secondary sexual development. Therefore, as with all girls her age who have not commenced breast development, a complete evaluation is required. Breasts that are Tanner stage I signify a lack of estrogen production. A serum FSH concentration would be most helpful in determining whether the estrogen deficiency is based on gonadal dysgenesis or a hypothalamic-pituitary disorder. Elevated FSH levels (>40 mIU/mL) indicate gonadal failure, whereas a low FSH level suggests a hypothalamic disorder. A random LH measurement is less helpful because episodic pulses may cause highly variable results. A pregnancy test and a karyotype are not indicated at present. A serum testosterone test is helpful when the patient is hirsute. In patients with a low FSH, consideration should be given to performing a GnRH stimulation test to determine the level of maturation of the hypothalamic-pituitary-ovarian axis.

13. **E,** Pages 1114–1115, 1062. A woman with secondary amenorrhea who does not respond to withdrawal of progesterone generally has low estrogen levels. This may be due to a uterine, ovarian, or hypothalamic-pituitary abnormality. Testing often reveals the most likely source. If the FSH and LH levels are high, ovarian failure is likely; if FSH is normal and LH is high, polycystic ovary syndrome is likely; if FSH and LH are normal or low and estrogen is normal or low, the disorder may be due to variations in GnRH pulses from the hypothalamus. In these situations, if the estradiol is greater than 40 pg/mL, the likely diagnosis is hypothalamic dysfunction, whereas if the estradiol is less than 40 pg/mL, hypothalamic failure is more plausible.

14. **D,** Pages 1106–1107. Both Rokitansky-Küster-Hauser syndrome and androgen insensitivity involve amenorrhea and breast formation; neither responds to progesterone withdrawal, and both involve a blind vagina. Only the karyotype is different.

15. **C,** Page 1113. Patients with anorexia nervosa have a hypothalamic disorder that interferes with normal GnRH release. Thus, both FSH and estrogen levels are extremely low. In addition, the peripheral conversion of T_4 to T_3 is impaired, resulting in low levels of T_3; however, T_4 levels are within the normal range. Patients with anorexia nervosa have low blood pressure and normal or elevated cortisol, which may help distinguish them from patients with hypopituitarism.

16. **C,** Page 1109. Patients with androgen insensitivity syndrome do not need breast augmentation because their breast development is usually adequate. They should be maintained in their female identity and given replacement estrogen after gonadectomy, which is performed after puberty to prevent testicular neoplasms. These patients should be treated with vaginal dilation to lengthen their often short vaginal canal.

17. **C,** Page 1109. Asherman syndrome is characterized by intrauterine adhesions that obliterate the endometrial cavity. The most frequent cause of Asherman syndrome is vigorous endometrial curettage, usually performed postpartum or after abortion, especially when endometritis is present; tuberculous endometritis is a rare cause. Patients with Asherman syndrome have secondary amenorrhea, despite normal FSH and serum estrogen levels. A uterine infection or intraperitoneal tuberculosis that leads to an endometrial infection can cause uterine synechiae or scarring, leading to amenorrhea. D&C is a common way that such adhesions are created.

18. **A,** Page 1105. Patients with Turner syndrome have gonadal dysgenesis and a karyotype of 45,X. In addition to primary amenorrhea and slight or absent breast development, these persons have other somatic abnormalities, the most prevalent being stature less than 5 feet (the gene for stature is located on the short arm of the X chromosome). In addition, a webbed neck, short fourth metacarpals, a shield chest, widely spaced nipples, and cubitus valgus are some of the more prevalent somatic anomalies. Because of the short stature and these morphometric features, the diagnosis is usually made before puberty. Arachnodactyly, which is found in Marfan syndrome, and clubbed feet are not commonly found in Turner syndrome.

19. **E,** Page 1116. Ovarian failure may result from deletion of genetic material on the X chromosome. When one X chromosome is entirely missing,

Turner syndrome results. However, various degrees of deletion have been described. If X chromosome material is missing, ovarian failure can occur. Persons with premature ovarian failure may have antibodies to other endocrine organs, suggesting an autoimmune cause. In such cases, patients are usually younger than 35 years and often have elevated antinuclear and antithyroid antibodies. Infectious etiologic conditions such as mumps oophoritis have also been observed. Patients with a 46,XX karyotype may suffer from ovarian failure on the basis of an autosomal recessive disorder such as 17-hydroxylase deficiency. Genetic males with a 46,XY karyotype may appear with "gonadal" failure on the basis of an X-linked recessive disorder. Because gonadal function is lost in utero, the external genitalia are not stimulated by androgens. As a result, the external genitalia appear to be female, and these persons are usually raised as girls. There is no secondary sexual development at the time of expected puberty. A karyotype should be obtained in all patients younger than 25 years who have ovarian failure. Ovarian failure can also be induced by chemotherapy or radiation. Birth order is not known to be associated with ovarian failure.

20. **A,** Page 1100. Persons with Rokitansky-Küster-Hauser syndrome do not have a uterus, and therefore this condition is not likely. Any entity such as imperforate hymen, transverse vaginal septum, or cervical agenesis could cause swelling of the uterus or vagina with a hematometra. Pregnancy is always a possible diagnosis in a 15-year-old, although an unlikely cause of primary amenorrhea.

21. **B,** Page 1110. Hysteroscopy is the most efficient way to make this diagnosis. Laparoscopy would be of no use. Ultrasound imaging, CT, and hysterography may all suggest the diagnosis; however, hysteroscopy with visualization of the intrauterine scarring is the most efficient method.

22. **D,** Pages 1113–1114. At least two of the following manifestations are common: (1) amenorrhea, (2) lanugo hair, (3) bradycardia, (4) periods of overactivity, and (5) episodes of spontaneous or self-induced vomiting after meals. Anorexia nervosa occurs in approximately 1 in 1000 Caucasian women. It is less common in African-American women and usually starts before the age of 25. Weight loss is usually about 25% of original body weight.

23. **C,** Pages 1110–1112. Amenorrhea associated with strenuous exercise is thought to be related to both stress and weight loss. Prolactin β-endorphin and catechol-estrogen levels are significantly higher and LH and FSH levels are significantly lower than normal in women who exercise strenuously. The α-endorphin levels are high.

24. **B,** Page 1104. Primary amenorrhea is relatively rare. Among those young women who have it, approximately half of cases are due to gonadal failure. One third of these patients have other abnormalities, mostly in the cardiac and renal areas. Absent uterus is probably the second most common cause, with approximately 15% of primary amenorrhea resulting from this. 17-Hydroxylase deficiency is extremely rare. Late-onset congenital adrenal hyperplasia would cause secondary amenorrhea. Pituitary tumors are very rare although still a possible cause of primary amenorrhea.

25. **A,** Pages 1113–1114. Although pregnancy is the most common cause of teenage amenorrhea, it is not a pathologic condition. Anorexia nervosa is common, at 1 per 1000, in Caucasian women, and is important because it is associated with a high suicide rate. The other options listed are all rare. Dysfunctional uterine bleeding or anovulation because of stress may result in amenorrhea but usually is associated with irregular bleeding.

26–30. 26, **A;** 27, **D;** 28, **C;** 29, **D;** 30, **B;** Pages 1104–1108, 1109–1116. Gonadal failure, which often occurs in Turner syndrome (XO), is the most common cause of primary amenorrhea. A 20-year-old with loss of smell has a variant of Kallmann syndrome, which is a hypothalamic disorder. The 30-year-old has a history suggestive of intrauterine adhesion formation or Asherman syndrome with intrauterine synechiae. The 22-year-old who weighs only 102 pounds probably has anorexia nervosa, which is one of the causes of hypothalamic dysfunction, which in turn is the most common nonphysiologic cause of amenorrhea. The patient with a chromophobe adenoma may have pituitary failure because of destruction of the pituitary gland by the tumor.

31. **B,** Page 1109. Reindollar's series of 262 cases of secondary amenorrhea reported 62% from hypothalamic disorders, 16% from pituitary disorders, 12% from ovary disorders, and 7% from uterine disorders.

32. **B,** Pages 1118–1119. Because this woman had menses and now has become amenorrheic with increasing her daily running distance, she should either be taking estrogen-progesterone replacement or she should decrease her running. Stopping running is probably not what this dedicated athlete wants to do or would be willing to do. Therefore, replacement estrogen-progesterone is probably the most practical solution. Karyotype is probably not indicated because normal menstrual function was present until the woman increased her physical activity. Clomiphene, which may be indicated to cause ovulation in a person who wishes to become pregnant, does not work

well if estrogen levels are low. Besides, this woman wants to run, not get pregnant. There is no need to replace cortisone.

33. **B,** Pages 1118–1119; Figure 38–15. In this 18-year-old phenotypic amenorrheic female without breast development, estrogen levels are low. Because she also has a low FSH level, concern exists about her hypothalamic-pituitary function, with the possibility of a hypothalamic or pituitary tumor. Therefore, this area should be imaged. Because her karyotype is 46,XX, gonadectomy would not be indicated since she does not have a Y chromosome and is unlikely to have a Y fragment. Testosterone levels are determined to rule out androgen insensitivity, but this patient has a uterus and has XX chromosomes, so this is not the problem. 17-Hydroxyprogesterone would be checked to detect a very rare deficiency of 17-hydroxylase. Patients with this deficiency have a high FSH level and a low estrogen level. A GnRH stimulation test should be performed if imaging does not detect a tumor.

34. **E,** Pages 1106–1107. Androgen resistance syndrome is due to the absence of a gene on the X chromosome that codes for testosterone receptors. In congenital adrenal hyperplasia, patients have hirsutism and virilization but they also have breasts and a uterus. Patients with gonadal dysgenesis have a uterus. 17-Hydroxylase deficiency is very rare. Patients with this deficiency have a uterus but no breasts because estrogen is not produced. Patients with prolactinomas have a uterus and breast tissue from the earlier effects of estrogen.

35. **B,** Pages 1104–1108. The lack of any secondary sexual characteristics by age 14 deserves some evaluation. Although this lack could be due to marked hypothalamic-pituitary-ovarian axis suppression (such as in an Olympic-level gymnast), this is a diagnosis of exclusion. Thus, doing nothing or reassuring the mother is not the optimal approach. Although oral contraceptive pills may be used, they should not be initiated until there is a diagnosis. The presence of a uterus helps determine the likelihood of a deficiency of 17 α-hydroxylase or 17,20-desmolase deficiency. Both of these are extremely rare, given that it is probably unreasonable to subject a 14-year-old to a pelvic examination at this point in the evaluation. A serum FSH level of greater than 40 mIU/mL indicates no functioning ovarian follicles in the gonadal tissue. Thus, in women with primary amenorrhea, the diagnosis of gonadal failure can be established if the FSH levels are abnormally elevated.

36. **D,** Page 1116. Amenorrhea and elevated FSH indicate ovarian follicular failure. This is hypergonadotropic-hypogonadism amenorrhea. Although this is occasionally transient, premature ovarian failure eventually results in a prolonged period of hypoestrogenemia with all of the complications of a premature and prolonged menopause. Since the patient underwent normal puberty, a karyotype is unlikely to reveal anything, and the cost is significant. With the diagnosis of premature ovarian failure, patient reassurance is not appropriate since she needs to be counseled regarding estrogen replacement and her infertility. If she does desire children, clomiphene citrate (Clomid) will not work since it requires functional follicles. The patient would have to adopt or use advanced reproductive technology with an ovum donor. Although an initial cycle with medroxyprogesterone will indicate whether the patient's estrogen status is already low by a withdrawal bleed, long-term cycling will not help since the patient will be hypoestrogenic. The patient needs to be started on estrogen replacement with a progestin since she has a uterus. Although menopausal preparations can be used, they are low enough in terms of dosage that the patient will likely not experience a withdrawal bleed. The oral contraceptives will provide more estrogen and monthly cycles, which often helps the patient emotionally.

Hyperprolactinemia, Galactorrhea, and Pituitary Adenomas

for Questions 1–26: Select the one best answer or completion.

1. A 37-year-old woman with galactorrhea has a prolactin level of 40 ng/mL on two occasions. Her thyroid function results are normal. The next step would be to

   A. observe for 3 months
   B. obtain anteroposterior and lateral coned-down views of the sella turcica
   C. perform magnetic resonance imaging (MRI)
   D. start bromocriptine
   E. refer for surgical resection

2. A patient who had been treated for a prolactin-secreting microadenoma has just delivered and wishes to breast-feed. You would advise her

   A. not to breast-feed
   B. to take bromocriptine while breast-feeding
   C. to take bromocriptine for 2 to 3 weeks after breast-feeding
   D. to undergo a serum prolactin determination before you decide what to advise
   E. to undergo computed tomography (CT) before you decide what to advise

3. All the following can cause galactorrhea and hyperprolactinemia except

   A. Cushing disease
   B. low-dose oral contraceptives
   C. chronic renal disease
   D. hyperthyroidism
   E. chest trauma

4. A 20-year-old gravida 0 complains of galactorrhea. She has no other complaints. Her periods are regular, occurring every 28 days. Her physical examination result is normal except for the galactorrhea. A serum prolactin level is reported to be 18 ng/mL. At this point you recommend

   A. CT
   B. hypocycloidal tomography
   C. pneumoencephalography
   D. visual field examination
   E. follow-up in 1 year

5. "Big-big" prolactin

   A. is the principal form of prolactin measured in bioassays
   B. is the principal form of prolactin measured in immunoassays
   C. is a dimer of the small monomeric form
   D. has reduced binding to mammary tissue membranes compared with the monomeric form
   E. constitutes 50% of the secreted form

6. Select the patient in Figure 39–1 whose serum prolactin level is most typical of the normal patient.

   A. patient A
   B. patient B
   C. patient C
   D. patient D
   E. patient E

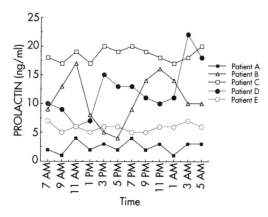

FIGURE 39-1

7. **In the healthy patient, lactation does not commence until after delivery because**

   A. prolactin is not secreted until after delivery
   B. placental lactogen is only weakly lactogenic
   C. β human chorionic gonadotropin (β-hCG) blocks the action of prolactin on the breast
   D. the increase in cortisol associated with the delivery process is important in the initiation of lactation
   E. estrogen inhibits the action of prolactin on the breast

8. **A 33-year-old woman, who is 5 feet 3 inches tall and weighs 180 pounds, has galactorrhea, oligomenorrhea, a serum prolactin level of 18 ng/mL, and a normal thyroid-stimulating hormone (TSH) level. At this point you would**

   A. do nothing for a year
   B. order an infusion of thyrotropin-releasing hormone (TRH) as a provocative stimulus of prolactin
   C. initiate bromocriptine therapy
   D. order MRI or CT
   E. order anteroposterior and lateral coned-down views of the sella turcica

9. **In which of the following patients with galactorrhea, all of whom might have an elevated serum prolactin level, are you most likely to find that the prolactin level actually is elevated?**

   A. a 20-year-old woman with low estrogen and amenorrhea
   B. a 30-year-old woman, 8 months' postpartum, breast-feeding, with amenorrhea, whose blood is drawn when the woman is in a basal state
   C. a 25-year-old woman with normal estrogen and oligomenorrhea
   D. a 30-year-old woman with normal estrogen and amenorrhea
   E. a 25-year-old woman with normal estrogen and normal menses

10. **In a woman who recently has had trouble breast-feeding her 7-month-old infant, the basal serum prolactin determination is 10 ng/mL. Having been asked for an opinion, you would state that**

    A. this is too low a level for successful lactation
    B. the woman is obviously under stress; if she relaxed, the prolactin would increase and she would be able to breast-feed
    C. the prolactin level is compatible with successful breast-feeding
    D. without knowing the conditions under which the result was obtained, you cannot offer an opinion
    E. the patient should be examined for Sheehan syndrome

11. **A 25-year-old single woman has oligomenorrhea, galactorrhea, and hyperprolactinemia (88 ng/mL). Thyroid function is normal. On MRI, a 3-mm microadenoma is noted. The oligomenorrhea and galactorrhea are not of concern to the patient. Recommended therapy for this patient is**

    A. bromocriptine
    B. external radiation therapy
    C. periodic progestin withdrawal
    D. surgical resection
    E. implantation of yttrium-90 rods

12. **The major mechanism by which elevated levels of prolactin inhibit ovulation appears to be**

    A. a direct action of big-big prolactin
    B. alterations in normal gonadotrophin-releasing hormone (GnRH) release
    C. direct inhibition of ovarian secretion of estradiol
    D. direct inhibition of ovarian secretion of progesterone
    E. interference with the positive estrogen effect on midcycle luteinizing hormone (LH) release

13. **True statements about prolactin include all the following except that it**

    A. is synthesized in chromophobe cells located in the pituitary gland
    B. is stored in chromophobe cells located in the pituitary gland
    C. is synthesized in decidual tissue
    D. is synthesized in endometrial tissue
    E. has a half-life of 20 hours

14. Pituitary tumors that mainly secrete adrenocorticotropic hormone (ACTH) or growth hormone frequently secrete prolactin. Hyperprolactinemia has been reported to occur in approximately what percentage of cases with the following conditions?

	Cushing disease	Acromegaly
A.	25%	10%
B.	10%	25%
C.	10%	10%
D.	25%	25%
E.	5%	10%

15. Findings commonly associated with patients who have hyperprolactinemia include all the following except

A. galactorrhea
B. amenorrhea
C. anovulation
D. oligomenorrhea
E. polymenorrhea

16. Bromocriptine (2-Br-α-ergocryptine mesylate)

A. is detectable in the circulation 24 hours after administration
B. frequently (40% to 50% of the time) causes orthostatic hypotension
C. frequently (40% to 50% of the time) causes insomnia
D. is a dopamine receptor agonist
E. is ineffective when administered other than by mouth

17. A 19-year-old college student experienced amenorrhea of 6 months' duration. A workup at the student health service revealed a normal physical examination result, including a normal pelvic examination result, a follicle-stimulating hormone (FSH) level in the low normal range, and an early morning serum prolactin level of 70 ng/mL. At this point you would order measurement of

A. quantitative β-hCG
B. TSH
C. repeat serum prolactin in the midafternoon
D. LH
E. MRI

18. A 28-year-old gravida 0 who consulted you because of infertility is found to have a prolactin microadenoma. In discussing bromocriptine treatment, you would tell this patient that

A. she will not become pregnant until her prolactin level is less than 20 ng/mL
B. she should notify you immediately if she is late for a period so that you can stop the medication (since there is evidence that it is teratogenic)
C. even with a dose of bromocriptine of up to 20 mg/day (about three times the average), prolactin levels fail to return to normal in 40% of patients with a microadenoma
D. bromocriptine is not associated with an increased risk of spontaneous abortion
E. if she stops bromocriptine during pregnancy, there is a 40% chance that she will develop visual field changes because of tumor growth

19. A 20-year-old Caucasian woman who is a long-distance track star has consulted you because of amenorrhea. Initially, you thought that the amenorrhea was due to her vigorous exercise. Then she experienced galactorrhea, and you obtained a serum prolactin level. Having diagnosed a prolactin-secreting microadenoma, you would inform the patient that if she is not treated she is very likely to experience

A. primary empty sella syndrome
B. osteoporosis
C. visual problems
D. hypothyroidism
E. adrenal insufficiency

20. The rationale for discontinuing bromocriptine in a woman who becomes pregnant and has a prolactin-secreting macroadenoma includes all the following except that

A. it suppresses fetal prolactin
B. more than 50% of such patients experience a decrease in visual fields during pregnancy
C. it crosses the placenta
D. prolactin levels increase during pregnancy
E. the long-term effects of bromocriptine on the newborn are unknown

21. A 40-year-old woman is found to have a prolactinoma. Her serum prolactin level is 250 ng/mL, and she gives a history of 3 years of amenorrhea and galactorrhea. The patient has inquired about surgical correction. In discussing the possible outcomes of transsphenoidal microsurgical resection, it would be correct to tell this patient that

    A. she will need to undergo radiation after operation
    B. the risk of permanent diabetes insipidus is greater than 40%
    C. the risk of hypopituitarism is 25%
    D. her age and the length of time she has had symptoms are unrelated to the likelihood of a cure
    E. the basic defect in dopamine regulation of prolactin secretion persists after removal

22. Prolactin stimulates the

    A. differentiation of mammary tissue
    B. secretion of milk into the alveoli of breast glands
    C. release of gonadotrophins
    D. milk ejection during nursing

23. Bromocriptine is best suited to the treatment of a prolactin-secreting macroadenoma in which of the following situations?

    A. prior to surgical resection
    B. after an irradiation failure
    C. only in patients without visual field impairment
    D. when the patient wishes to preserve the possibility of future breast-feeding

24. Physiologic stimuli that increase prolactin release include

    A. stress
    B. reduced exercise
    C. sleep deprivation
    D. orgasm
    E. menstruation

25. A decrease in serum prolactin is usually noted with

    A. an infusion of thyrotropin-releasing hormone
    B. a craniopharyngioma
    C. the empty sella syndrome
    D. sarcoidosis
    E. bromocriptine

26. Which of the following statements about hyperprolactinemia without macroadenoma is true?

    A. Therapy is not required unless estrogen levels are low.
    B. Pregnancy is contraindicated.
    C. Macroadenomas develop in the majority of patients with hyperprolactinemia.
    D. Galactorrhea is rare.

DIRECTIONS:

for Questions 27–31: For each numbered item, select the one heading most closely associated with it. Each lettered heading may be used once, more than once, or not at all.

27–28. Physiologic action

  (A) dopamine
  (B) epinephrine
  (C) serotonin
  (D) 2-Br-α-ergocryptine mesylate
  (E) estradiol

27. Prolactin-inhibiting factor (PIF)

28. Prolactin-releasing factor (PRF)

29–31. Several pharmacologic agents are associated with galactorrhea and hyperprolactinemia. The pathophysiologic condition depends on the agent. Match the mechanism with the medication.

  (A) blocks dopamine uptake
  (B) blocks hypothalamic dopamine receptors
  (C) depletes catecholamines
  (D) blocks the conversion of tyrosine to dopa
  (E) blocks the conversion of tryptophan to serotonin

29. Reserpine

30. Haloperidol

31. Tricyclic antidepressants

DIRECTIONS:

for each numbered item 32–33, indicate the condition for which the test is appropriate.

(A) prolactin-secreting macroadenoma
(B) prolactin-secreting microadenoma
(C) both (A) and (B)
(D) neither (A) nor (B)

32. Visual field test

33. Insulin tolerance test

ANSWERS

1. **C,** Pages 1132–1133. In cases with borderline elevations of prolactin (20 to 60 ng/mL), MRI should be performed.

2. **C,** Page 1139. After delivery, breast-feeding may be initiated without adverse effects on the tumor. After completion of nursing, bromocriptine should be taken for 2 to 3 weeks and then discontinued. At that time, a serum prolactin measurement and repeat MRI or CT should be performed if prolactin is elevated so that the need for further treatment can be reassessed.

3. **D,** Pages 1128–1129. Pathologic causes of hyperprolactinemia, in addition to a prolactin-secreting pituitary adenoma, include other pituitary tumors that produce acromegaly and Cushing disease. Additional causes are hypothalamic disease, various pharmacologic agents, hypothyroidism (not hyperthyroidism), chronic renal disease, or any chronic type of breast nerve stimulation, such as may occur with a thoracic operation, herpes zoster, or chest trauma. Ingestion of oral contraceptive steroids can also increase prolactin levels, with a greater incidence of hyperprolactinemia occurring with higher-estrogen formulations. Nevertheless, galactorrhea does not usually occur during oral contraceptive ingestion because the exogenous estrogen blocks the binding of prolactin to its receptors.

4. **E,** Pages 1132–1133. In most laboratories, a normal serum prolactin level is less than 22 ng/mL. Women with regular menses, galactorrhea, and normal prolactin levels do not have prolactinomas, and therefore radiologic studies are unnecessary in such women. There would certainly be no suspicion of a macroadenoma, and so visual fields would not be warranted. Since 3% to 5% of patients with hyperprolactinemia have hypothyroidism, a TSH assay is warranted at the time the prolactin is drawn. Since this patient does not have hyperprolactinemia, only follow-up is indicated.

5. **D,** Pages 1125–1126. Big-big prolactin (100,000 daltons) may represent an aggregation of many monomeric molecules of prolactin (22,000 daltons). The small form is biologically active, and about 80% of the hormone is secreted in the small form. The larger forms of prolactin, big and big-big, are immunoreactive, but most of the immunoassayable prolactin is in the small form. Big-big prolactin has reduced binding to mammary tissue membranes compared with the monomeric form and is thus inactive in some bioassays. Specific receptors for prolactin are present in the plasma membrane of mammary cells and in many other tissues.

6. **D,** Page 1126. Prolactin levels normally fluctuate throughout the day, with maximum levels observed at night during sleep and a smaller increase occurring in the early afternoon.

7. **E,** Page 1126. During pregnancy, the levels of prolactin increase, reaching about 200 ng/mL in the third trimester, and the rise is directly related to the increase in circulating levels of estrogen. Despite the elevated prolactin levels noted during pregnancy, lactation does not occur because estrogen inhibits the action of prolactin on the breast, most likely blocking prolactin's interaction with its receptor. One or 2 days after delivery of the placenta, both estrogen levels and prolactin levels decline rapidly and lactation is initiated. Prolactin levels reach basal levels in nonnursing women in 2 to 3 weeks.

8. **E,** Page 1132. A prolactinoma and hypothyroidism have been ruled out in this patient with oligomenorrhea, normal prolactin, and normal TSH. Because a few patients with galactorrhea, abnormal menstrual function, and normal prolactin levels have been found to have the empty sella syndrome, the diagnosis should be confirmed by CT or MRI.

9. **A,** Pages 1127–1128. Hyperprolactinemia has been reported to be present in 15% of all anovulatory women and in 20% of women with amenorrhea of undetermined cause. The incidence of galactorrhea in women with hyperprolactinemia has been reported to range from 30% to 80%. The incidence of hyperprolactinemia is higher (88%) in those women with galactorrhea who have amenorrhea and low estrogen levels than in women with galactorrhea and normal menses, oligomenorrhea, or amenorrhea with normal estrogen levels (49%). Basal levels of circulating prolactin decline to the nonpregnant range about 6 months after parturition in nursing women.

10. **C,** Page 1126. Prolactin levels reach normal nonpregnant concentrations in nonnursing women in 2 to 3 weeks. Although basal levels of circulating prolactin decline to the nonpregnant range about 6 months after parturition in nursing women, prolactin levels increase markedly after each act of sucking and stimulate milk production for the next feeding. A level of 10 ng/mL is in the normal range. Since the patient had established breast-feeding, Sheehan syndrome is not a consideration. Stress should increase (not decrease) the release of prolactin.

11. **C,** Pages 1133–1137. Bromocriptine therapy is used primarily in women with microadenomas who wish to conceive or who are disturbed by their symptoms. This patient is not married and did not indicate that conception was an objective. She is not bothered by either the galactorrhea or the oligomenorrhea. Since she experiences some menses, she is producing estrogen. Thus, she does not appear to be at increased risk for osteoporosis and should be treated with periodic progestin withdrawal (medroxyprogesterone acetate, 10 mg/day for 10 days) to prevent endometrial hyperplasia. A barrier type of contraception is advisable. Cabergoline may be a medical option with fewer side effects. Surgical resection is an option for patients with larger tumors. Radiation is not a primary mode of treatment for this lesion. Results have been inconsistent, and there is a delay of several months between treatment and resumption of ovulation.

12. **B,** Page 1127. The mechanism, which best explains why elevated prolactin levels interfere with gonadotrophin release, has not been completely elucidated, but the major factor appears to be alterations in normal GnRH release. It has also been shown that elevated levels of prolactin directly inhibit basal and gonadotrophin-stimulated ovarian secretion of both estradiol and progesterone. However, this mechanism is probably not the primary cause of anovulation because women with hyperprolactinemia can be stimulated to ovulate with various agents, including pulsatile GnRH. Some patients with moderate hyperprolactinemia have a greater-than-normal proportion of the big-big form of prolactin. Because this form of prolactin has reduced bioactivity, such persons can have normal pituitary and ovarian function.

13. **E,** Pages 1125–1126. Prolactin is synthesized and stored in the pituitary gland in chromophobe cells called *lactotrophs,* which are located mainly in the lateral areas of the gland. In addition, prolactin is synthesized in decidual and endometrial tissue. Prolactin circulates in unbound form and has a 20-minute half-life.

14. **B,** Pages 1128–1129. Pituitary tumors that secrete mainly ACTH or growth hormone frequently secrete prolactin. Hyperprolactinemia has been reported to occur in about 10% of patients with Cushing disease and 25% of patients with acromegaly.

15. **E,** Page 1127. Hyperprolactinemia is usually associated with galactorrhea and can produce disorders of menstrual function, including amenorrhea, oligomenorrhea, and anovulation. Polymenorrhea is not a finding associated with increased serum prolactin.

16. **D,** Pages 1133–1136. Bromocriptine directly stimulates dopamine receptors; as a dopamine receptor agonist, it inhibits prolactin secretion both in vitro and in vivo. After ingestion, bromocriptine is rapidly absorbed, with peak blood levels reached 1 to 3 hours later. It is not detectable in the serum after 14 hours. For this reason, the drug is usually given at least twice daily. The most frequent side effect is orthostatic hypotension, which occurs in about 15% of patients. To minimize the effects of orthostatic hypotension, the initial dose should be taken at bedtime with food. Less common adverse symptoms include headache, nasal congestion, fatigue (not insomnia), constipation, and diarrhea. About 10% of women cannot tolerate oral bromocriptine because of severe side effects. Vermesh and associates reported that the drug was very well absorbed vaginally without the presence of side effects. A long-acting injectable form of bromocriptine that is effective for 1 month has also been developed, but it is not yet available for clinical use.

17. **B,** Page 1129. About 3% to 5% of persons with hyperprolactinemia have hypothyroidism. This is the result of the decreased negative feedback of thyroxine (T_4) on the hypothalamic-pituitary axis. The resulting increase in TRH stimulates prolactin secretion and TSH secretion from the pituitary. Thus, a TSH assay should be obtained for all patients with hyperprolactinemia. If the TSH level is elevated, triiodothyronine (T_3) and T_4 should be

measured to confirm the diagnosis of primary hypothyroidism. This is necessary because occasionally the TSH is elevated because of a TSH-secreting pituitary adenoma. In this patient, with a normal pelvic examination result, quantitative β-hCG measurement is not indicated. One might have taken a qualitative β-hCG level as an initial screening test. Measuring the level of LH would not help in establishing a diagnosis. A serum prolactin obtained in midafternoon would be about the same or higher, not lower. MRI is indicated if the TSH is normal.

18. **D, Pages 1133–1136.** The usual therapeutic dose of bromocriptine is 2.5 mg two or three times a day. In about 10% of patients with microadenomas, prolactin levels fail to return to normal despite administration of up to 20 mg/day. Despite the persistently elevated prolactin levels, many of these patients ovulate and conceive. There is no evidence that the drug is teratogenic or adversely affects pregnancy outcome. The incidence of spontaneous abortion and multiple pregnancy is not increased. Less than 1% of patients with microadenomas experience changes in visual fields. About 20% of patients with macroprolactinomas experience adverse changes in visual fields and polytomographic or neurologic signs during pregnancy. Some of these patients require bromocriptine or operative treatment during pregnancy or shortly postpartum.

19. **B, Page 1133.** Several studies have demonstrated the benign course of untreated microadenomas. These tumors seldom enlarge. Therefore, treatment may not be necessary if the patient is not bothered by the amenorrhea or galactorrhea. In this case, the patient is at increased risk for osteoporosis because of the low estrogen levels associated with prolactin elevations and her long-distance running. For this reason, she should receive exogenous estrogen. Macroadenomas, not microadenomas, are likely to enlarge and cause visual field distortion or disturbance of pituitary function. A cause, not a consequence, of hyperprolactinemia is the primary empty sella syndrome. This is a clinical situation in which an intrasellar extension of the subarachnoid space results in compression of the pituitary gland and an enlarged sella turcica.

20. **B, Pages 1138–1139.** Twenty percent, not 50%, of patients with macroadenomas experience adverse changes in visual fields and polytomographic or neurologic signs during pregnancy. Bromocriptine crosses the placenta and does suppress fetal prolactin, but it does not suppress placental hormone production. Its long-term effects on the newborn are unknown, although the risk of congenital anomalies, spontaneous abortion, and

multiple gestation does not appear to increase. Postnatal surveillance of more than 200 children born after their mothers had been taking bromocriptine revealed no adverse effects to date. If stopped at the onset of pregnancy, bromocriptine should be reinstated in those pregnant patients who experience visual impairment. During pregnancy, women with a macroadenoma should undergo monthly visual fields and neurologic testing.

21. **E, Page 1138.** Radiation therapy should be used only as adjunctive management after incomplete operative removal of large tumors. A prolactin level of 250 ng/mL is high, but this factor alone does not mean that the lesion is so large that it cannot be completely removed at operation. Transsphenoidal operations carry a mortality rate of less than 0.5%. The risk of permanent diabetes insipidus and hypopituitarism is less than 2%. The initial cure rate for patients with a serum prolactin level above 200 ng/mL is 35%. Operative treatment of tumors in patients older than 26 with amenorrhea for more than 6 months carries a poorer prognosis than does such treatment of tumors in younger patients with a shorter duration of amenorrhea. In patients with prolactinomas, there is a defect in dopamine regulation of prolactin secretion that persists even after surgical removal of the adenoma. This loss of dopaminergic inhibition of prolactin that persists for years after tumor removal is thought to explain the high rate of recurrence of tumors in the long-term follow-up of patients.

22. **B, Page 1127.** The main functions of prolactin are the stimulation of growth of mammary tissue and the production and secretion of milk into the alveoli. Prolactin interferes with gonadotrophin release. Women with hyperprolactinemia have abnormalities in the frequency and amplitude of LH pulsations, with a normal or increased gonadotrophin response following GnRH infusion.

23. **A, Pages 1137–1138.** Bromocriptine shrinks 80% to 90% of all macroadenomas, and although the recurrence rate after cessation of therapy is high, long-term therapy has been successful in some patients. This medication is expensive, and a number of women, especially those taking higher doses, experience unpleasant side effects. Cabergoline is a long-acting dopamine receptor agonist that is taken twice weekly. The effectiveness of cabergoline was greater than bromocriptine and adverse effects were less frequent, less severe, and of shorter duration than with bromocriptine. Therefore, some patients prefer surgical treatment. If given preoperatively to shrink the tumor, the drug should be continued until the time of operation because, after withdrawal of the drug, the tumor size may increase

just as rapidly as it decreased. Bromocriptine has been successfully used to treat patients with failure of, or recurrence after, operation or irradiation therapy. Visual field impairment has disappeared with bromocriptine treatment.

24. **A,** Pages 1126–1127. Nipple and breast stimulation increases prolactin levels in the nonpregnant female. Other stimuli include stress, exercise, and sleep. Although there are small changes in prolactin secretion throughout the menstrual cycle, these are minor.

25. **E,** Pages 1129–1130. TRH can cause the release of prolactin. The normal response to an infusion of 500 mg is greater than three times the baseline prolactin. A craniopharyngioma can produce hyperprolactinemia, as can an infiltration of the hypothalamus by sarcoidosis, histiocytosis, leukemia, or carcinoma. The empty sella syndrome is a condition in which an intrasellar extension of the subarachnoid space results in compression of the pituitary gland and an enlarged sella turcica that may be associated with galactorrhea and hyperprolactinemia. Therefore, in patients with radiologic evidence of an enlarged sella, CT or MRI should be obtained to establish or rule out the presence of empty sella syndrome. Bromocriptine is useful for decreasing prolactin in most cases of elevation.

26. **A,** Pages 1133–1135. Almost all patients with hyperprolactinemia experience a benign course and require no treatment unless pregnancy is desired or estrogen levels are low. Studies indicate that patients may actually benefit from pregnancy, with roughly half of pregnant women experiencing a reduction of their prolactin levels. Patients with hyperprolactinemia rarely experience macroadenomas or other gross changes. Even in patients with known macroadenomas, progression is unusual. The symptom of galactorrhea varies highly, and its presence or absence cannot be used to predict the presence of a macroadenoma.

27–28. 27, **A;** 28, **C;** Pages 1126–1127. Prolactin synthesis and release are controlled by central nervous system neurotransmitters. The major control mechanism is inhibition. It appears that the major physiologic inhibitor of prolactin release is the neurotransmitter dopamine, which acts directly on the pituitary gland. Dopamine appears to be the prolactin-inhibiting factor. Both serotonin and TRH stimulate prolactin release. Since the latter stimulates prolactin release only minimally (unless infused), it appears that serotonin is a prolactin-releasing factor. The rise in prolactin levels during sleep appears to be controlled by serotonin. Bromocriptine, 2-Br-α-ergocryptine mesylate, is a semisynthetic ergot alkaloid that is a dopamine receptor agonist. It is used to treat hyperprolactinemia. Estrogen stimulates prolactin production and release and is especially important in this regard at the time of puberty and during pregnancy. It is not, however, considered a prolactin-releasing factor.

29–31. 29, **C;** 30, **B;** 31, **A;** Pages 1126–1127. One of the most frequent causes of galactorrhea and hyperprolactinemia is the ingestion of pharmacologic agents. The antihypertensive agent reserpine depletes catecholamines, and methyldopa blocks the conversion of tyrosine to dihydroxyphenylalanine (dopa). The tricyclic antidepressants block dopamine uptake, and haloperidol and phenothiazines block hypothalamic dopamine receptors. Amphetamines stimulate the serotoninergic system.

32–33. 32, **A;** 33, **A;** Pages 1132–1133. Visual field determination and tests of ACTH and thyroid function are not necessary in patients with microadenomas because these small tumors do not interfere with overall pituitary function and do not extend beyond the sella. However, these evaluations should be performed in persons with macroadenomas. An insulin tolerance test is a test of ACTH reserve.

CHAPTER
40

Hyperandrogenism

DIRECTIONS:

for Questions 1–31: Select the one best answer or completion.

1. **Typical clinical features of virilization include all the following** *except*

   A. decreased breast size
   B. dryness of the vagina
   C. development over a relatively long time (more than 2 years)
   D. increase in muscle mass
   E. secondary amenorrhea

2. **The majority of the peripheral clinical manifestations of hirsutism are caused by**

   A. increased circulating levels of androstenedione
   B. increased circulating levels of dehydro-epiandrosterone (DHEA)
   C. increased levels of 5α-reductase
   D. increased levels of free testosterone
   E. increased levels of sex hormone–binding globulin (SHBG)

3. **To exert a biologic effect such as hirsutism, testosterone is metabolized peripherally in target tissues to**

   A. 5α-dehydrotestosterone (DHT)
   B. dehydroepiandrosterone sulfate (DHEA-S)
   C. androstenedione
   D. free testosterone
   E. etiocholanolone

4. **In the severe form of congenital adrenal hyperplasia with complete 21-hydroxylase deficiency, clinical manifestations become apparent in a female**

   A. at the time of birth
   B. at the time of menarche
   C. sometime between childhood and adolescence
   D. in the late teens
   E. in the fourth decade and present as hirsutism

5. **Biochemical characteristics of polycystic ovary syndrome (PCOS) include all the following** *except*

   A. increased gonadotrophin-releasing hormone (GnRH) pulse amplitude
   B. tonically elevated levels of luteinizing hormone (LH)
   C. decreased levels of follicle-stimulating hormone (FSH)
   D. increased levels of circulating ovarian androgens
   E. decreased levels of biologically active (non-SHBG-bound) estradiol

6. **A 26-year-old woman who is 5 feet 3 inches tall and weighs 220 pounds has biochemically proven PCOS. In addition, she is most likely to have**

   A. hypothyroidism
   B. congenital adrenal hyperplasia
   C. Addison disease
   D. impaired glucose tolerance
   E. primary hyperparathyroidism

7. **Increased terminal hair growth in a patient is consistent with each of the following** *except*

   A. clinical hirsutism
   B. elevated levels of circulating androgen
   C. increased activity of 5α-reductase
   D. an increased amount of vellus hair
   E. a prolonged length of anagen

8. The major clinical difference between PCOS and stromal hyperthecosis is a

   A. greater ovarian enlargement in stromal hyperthecosis
   B. thickened ovarian capsule in stromal hyperthecosis
   C. higher levels of circulating free estradiol in stromal hyperthecosis
   D. progressive androgen stigmata including virilization in stromal hyperthecosis
   E. anovulation in stromal hyperthecosis

9. A 28-year-old gravida 1, para 0, who is approximately 32 weeks pregnant has had an acute onset of progressive, bothersome hirsutism of the upper lip and chin. During this time she has developed acne. The most likely reason is that the patient

   A. has an increased rate of androgen conversion from placental progesterone
   B. has androgenic manifestations because of increased peripheral 5α-reductase activity
   C. has increased ovarian testosterone production
   D. has increased maternal adrenal DHEA-A production
   E. has increased peripheral conversion to DHT

10. A 22-year-old, gravida 1, para 1, 125-pound woman is referred with bothersome central hirsutism. She has regular menstrual periods, and the referring physician has obtained both serum testosterone and DHEA-S levels, which are normal. The most likely source of her problem is increased

    A. free testosterone
    B. androstenedione
    C. androsterone
    D. 5α-reductase activity
    E. etiocholanolone

11. The best treatment for the patient in Question 10 is

    A. spironolactone
    B. dexamethasone
    C. conjugated estrogens
    D. oral contraceptives
    E. electrolysis

12. In evaluating a 30-year-old oligomenorrheic, hirsute woman, the DHEA-S level of 4 ng/mL (normal = 0.8 to 3.4 ng/mL). An adrenocorticotropic hormone (ACTH) stimulation test is performed to rule out primary adrenal disease, and the DHEA-S is found to triple. This is consistent with the diagnosis of

    A. Cushing disease
    B. acromegaly
    C. adrenal carcinoma
    D. PCOS
    E. androgen-secreting ovarian tumor

13. Symptoms of androgen excess in patients with congenital adrenal hyperplasia are the result of excessive

    A. adrenal production of free testosterone
    B. peripheral conversion of C_{19} steroids to testosterone
    C. adrenal production of free DHEA-S
    D. adrenal production of free androstenedione
    E. adrenal cortisol production

14. A 24-year-old oligomenorrheic nulligravida is diagnosed as having PCOS. The patient is not anxious to become pregnant at this time. The best treatment is cyclic

    A. medroxyprogesterone acetate
    B. conjugated estrogens
    C. norethindrone
    D. levonorgestrel acetate
    E. combination oral contraceptives

15. A 30-year-old, 5 feet 1 inch, 110-pound gravida 2, para 2, is referred to you for treatment of slowly progressive hirsutism. She has regular monthly menstrual periods. Her serum testosterone is 0.5 ng/mL (normal = 0.2 to 0.8 ng/mL) and serum DHEA-S is 1.2 ng/mL (normal = 0.8 to 3.4 ng/mL). The most likely diagnosis is

    A. Cushing syndrome
    B. idiopathic hirsutism
    C. PCOS
    D. congenital adrenal hyperplasia
    E. stromal cell hyperthecosis

16. The best treatment of the patient in Question 15 is

    A. dexamethasone
    B. combination oral contraceptives
    C. conjugated estrogens
    D. medroxyprogesterone acetate
    E. spironolactone

17. A 28-year-old slender, athletic-looking, normotensive woman has an 18-month history of oligomenorrhea and a 6-month history of progressive central hirsutism and clitoromegaly. Her serum testosterone is 0.8 mg/mL (normal = 0.2 to 0.8 ng/mL). The DHEA-S is 10 mg/mL (normal = 0.8 to 3.4 ng/mL). The pelvic examination is normal. This patient should undergo

    A. CT of the adrenal glands
    B. ACTH stimulation testing
    C. overnight dexamethasone suppression testing
    D. complete dexamethasone suppression testing
    E. laparoscopic examination of the ovaries

18. The best laboratory test to confirm a suspected diagnosis of congenital adrenal hyperplasia is a

    A. serum testosterone
    B. serum DHEA-S
    C. serum pregnanetriol
    D. serum 17-hydroxyprogesterone
    E. urinary 17-ketosteroids

19. A 26-year-old infertile woman has oligo-menorrhea. She is 5 feet 7 inches tall and weighs 160 pounds. The ovaries are bilaterally enlarged. She does *not* have hirsutism. Of the following, the most likely to be normal is

    A. DHEA-S
    B. 3α-diol-G
    C. testosterone
    D. androstenedione
    E. LH

20. A 25-year-old woman delivers a 3200-g infant at term after an uncomplicated pregnancy. Newborn examination is normal except for the presence of ambiguous genitalia, including an enlarged clitoris, a vaginal dimple, and an incompletely developed scrotum. The most likely diagnosis is

    A. congenital adrenal hyperplasia
    B. androgen insensitivity syndrome (testicular feminization)
    C. Cushing syndrome
    D. Turner syndrome
    E. adrenal carcinoma

21. A 26-year-old woman is referred for evaluation of bothersome hirsutism. The referring physician has obtained a serum testosterone level, which is 1.0 ng/mL (normal = 0.2 to 0.8 ng/mL). Further information can be best gained by ordering a test for the level of

    A. serum androstenedione
    B. serum androsterone
    C. serum etiocholanolone
    D. serum DHEA-S
    E. urinary 17-ketosteroids

22. Which of the following characterizes late-onset 21-hydroxylase deficiency?

    A. phenotype apparent at birth
    B. most common in the Ashkenazi Jewish population
    C. homozygous condition with two severely defective alleles
    D. most common X-linked disorder in humans

23. Late-onset 21-hydroxylase deficiency is best differentiated from PCOS by

    A. a basal serum 17-hydroxyprogesterone level
    B. urinary 17-hydroxyprogesterone
    C. urinary 17-ketosteroids
    D. AM and PM cortisol levels

24. Historic features helpful in identifying the source of androgen in a 21-year-old woman complaining of progressive hirsutism for the past year include all of the following *except*

    A. her menstrual history
    B. her prepubertal and pubertal linear growth history
    C. rapidity of hair growth
    D. age of onset
    E. all the above

25. In treating hirsutism with various pharmacologic agents, patients should be told all of the following *except*

    A. they will need to continue therapy for approximately 4 years
    B. a response may take at least 3 months to become apparent
    C. approximately three quarters of patients will have a favorable response with 1 year of treatment
    D. ovarian failure is a common side effect

26. Biochemical characteristics associated with the ovarian histologic pattern shown in Figure 40–1 include all the following *except*

    A. increased pulsatility of GnRH
    B. tonically elevated LH
    C. increased total circulating estrogens
    D. reduced testosterone

27. True statements concerning circulating testosterone include all the following *except*

    A. most is biologically inactive
    B. it is metabolized in the periphery to 5α-dihydrotestosterone
    C. a laboratory report typically reflects total testosterone
    D. it is biologically active as testosterone

28. which of the following is elevated in women with PCOS?

    A. total serum estradiol
    B. unbound circulating estradiol
    C. estriol
    D. all the above

FIGURE 40–1

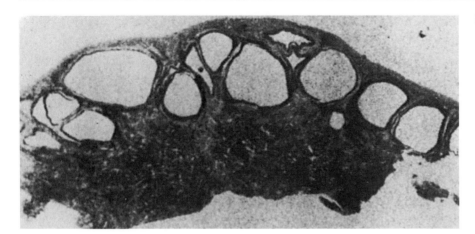

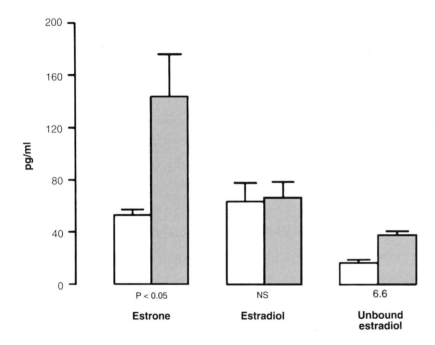

FIGURE 40–2 Serum estrogen concentrations in 13 normal women and 22 patients with polycystic ovarian syndrome *(shaded areas).* (From Lobo RA, Granger L, Goebelsemann U, et al: J Clin Endocrinol Metab 52:156, 1981. Copyright by The Endocrine Society, 1981.)

29. The estrogen milieu in a patient with PCOS as represented in Figure 40–2 encompasses all of the following *except*

    A. an increase in total circulating levels of estradiol
    B. an increase in biologically active estradiol
    C. a decrease in total serum estrone
    D. reduced estriol

30. Which of the following characteristics is the most controversial in describing PCOS?

    A. ovulatory dysfunction
    B. hyperandrogenism
    C. hyperandrogenemia
    D. morphologic changes of ovary

31. All of the following are accurate statements regarding the oral antihyperglycemic agent metformin *except*

    A. suppresses ovulation
    B. increases insulin sensitivity
    C. decreases insulin levels
    D. lowers free testosterone levels

ANSWERS

1. **C,** Page 1144. Virilization is a relatively uncommon clinical finding, and its presence is usually associated with markedly elevated levels of circulating testosterone (2 ng/mL or greater). In contrast with the gradual development of hirsutism, signs of virilization usually occur over a relatively short period. These signs are due to both the masculinizing and the determinizing action of testosterone and include temporal balding, clitoral hypertrophy, decreased breast size, dryness of the vagina, and increased muscle mass. Women with virilization are nearly always amenorrheic, and the presence of an androgen-secreting neoplasm should always be suspected in this clinical situation.

2. **D,** Pages 1145–1147. Androstenedione and DHEA do not have androgenic activity but are peripherally converted at a slow rate to a biologically active androgen, testosterone. About two thirds of the daily tetosterone produced in a woman originates from the ovaries. Thus, increased circulating levels of testosterone usually indicate abnormal ovarian androgen production. Most testosterone in the circulation (about 85%) is tightly bound to SHBG and is thought to be biologically inactive. An additional 10% to 15% is loosely bound to albumin with only about 1% to 2% not bound by any protein (free testosterone). Both the free and albumin-bound fraction are biologically active. Serum testosterone can be measured as the total amount, the amount that is believed to be biologically active (non–SHBG-bound), and the free form.

3. **A,** Pages 1147–1148. To exert a biologic effect, testosterone is metabolized peripherally in targeted tissues to the more androgenic DHT by the enzyme 5α-reductase. Even with normal circulatory levels of androgen, increased 5α-reductase activity in the pilosebaceous unit will result in increased androgenic activity, producing hirsutism. In evaluating hirsute women, it is important to remember that serum levels of total testosterone may be similar in both normal and hirsute women but that there are significant differences in the amounts of non–SHBG-bound testosterone and 3α-diol-G (a breakdown product of 5α-reductase). Thus, the clinician should remember there are three markers of androgen production in the serum, one for each compartment where androgens are produced: (1) ovary—testosterone; (2) adrenal gland—DHEA-S; and (3) periphery—3α-diol-G.

4. **A,** Page 1156. Congenital adrenal hyperplasia is an inherited disorder caused by an enzymatic defect (usually 21-hydroxylase deficiency) or, less often, an 11β-hydroxylase deficiency resulting in decreased cortisol biosynthesis. The increased production of C_{19} steroids is in turn peripherally converted to testosterone, which produces signs of androgen excess. Because the enzymatic defects are congenital, the classic severe form (complete block) usually becomes manifest in fetal life and is the most common cause of sexual ambiguity in the newborn. The more attenuated (mild) block of 21-hydroxylase deficiency does not produce physical signs until after puberty, making it a more common source of hirsutism and virilization in the second or early third decade of life.

5. **E,** Pages 1150–1151. PCOS is a relative common endocrinologic disorder that begins soon after menarche and consists of a series of biochemical abnormalities, including an increased GnRH pulse amplitude and tonically elevated levels of LH. Follicle-stimulating hormone typically is normal or low elevated in this disorder. In addition, there are increased circulating levels of androgen produced by both the ovaries and the adrenal glands. It has been shown that the peripheral manifestations of hirsutism associated with this disorder are more likely related to the patient's ability to peripherally convert the increased androgen load by 5α-reductase. Thus, the hirsutism often found with this disorder is peripherally mediated. Interestingly, most patients with polycystic ovary syndrome have increased levels of biologically active (non–SHBG-bound) estradiol, although total circulating levels of estradiol are not increased.

6. **D,** Page 1152. Hyperinsulinemia occurs in women with PCOS whether or not they are obese. Only obese women with PCOS have impaired glucose tolerance, however. Thus the negative impact of obesity and polycystic ovary syndrome on insulin resistance is additive. Although the other endocrinopathies may occur with PCOS, they are not necessarily found in association with this disorder. Some investigators have suggested that hyperandrogenism causes insulin resistance, whereas others have presented data indicating that the reverse is true: hyperinsulinemia produces hyperandrogenism in women with PCOS. This relationship remains controversial.

7. **D,** Page 1144. There are two types of hair—vellus hair, which is soft, fine, and unpigmented, and terminal hair. Terminal hair growth undergoes three phases: *anagen*, which is the growth phase; a transitional phase called *catagen*; and a resting phase called *telogen*, after which the hair sheds. Androgen is necessary to produce the development

of terminal hair, and the time spent in anagen is governed by circulating androgen levels. The level of activity of the enzyme 5α-reductase in the hair follicle influences the degree to androgenic activity. With elevated levels of androgen or increased activity of 5α-reductase, terminal hair appears where normally vellus hair is present. In this situation, the length of anagen is prolonged. The presence of hirsutism, without other signs of virilization, is associated with relatively mild disorders of androgen production with circulating levels of testosterone either normal or mildly elevated (<1.5 ng/mL). Hirsutism usually has a gradual onset and is not caused by a severe enzymatic defect or neoplasm.

8. **D,** Pages 1155–1156. Stromal hyperthecosis is an uncommon benign ovarian disorder in which the ovaries are bilaterally enlarged and histologically have nests of luteinized theca cells within the stroma (Figure 40–17 in Stenchever). The size of the ovaries and capsular thickening are similar to those found in PCOS. Anovulation is characteristics of both syndromes. This disorder is similar to polycystic ovary syndrome in that it is gradual and likely to be associated with amenorrhea and hirsutism. However, unlike PCOS, with increasing age stromal hyperthecosis is associated with progressively increasing amounts of testosterone secretion. By the time a woman reaches her fourth decade of life, the severity will have gradually progressed to cause virilization. Serum testosterone levels may reach those found usually in testosterone-secreting tumors (> 2 ng/mL).

9. **C,** Page 1148. Signs of androgen excess during this pregnancy are most likely caused by increased ovarian testosterone production. This is usually caused by either a luteoma of pregnancy or hyperreactio luteinalis. The former is a unilateral or bilateral solid ovarian enlargement, whereas the latter is bilateral cystic ovarian enlargement. After pregnancy excessive ovarian androgenic production resolves spontaneously and the androgenic signs regress.

10. **D,** Pages 1148–1149. Idiopathic hirsutism (a peripheral disorder of androgen metabolism) is the most common type of androgenic disorder. This usually occurs in regularly menstruating women and is associated with normal levels of serum testosterone and DHEA-S. It has recently been shown that nearly all these persons have increased levels of 3α-diol-G, indirectly indicating that the cause of hirsutism could be increased 5α-reductase activity, which converts normal levels of testosterone to increased amounts of biologically active androgens DHT and 3α-diol-G. If measured, serum androstenedione is usually normal. The other two androgens, androsterone

and etiocholanolone, are both 17-ketosteroids and are the metabolic breakdown products of androstenedione.

11. **A,** Page 1149. Idiopathic hirsutism is related to abnormalities in the excessive peripheral production of 3α-diol-G and DHT. It has been shown that there is a localized increase in the activity of 5α-reductase. This is considered a condition of peripheral androgen metabolism in the pilosebaceous apparatus of the skin. Antiandrogens that block peripheral testosterone action or interfere with 5α-reductase activity are moderately effective therapeutic agents. The most widely used agent in this country is spironolactone. The other agents do not exert a direct end-organ effect because they are not associated with appreciable changes in 5α-reductase activity. Electrolysis may improve the cosmetic appearance in select areas, but it does not treat the underlying problem.

12. **D,** Pages 1149–1152. Approximately half of the women with polycystic ovary syndrome have elevated levels of DHEA-S, with one third of them having levels greater than 4 ng/mL. Although ACTH levels are normal in these women, infusions of ACTH produce an exaggerated response of DHEA-S, indicating that perhaps the adrenal gland in some patients with PCOS has increased sensitivity to ACTH and that the adrenal gland may be involved in the pathogenesis of this syndrome. Cushing disease is the result of excessive adrenal production of glucocorticoids caused by increased secretion of ACTH. When the signs and symptoms are due to excessive glucocorticoids secondary to adrenal tumors, the problem is referred to as Cushing syndrome. These disorders are best evaluated by studies of adrenal suppression such as the overnight dexamethasone suppression test. The findings of androgen excess and exaggerated androgen response in this patient are unrelated to the manifestations associated with acromegaly. Likewise, extremely high levels of DHEA sulfate found with rare adrenal carcinomas are relatively unaffected by the ACTH stimulation test. One would not expect to uncover an androgen-secreting ovarian tumor by this test because ACTH has no effect on the ovary.

13. **B,** Page 1156. Congenital adrenal hyperplasia involves an enzymatic defect of either 21-hydroxylase or 11β-hydroxylase, resulting in decreased cortisone synthesis. ACTH production is thereby increased, and there is a progressive buildup of cortisol precursors, including 17-hydroxyprogesterone and 17-hydroxypregnenolone. These steroids are then converted to DHEA and androstenedione, which in turn are peripherally converted to testosterone, causing hirsutism or virilization,

depending on the severity of the enzymatic block. Testosterone is normally not produced in high amounts directly from the adrenal gland, and there is not an excessive amount of endogenously produced (adrenal) DHEA-S. The excessive amount of androstenedione produced is secondary to the enzymatic block or exerts its androgenic effect through peripheral conversion to testosterone.

14. **E,** Pages 1160–1161. The treatment of PCOS depends on which complaints are most bothersome to the patient. If hirsutism and irregular or infrequent bleeding are most bothersome and if the patient is not desirous of becoming pregnant, combination oral contraceptives containing low androgenic progestins are best. Oral contraceptives are preferable because these agents inhibit LH secretion, decrease circulating testosterone levels, and increase the levels of sex hormone--binding globulin (SHBG), thus binding and inactivating more of the testosterone in circulation. Medroxyprogesterone acetate, conjugated estrogens, and norethindrone acetate do not inhibit LH or decrease circulating testosterone levels to the same extent that cyclic combination oral contraceptives do.

15. **B,** Page 1148. The case exemplifies a patient with idiopathic hirsutism. She has normal adrenal and ovarian androgen levels and is experiencing regular menstrual periods. Fertility has not been a concern. It can be assumed that this patient has increased peripheral androgen activity and, if measured, would have a high 3α-diol-G value. This metabolite is not routinely measured because the presumptive diagnosis is one of exclusion (made by excluding the other possibilities). This woman did not have additional findings suggestive of Cushing disease such as centripetal obesity, dorsal neck fat pads, abdominal striae, or muscle wasting and weakness. Likewise, she does not have the oligomenorrhea that most patients with polycystic ovarian syndrome do, and she does not have the associated modestly elevated serum testosterone. Congenital adrenal hyperplasia is not suspect because of normal DHEA-S levels and an absence of menstrual irregularity and true virilization. Similarly, stromal cell hyperthecosis is ruled out by the lack of menstrual irregularity and a normal testosterone level.

16. **E,** Page 1149. The best treatment for idiopathic hirsutism is an agent that inhibits peripheral androgen activity. Of the drugs approved for use in the United States, the most efficacious is spironolactone. Cimetidine has also been used successfully. In Europe, cyproterone acetate has been used successfully, but it is not available in the United States. It has been reported that hair shaft density and the rate of hair growth decrease after 2 months of spironolactone therapy in doses in excess of 100 mg/day. Medroxyprogesterone acetate is also an antiandrogen.

17. **A,** Page 1156. Patients with rapidly progressive signs of androgen excess, including virilization, who have modestly elevated testosterone values but markedly elevated DHEA-S values should be suspected of having an androgen-producing adrenal tumor. These tumors secrete a large amount of C_{19} steroids, which are normally produced by the adrenal gland; C_{19} steroids include DHEA-S, DHEA, and androstenedione. The peripheral conversion of these relatively weak androgens to testosterone produces the androgen stigmata. Because of the potential severity of this problem, patients with these laboratory findings and a history of rapid onset signs of androgen excess should undergo CT of the adrenal glands to confirm the diagnosis. An ACTH stimulation test would be of little value since one is not concerned with measuring cortisol precursors secondary to an enzymatic block. Similarly, dexamethasone suppression tests are not indicated because this patient did not have the stigmata of Cushing disease. Since the markedly excessive androgen in this case is of adrenal origin and since the testosterone level is only mildly elevated, there should be little concern that there is a potential ovarian source, so laparoscopy is not indicated.

18. **D,** Page 1158. The diagnosis of congenital adrenal hyperplasia is established if serum levels of 17-hydroxyprogesterone are greater than 8 ng/mL. This test has replaced the less precise measurement of its metabolite, pregnanetriol. Since one is measuring metabolic product resulting from an enzymatic block, obtaining serum testosterone or DHEA-S will not reveal the source of the problem. Although urinary 17-ketosteroid levels may be elevated, this test is less specific, and awkward collection techniques make interpretation of test results difficult in the newborn.

19. **B,** Pages 1149–1155. PCOS should be thought of as a disorder of hyperandrogenism with chronic anovulation. Serum testosterone levels and serum androstenedione levels are usually mildly to moderately elevated. In addition, about half of the women with this syndrome have elevated DHEA-S. It is estimated that approximately 30% of women with PCOS do not have hirsutism, even though nearly all of them have elevated circulating androgen levels. The presence or absence of hirsutism depends on whether those androgens are converted peripherally by 5α-reductase to the more potent androgens dihydrotestosterone and 3α-diol-G. This 5α-reductase activity is reflected by increased levels of 3α-diol-G. In this patient,

with no hirsutism, it would be expected that her 3α-diol-G level would be normal. In the polycystic ovary syndrome, LH levels are tonically elevated, usually above 20 mIU/mL.

20. **A,** Page 1156; Table 40–6 in Stenchever. Congenital adrenal hyperplasia is the most common cause of sexual ambiguity in the newborn. This is usually caused by a severe 21-hydroxylase block with a resultant increase in ACTH secretion and increased adrenal production of cortisol precursors proximal to the enzymatic block. These precursors include both 17-hydroxypregnenolone and 17-hydroxyprogesterone. These steroids are then converted to DHEA and androstenedione, which in turn are peripherally converted to testosterone, resulting in masculinization of the female external genitalia. The associated fluid and electrolyte changes occurring in these infants can be severe and lead to death. Cushing syndrome results in excessive adrenal production of glucocorticoids caused by increased ACTH secretion and is generally not manifest in the newborn. Likewise, androgen insensitivity syndrome and Turner syndrome are generally disorders appreciated in girls at about the time of menarche or in midadolescence because of their amenorrhea. Adrenal carcinoma is extremely rare in any age group and especially in the newborn. This would be suspected with markedly elevated levels of DHEA-S as opposed to the elevated levels of cortisol precursors one would find in congenital adrenal hyperplasia.

21. **D,** Page 1145. This patient's hirsutism has been partially investigated by the mildly elevated testosterone of 1.0 ng/mL. This is indicative of ovarian androgenic hyperfunction and may be the only source of hyperandrogenism in this patient. However, the other major source for androgen production, the adrenal gland, has not been investigated. The best test to measure the other major androgen source is to obtain DHEA-S. This gives more complete information as to whether the patient has a combined source of androgen excess. This test is much better than urinary 17-ketosteroids because it gives a direct assessment of potential adrenal androgen excess. Androsterone and etiocholanolone are both 17-ketosteroids and represent metabolic breakdown patterns of androstenedione. This in turn is produced in part from the metabolism of testosterone, which is not a 17-ketosteroid. Therefore, in investigating patients with complaints of hirsutism, the two basic tests of androgen hyperfunction should represent the two major sources for female androgen production, the adrenal gland and the ovary.

22. **B,** Page 1156. Estimates by geneticists indicate that late-onset 21-hydroxylase deficiency varies in incidence among different ethnic groups but that overall it is probably the most frequent autosomal genetic disorder in humans (Table 40–1). Both

---

TABLE 40–1
Genotypic Characterization of Forms of 21-Hydroxylase Deficiency

Form of 21-Hydroxylase Deficiency	Clinical Phenotype	Hormonal Phenotype (in Response to ACTH)	Genotype
Classic (congenital adrenal hyperplasia)	Prenatal virilization, fully symptomatic	Marked elevation of precursors (serum 17-hydroxyprogesterone and Δ-androstenedione)	$\dfrac{21\text{-}OH\text{-}def^{severe}}{21\text{-}OH\text{-}def^{severe}}$
Nonclassic (late-onset 21-hydroxylase deficiency [LOHD])	Symptomatic: later development of virilization; milder symptoms / Asymptomatic: no virilization or other symptoms	Moderate elevation of precursors	$\dfrac{21\text{-}OH\text{-}def^{severe}}{21\text{-}OH\text{-}def^{mild}}$ $\dfrac{21\text{-}OH\text{-}def^{mild}}{21\text{-}OH\text{-}def^{mild}}$
Carrier	Asymptomatic	Precursor level greater than normal	$\dfrac{21\text{-}OH\text{-}def^{severe}}{21\text{-}OHase\ (normal)}$ $\dfrac{21\text{-}OH\text{-}def^{mild}}{21\text{-}OHase\ (normal)}$
Normal	Asymptomatic	Lowest levels—some overlap seen with carriers	$\dfrac{21\text{-}OHase\ (normal)}{21\text{-}OHase\ (normal)}$

From New MI, White PC, et al: The adrenal hyperplasias. In Scriver CR, Beaudet AL, Sly S, et al., eds: Metabolic Basis of Inherited Diseases, 6th ed. New York, McGraw-Hill, 1989.

classic congenital adrenal hyperplasia and late-onset 21-hydroxylase deficiency are transmitted in an autosomal recessive manner at the CYP21B locus. There are three possible manifestations of CYP21Y alleles (normal, mildly defective, or severely defective). Late-onset 21-hydroxylase deficiency is a phenotype that is symptomatic after adolescence. Affected persons may be homozygous for alleles yielding mildly abnormal enzymatic activity or compound heterozygotes with a combination of defective alleles.

Patients with compound heterozygotes may have one mildly defective and one severely defective allele, or they may be homozygous with two mildly defective alleles. If they were homozygous with two severely defective alleles, they would have had ambiguous genitalia at birth. The incidence of late-onset 21-hydroxylase deficiency is highest in the Ashkenazi Jewish population.

23. **A,** 1158. To differentiate late-onset 21-hydroxylase deficiency from polycystic ovary syndrome, basal (early morning) serum 17-hydroxyprogesterone levels should be measured. This test has replaced less precise measurement of the urinary metabolite pregnanetriol. If basal levels of 17-hydroxyprogesterone are greater than 8 ng/mL, the diagnosis of late-onset 21-hydroxylase deficiency is established. If 17-hydroxyprogesterone is above normal (2.5–3.3 ng/mL) but less than 8 ng/mL, an ACTH stimulation test should be performed. After infusion of 25 μg of synthetic ACTH as a single bolus, a serum sample for 17-hydroxyprogesterone is obtained in 1 hour and if the level increases more than 10 ng/mL, the diagnosis of the late-onset 21-hydroxylase deficiency is established. The 17-ketosteroid level was formerly used to measure metabolites of androgen production, but it has largely been replaced by serum androgens or plasma androgens. Measurement of androgens is of more value in identifying cases of hirsutism or virilism, which are not associated with 21-hydroxylase enzymatic block.

24. **D,** Page 1159. The three androgenic disorders most likely to be the source of this patient's problem are PCOS; late-onset 21-hydroxylase deficiency, and idiopathic hirsutism. They all may be associated with a similar history and physical findings. Menstrual irregularity is an uncommon finding in women with idiopathic hirsutism. These women will have normal testosterone and DHEA-S levels. Patients with late-onset 21-hydroxylase deficiency may have a history of prepubertal accelerated growth (ages 6 to 8 years) with later decreased growth and a short ultimate height. The age at which hair growth became noticeable is not helpful in differentiating the source of the androgen. The rapidity with which the hirsutism

appeared is pertinent. Tumors are associated with rapid onset.

25. **D,** Page 1162. After the source of androgen excess in patients who are hirsute has been identified, an explanation about the likelihood of the success of the proposed treatment is appropriate. Because of the length of the hair growth cycle, response to treatment should not be expected within the first 3 months. Objective methods of assessing changes of hair growth, such as photographs, are useful. With the use of varying antiandrogenic agents (oral contraceptives, dexamethasone, sprionolactone), successful response should occur in about 70% of patients within 1 year of treatment. The remaining excess hair can be removed by electrolysis. Treatment should be continued for 2 years and then stopped to determine if the hirsutism recurs and, if so, therapy can be reinstated.

26. **D,** Pages 1149–1155. (Figure 39–1 from Wilroy RS Jr, Given JR, Wiser WL, et al: Hyperthecosis: an inheritable form of polycystic/ovarian disease. In Bergsma D, ed: Genetic Forms of Hypogonadism. Miami, Symposia Specialists for the National Foundation–March of Dimes, 1975, BD: OAS XI[4]: 81.) This photomicrograph depicts a histologic picture typical of polycystic ovarian syndrome. There are characteristic multiple subcapsular cysts, and there are numerous premature atretic follicles. Biochemical associations with these findings include increased pulsatility of GnRH, which produces tonically elevated LH levels and increased ovarian androgen production. In addition, because of increased peripheral conversion of androstenedione to estrone in conjunction with decreased SHBG levels, there is tonic hyperestrogenism.

27. **D,** Pages 1145–1147. Most testosterone in the circulation (about 85%) is tightly bound to SHBG and is thought to be biologically inactive. Only about 10% to 5% is loosely bound to albumin. About 1% to 2% is *not* bound to any protein, representing free testosterone. The measured concentration of free testosterone as a sample is generally reported only on request. Serum testosterone can be measured in any of these forms. To exert a biologic effect, testosterone is metabolized peripherally in the target tissues to the more potent androgen, DHT. It has been shown that although serum levels of total testosterone are similar in normal and hirsute women, there are significant differences in the amount of non–SHBG-bound testosterone, which is elevated in about 60% to 70% of hirsute women.

28. **B,** Page 1151. Women with PCOS have increased levels of biological active (non-sex-hormone–binding globulin, or non-SHBG) estradiol, although total circulating levels of estradiol are not increased. The increased amount of non–SHBG-bound

estradiol is caused by a decrease in SHBG, which is produced primarily by increased levels of androgens and secondarily by the obesity present in many of these women. Even though the polycystic ovary does not secrete increased amounts of estrogen or estadiol, the increased levels of androstenedione are peripherally converted to estrone, causing increased circulating estrone levels. Appreciable amounts of estriol are present only in pregnancy as a function of the metabolism of the fetal placenta complex.

29. **D,** Page 1151. In addition to increased levels of circulating androgens, women with polycystic ovary syndrome have increased levels of biologically active (non–SHBG-bound) estradiol, although total circulating levels of estradiol are not increased (Figure 40–2). The increased amount of non–SHBG-bound estradiol is caused by a decrease in SHBG levels, which is produced primarily by the increased levels of androgens and

secondarily by the obesity present in many of these women. Serum estrone is also increased, but it is not as biologically active.

30. **D,** Page 1149. There is not a universally accepted definition of PCOS. Most authors agree that it should be described with the presence of ovulatory dysfunction, clinical evidence of hyperandrogenism and/or hyperandrogenemia, and exclusion of related disorders such as late-onset hydroxylase deficiency. Controversy exists as to whether the presence of the morphologic changes of polycystic ovaries need to be present in order to establish the diagnosis of PCOS.

31. **A,** Pages 1153, 1160. It has been shown that hyperinsulinemia produces hyperandrogenism in women with PCOS. Administration of the antihypoglycemic agent metformin decreases insulin levels yet increases insulin sensitivity, lowers serum androgen levels, and in many women induces ovulation.

Infertility

for Questions 1–32: Select the one best answer or completion.

1. During the evaluation of an infertile couple, the husband's initial semen analysis is received. The report information is listed below. The abnormal parameter is

   A. volume: 2.5 mL
   B. pH: 7.5
   C. sperm density: 15 million/mL
   D. sperm motility: 75% have good to excellent motility
   E. sperm morphologic features: 65% normal

2. Based on the previous semen analysis results, and assuming that the husband has a normal medical history, the most appropriate recommendation is

   A. repeat the semen analysis immediately
   B. repeat the semen analysis in 1 month
   C. begin clomiphene citrate therapy
   D. begin tetracycline therapy
   E. refer the patient to a urologist

3. The only direct evidence of ovulation is

   A. a serum progesterone level of 10 ng/mL
   B. a history of regular menstrual cycles
   C. an endometrial biopsy revealing a secretory endometrium
   D. a biphasic basal body temperature (BBT) chart
   E. pregnancy

4. A 25-year-old gravida 1, para 1, is undergoing laparoscopy for infertility of 2 years' duration. You notice four 1-mm superficial implants of endometriosis on the left ovary and a few filmy adhesions around both ovaries. If it is assumed that the rest of her workup is normal, the most appropriate treatment for this patient is to

   A. perform laparotomy immediately
   B. perform laparotomy in 6 months
   C. begin danazol postoperatively
   D. recommend in vitro fertilization (IVF)
   E. fulgurate and delay medical or other surgical intervention at least 12 months

5. The poorest prognosis for conception is associated with

   A. intrauterine adhesions
   B. leiomyoma
   C. a bicornuate uterus
   D. in utero DES exposure
   E. pelvic tuberculosis

6. A couple with primary infertility inquires about possible sexually transmitted diseases associated with artificial insemination with a donor's semen (AID). You should inform them that semen is frozen for 6 months to allow the detection of

   A. *Chlamydia trachomatis*
   B. human immunodeficiency virus (HIV)
   C. *Neisseria gonorrhoeae*
   D. syphilis
   E. serum hepatitis B

7. A 28-year-old nulligravida is scheduled to begin clomiphene citrate treatment for anovulation. She should be informed that, compared with the general population, conception following clomiphene treatment is associated with an increased incidence of

A. spontaneous abortion
B. ectopic pregnancy
C. multiple gestation
D. congenital malformation
E. intrauterine fetal death

8. A 23-year-old with a history of 2 years of infertility undergoes hysterosalpingography, which is reproduced in Figure 41–1. The most efficacious treatment for this problem would be

A. transcervical balloon tuboplasty
B. intrauterine insemination (IUI)
C. gamete intrafallopian transfer (GIFT)
D. tubal reanastomosis
E. IVF

9. As used in the past, IUI with washed semen would be most appropriate for couple with

A. cervical stenosis
B. oligospermia
C. inadequate mucus
D. small semen volume
E. bilateral cornual obstruction

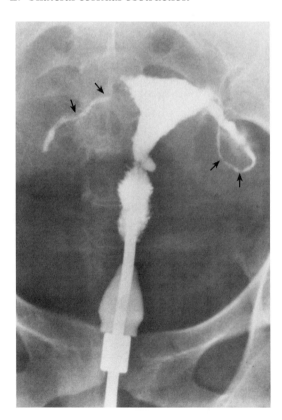

FIGURE 41–1

10. A 30-year-old gravida 1, para 1, is receiving clomiphene citrate, 50 mg/day, on days 5 through 9 of the cycle for the treatment of anovulation. A serum progesterone drawn on day 23 is 16 ng/mL. During the next cycle, the dose of clomiphene prescribed per day on days 5 through 9 should be

A. 50 mg
B. 100 mg
C. 150 mg
D. 200 mg
E. 250 mg

11–12. Match the infertility investigation with the best menstrual cycle day to perform it.

(A) 1
(B) 7
(C) 13
(D) 17
(E) 26

11. Hysterosalpingogram

12. Endometrial biopsy

13. Asthenospermia is defined as

A. abnormal sperm morphologic features
B. low sperm count
C. reduction of sperm motility
D. inability of sperm to fertilize egg

14. Clomiphene citrate is classified as a

A. natural estrogen
B. natural progesterone
C. synthetic testosterone
D. synthetic progestin
E. synthetic estrogen

15. The most ominous sequela of ovarian hyperstimulation syndrome (OHSS) is

A. abdominal distention
B. ascites
C. oliguria
D. pleural effusion
E. hypercoagulability

16. Which of the following treatments has improved the fecundability rates in couples with unexplained infertility?

A. controlled ovarian hyperstimulation
B. IUI
C. IVF
D. all the above

17–20. Match the etiologic factor with its reported frequency as a cause of infertility.

(A) 5%
(B) 15%
(C) 35%
(D) 50%
(E) 75%

17. Anovulation

18. Abnormal semen

19. Impairment of tubal motility

20. Abnormal sperm transport through the cervix

21. All test results from a couple undergoing infertility evaluation are normal. What instructions regarding coitus should they be given?

A. every other day over 6 days at midcycle
B. daily for 3 consecutive days at midcycle
C. weekly throughout the month
D. every other day during the middle 2 weeks of the month

22. Which of the following is the best method to predict ovulation?

A. BBT
B. serum progesterone
C. symptoms of mittelschmerz
D. urinary luteinizing hormone (LH)

23. What is the minimum number of hours of sleep recommended to provide accurate information for a BBT chart?

A. 4 hours
B. 6 hours
C. 8 hours
D. 10 hours

24. If follicle-stimulating hormone is drawn, when is the optimal time in the cycle?

A. days 1–3
B. days 8–10
C. days 13–15
D. days 24–26

25. Oil-soluble contrast media are preferable to water-soluble media in performing hysterosalpingography in what cases?

A. older patients
B. known tubal disease
C. unexplained infertility
D. history of endometriosis

26. Which of the following is considered a regular part of the infertility workup?

A. postcoital test
B. hysterosalpingography
C. diagnostic laparoscopy
D. hamster egg sperm penetration test

27. The most effective method of detecting ovarian hyperstimulation in a patient undergoing human menopausal gonadotrophin therapy is

A. midcycle daily ultrasonography
B. urinary LH measurement
C. monitoring of serum estradiol
D. late luteal serum progesterone measurement

28. A hysterosalpingogram is interpreted as normal. It would be correct to inform the patient that

A. there are no pelvic adhesions
B. there is no evidence of salpingitis isthmica nodosa
C. there is no endometriosis
D. she has normal fertility

29. A 25-year-old patient has undergone an infertility investigation, including serum progesterone, semen analysis, postcoital test, and hysterosalpingogram. All test results were normal. A diagnostic laparoscopy is now scheduled. Tests performed at the time of laparoscopy that would likely provide additional information about the etiologic complex of infertility include

A. hysteroscopy
B. a cervical culture
C. transcervical insufflation with indigo carmine
D. ovarian biopsy

30. Under what circumstances is treatment of hyperprolactinemia helpful in managing infertility?

A. The patient is 35 years old or older.
B. The male partner has a low sperm count.
C. The patient is anovulatory.
D. The prolactin is above 100 ng/mL.

31. Hysterosalpingography shows patency of one oviduct in a patient being evaluated for infertility. All other study results are normal. Based on this finding, the next most appropriate step in the management of this patient is

A. advise continued timed intercourse
B. schedule diagnostic laparoscopy
C. schedule reconstructive surgery
D. advise egg retrieval and IVF

32. **When two embryos are transferred into women who are younger than 35, the rate of twinning is approximately**

    A. 5%
    B. 10%
    C. 15%
    D. 20%

ANSWERS

1. **C,** Page 1175. Although there are no absolute standards for a normal semen sample, there are some recommended guidelines (Table 41–1).

2. **B,** Page 1175. Given a semen sample that shows normal parameters except for a low count, this specimen might merely reflect one extreme in the wide normal variability in a man's semen sample. Repeating the test in 1 month with an appropriate abstinence period of 2 to 3 days preceding collection would be the appropriate next step. Immediately repeating the test might be stressful or might provide an abnormally low value. It should be recalled that it takes 74 days for germ cells to become mature sperm. Therefore, the appropriate timing of a repeat semen analysis is important. Clomiphene citrate and tetracycline therapy would be inappropriate until a specific diagnosis is made. A physical examination by a qualified urologist or reproductive gynecologist is a part of the workup of a male with a semen abnormality, but at this point there is no evidence that it is needed.

3. **E,** Pages 1174–1175. The first diagnostic step in the evaluation of infertility is to obtain presumptive evidence that the woman is ovulating. A history of regular menses constitutes presumptive evidence of ovulation, and a midluteal serum progesterone

level greater than 10 ng/mL is also indirect evidence of adequate ovulation. Both endometrial biopsy and BBT charts reflect response to progesterone but are not direct evidence of ovulation. The only direct evidence of ovulation is pregnancy.

4. **E,** Pages 1198–1199; Figure 41–26. Based on the American Society of Reproductive Medicine classification of endometriosis, the patient has minimal endometriosis (stage I). No therapy, either medical or surgical, has been shown to be efficacious in patients with less than moderate endometriosis (stage III). Since no other cause of infertility has been identified, it is advisable to delay medical or surgical intervention for at least 12 months. In all likelihood, at the time of laparoscopy the laparoscopist would fulgurate the implants and lyse the adhesions.

5. **E,** Page 1191. Women with pelvic tuberculosis should be considered "sterile" because pregnancies after chemotherapy are rare. On the other hand, if intrauterine adhesions are the sole abnormality and not overly extensive, the prognosis for conception after lysis of adhesions is good. Congenital uterine defects such as a bicornuate uterus are a cause of infertility, but these patients are not sterile. Maternal ingestion of DES has not been clearly shown to be a cause of infertility. There are fairly uncommon circumstances in which leiomyoma can be associated with infertility. In selected cases, myomectomy has been reported to achieve pregnancy rates as high as 50%.

6. **B,** Page 1190. Donors for AID should be carefully screened to ascertain that they are in good health, do not have a potentially inheritable disorder, and will not transmit an infectious agent in the semen. Screening must be performed to rule out hepatitis B, syphilis, *Neisseria gonorrhoeae*, and *Chlamydia trachomatis*. Since cultures for HIV may not turn positive for several months after the infection is acquired, it is suggested that only frozen semen stored for at least 6 months be used. The donor is then tested for HIV after the 6-month storage period.

7. **C,** Page 1184. When conception occurs after ovulation has been induced with clomiphene, the

TABLE 41–1
Recommended Standards for Semen Analysis

Parameter	Recommended Normal Value
Volume	2.0 mL or more
pH	7.2–7.8
Sperm density	$\geq 20 \times 10^6$/mL
Total sperm count	$\geq 40 \times 10^6$/mL
Sperm motility	$\geq 50\%$ with progressive motility
Vital staining	$\geq 50\%$ live (exclude dye)
Sperm morphologic features	$\geq 50\%$ or more
White blood cell count	$<10^6$/mL

Modified from Aitken RJ, Comhaire FH, Eliasson R, et al: WHO Laboratory Manual for the Examination of Human Semen and Semen-Cervical Mucus Interaction. Cambridge, MA, Cambridge University Press, 1987.

incidence of multiple gestation increases to 5%. The rates of spontaneous abortion, ectopic gestation, intrauterine fetal death, and congenital malformation are not significantly increased over those of the general population.

8. **E,** Pages 1191–1198; Figure 40–1 from Mishell DR Jr, Davajan V: Infertility, Contraception and Reproductive Endocrinology, 2nd ed. Oradell, NJ, Medical Economics, 1986. The hysterosalpingogram shown demonstrates bilateral hydrosalpinges with dilation, clubbing, and obstruction at the fimbriated ends. Since the prognosis for a term pregnancy after repair of this disease is poor, the patient would best be advised to consider IVF. Transcervical balloon tuboplasty is reserved for proximal tubal disease. IUI would be inappropriate because, with extensive tubal disease, sperm would still not have access to the egg. GIFT is inappropriate because of the extensive tubal disease. Tubal reanastomosis is suitable only if previous surgical sterilization of the tubes has occurred. The anatomy should otherwise be normal.

9. **B,** Page 1189. Washed IUI is a technique in which sperm are inseminated into the uterus after they have been separated from the semen by centrifugation. The technique is used in several different circumstances: if the amount of mucus is small or the mucus is not thin and watery with good spinnbarkeit; if the patient has undergone conization with resultant scant mucus; if the male is oligospermic; if the semen volume is small (<2 mL) or large (>8 mL); or if the semen is of high viscosity. While useful in each of these circumstances, the largest benefit is likely to be obtained when the number of sperm is the lowest. Current therapy for oligospermia is more often IVF or intracytoplasmic injection of the sperm. Insemination of sperm into the uterus is of no benefit if there is no access to the egg. There is therefore no role for IUI in the treatment of bilateral cornual obstruction.

10. **A,** Pages 1183–1184. Serum levels of progesterone in patients in whom ovulation is induced by clomiphene citrate are consistently greater than 15 ng/mL. These levels are higher than the 10 ng/mL seen in spontaneous ovulatory cycles because clomiphene induces more than one follicle to mature and luteinize. Because this patient demonstrates a sufficient response on 50 mg/day, clomiphene should be continued at the same dose in the next cycle.

11–12. 11, **B;** 12, **E;** Pages 1173–1178. Certain infertility tests should be performed at specific times of the cycle to avoid potential complications and to maximize the information obtained. The hysterosalpingogram should be obtained during the week after menses to avoid either irradiating a possible pregnancy or inducing iatrogenic endometriosis. An endometrial biopsy late in the luteal phase will reflect the maximal effect from the sex steroids produced by the corpus luteum.

13. **C,** Page 1169. Asthenospermia is defined as loss or reduction of the motility of the spermatozoa.

14. **E,** Page 1183. Clomiphene citrate is a weak synthetic estrogenic compound with three benzene rings given orally to induce ovulation in anovulatory women with circulating estradiol levels greater than 40 pg/mL.

15. **E,** Page 1170. OHSS refers to ovarian enlargement to a diameter of more than 6 cm as a result of stimulation of multiple follicles. In the mild form, there is abdominal pain, distention, and weight gain. In the moderate form, ovarian enlargement is more than 10 cm with ascites, nausea, and vomiting. Severe OHSS is associated with hemoconcentration, oliguria, and elevated serum creatine. Pleural effusions and ascites can be present. OHSS becomes critical when hypercoagulability and hypotension occur. This condition may be fatal.

16. **D,** Page 1172. Several studies have reported the incidence of spontaneous conception among infertile couples without a specifically diagnosed cause of infertility (unexplained infertility). The cumulative pregnancy rates at the end of 2 to 7 years without any treatment ranged from 43% to 87%. For couples with unexplained infertility, controlled ovarian hyperstimulation, IUI, and IVF have all been shown to increase fecundability rates compared with no treatment.

17–20. 17, **B;** 18, **C;** 19, **C;** 20, **B;** Page 1173. The exact incidence of the various factors causing infertility varies among different populations and cannot be precisely determined. In general, however, 10% to 15% of infertility results from anovulation; 30% to 40% is caused by pelvic factors, such as adhesions from endometriosis or infection, or tubal occlusion that interferes with normal ovum transport; about 30% to 40% is associated with abnormalities in the male reproductive system, which are associated with oligozoospermia, high viscosity of semen, low sperm motility, or low volume of semen (male factor); and an additional 10% to 15% is associated with abnormal sperm-cervical mucous penetration (cervical factor).

21. **B,** Page 1174. Unless the husband has oligospermia, daily intercourse for 3 consecutive days at midcycle should be encouraged. Since the egg disintegrates within a few hours after it reaches the ampulla of the oviduct, it is best that sperm be present in this area when the egg arrives so that fertilization can occur. Sperm transport to the oviduct from the cervix normally occurs from 5 minutes to more than 1 day after coitus. Therefore, coitus should occur before ovulation.

22. **D,** Pages 1174–1175. Since the day of ovulation usually occurs 1 to 3 days after the BBT nadir, which cannot be determined prospectively, as well as 1 day after the day of the urinary LH peak, measurement of the urinary LH surge by rapid immunoassay can be used to predict more precisely the day of ovulation and the optimal time for coitus. Serum progesterone reflects ovulation and therefore cannot be used to predict ovulation. Mittelschmerz, or the pain associated with ovulation, is too variable and cannot be used prospectively.

23. **B,** Pages 1174–1175. Daily BBT measurement provides indirect evidence that ovulation has taken place. The BBT graph also provides information concerning the approximate day of ovulation and duration of the luteal phase. The BBT should be taken shortly after awakening only after at least 6 hours of sleep and before ambulating, with oral sublingual placement of a special thermometer with gradients between 96°F and 100°F.

24. **A,** Pages 1175–1176. The initial laboratory tests performed on the female partner should include a complete blood count, urine analysis, cervical cytologic testing, and a fasting blood glucose determination. If the woman is older than 35, a serum FSH level should be measured in one of the first 3 days of the cycle. An elevated FSH level (>20 mIU/mL) provides indirect evidence of impending ovulatory failure. In one study of IVF, all eggs aspirated from ovarian follicles of women with FSH levels higher than 24 mIU/mL in that cycle could not be fertilized when incubated with sperm.

25. **C,** Page 1176. It is best to schedule the hysterosalpingogram during the week following the end of menses to avoid irradiating a possible pregnancy. The examination should be performed with use of a water-soluble contrast medium and image-intensified fluoroscopy. A water-soluble contrast medium enables better visualization of the tubal mucosal folds and vaginal markings than does an oil-based medium. Prior studies had indicated that there was an increase in pregnancy rates in patients with unexplained infertility when an oil-soluble media was used. Recent studies call this into question, although oil-soluble contrast media are still used in some centers. Watson and colleagues performed a meta-analysis of clinical studies, including four randomized trials, and reported that a therapeutic benefit is more likely when oil-soluble contrast media are used during hysterosalpingography for the diagnostic evaluation of infertility; this is because the odds of pregnancy occurring after the procedure were twofold higher when oil-soluble media were used compared with water-soluble media. The greatest increase in pregnancy rates occurred in the group with unexplained infertility. Because oil-soluble contrast media have a greater number of complications, including pain resulting from peritoneal irritation and formation of granulomas, than water-soluble media, it may be best to obtain routine hysterosalpingograms with water-based media. Then, if the couple is found to have unexplained infertility, a trial of therapeutic flushing of the oviducts with oil-contrast media may be used as the initial treatment.

26. **B,** Pages 1177–1178. It was previously advised to perform a postcoital test and a laparoscopy as part of the initial infertility evaluation. The treatment of an abnormal postcoital test is controlled ovarian hyperstimulation and IUI. Since this is the same therapy for infertile couples with a normal postcoital test result and tubal patency, it does not appear to be cost-effective or necessary to continue to perform a postcoital test. Routine diagnostic laparoscopy was previously advised as part of the diagnostic evaluation of all women with infertility. Since this invasive procedure usually requires general anesthesia and is costly, it should be performed only if there is a likelihood of visualizing peritubal adhesions or endometriomas. Endometriomas usually can be visualized by pelvic sonography. If the sonographic appearance of the ovaries is normal and the hysterosalpingogram appears normal, it is unlikely that peritubal adhesions that restrict ovarian pickup are present in a woman who also has a negative *Chlamydia* antibody titer. The probability that peritubal adhesions of sufficient severity to cause infertility will be found at the time of laparoscopy is therefore much less than 5% in a woman with no history of salpingitis or symptoms of dysmenorrhea, a normal bimanual pelvic examination result, a normal CA-125 level, and absence of antibodies to *Chlamydia trachomatis*. Therefore, it is not cost-effective to perform a diagnostic laparoscopy as part of the initial infertility evaluation in women in whom these laboratory test results, pelvic sonographic results, hysterosalpingographic results, history, and physical examination results are all normal.

27. **D,** Page 1185. Although IVF was originally intended for women with severe tubal disease, it is now being used for women with severe endometriosis and couples with male factor or unexplained infertility. Nearly all centers use some type of ovarian hyperstimulation because the rate of pregnancy is related to the number of embryos placed in the uterine cavity. Because of the use of hyperstimulation, daily midcycle ultrasonography and estrogen measurements must be performed. The most sensitive of these tests for the

detection of ovarian hyperstimulation is the daily ultrasonography.

28. **B,** Page 1177. A normal hysterosalpingogram demonstrates bilateral tubal patency and thus excludes the presence of salpingitis isthmica nodosa (diverticula of the endosalpinx into the muscularis of the isthmic portion of the tube). Although tubal patency is documented, the presence of peritubal pelvic adhesions cannot be completely ruled out by hysterosalpingography alone. Laparoscopy is necessary to rule out pelvic adhesions or endometriosis. This patient's fertility status is still unknown at this time.

29. **C,** Page 1177. When diagnostic laparoscopy is performed for infertility, indigo carmine should be introduced through the cervix to confirm tubal patency. If the hysterosalpingogram appears normal, hysteroscopy is not indicated. A cervical culture should have been performed earlier in the workup if there had been any suspicion of cervical infection. Cervical culture is obviated when postcoital tests show no white blood cells and an ample number of motile sperm. Care should be taken to handle the ovaries and tube carefully at the time of laparoscopy to avoid trauma that might lead to adhesion formation. For this reason, random biopsy is not only unlikely to yield useful information, it might lead to adhesion formation, bleeding, or other complications that could further impede fertility.

30. **C,** Page 1135. If women with anovulation have hypothyroidism or hyperprolactinemia, treatment with thyroid replacement or bromocriptine, respectively, has been shown to cause resumption of ovulation and enhanced fecundity. However, Glazener and colleagues reported that in women with regular ovulatory cycles and hyperprolactinemia, pregnancy rates 1 year after clinical evaluation without treatment are similar to those of ovulatory women without hyperprolactinemia. Several investigators have performed randomized clinical trials with bromocriptine and placebo that have shown that treatment with bromocriptine does not increase fecundity rates in ovulatory infertile women. A prolactin level of 100 mg/mL or greater is generally associated with large pituitary tumors necessitating aggressive therapy, relegating fertility concerns to a secondary role. It is unlikely that these patients are ovulatory. It is the presence of ovulation, not the absolute serum level of prolactin, that is most predictive of the benefit of medical therapy.

31. **B,** Page 1177. Studies by Mol and associates have indicated that when one oviduct is patent, there is only a minimal reduction in fecundability. As a result, assisted reproductive technologies and tubal reconstruction are not indicated. Because hysterosalpingography cannot reliably assess the possibility of pelvic adhesions that might interfere with fertilization, diagnostic laparoscopy is the next most appropriate step in the treatment of this patient.

32. **D,** Page 1205. The rate of twin pregnancies for women under the age of 35 is roughly 20% when two embryos are transferred as part of IVF techniques.

Menopause

for Questions 1–24: Select the one best answer or completion.

1. A 45-year-old diabetic, hypertensive patient complains of severe hot flashes following a recent hysterectomy and bilateral salpingo-oophorectomy performed for large uterine leiomyomata. Without medication, the patient's blood pressure is 145/95. This woman has a history of thrombophlebitis at age 30 due to a femur fracture during a motor vehicle accident. Prior to her surgery, her blood lipids were measured. This woman's low-density lipoprotein (LDL) cholesterol was high, and her high-density lipoprotein (HDL) cholesterol low. You would

   A. prescribe estrogen
   B. prescribe a regimen of estrogen and progesterone
   C. not prescribe estrogen because of her blood lipid profile
   D. not prescribe estrogen because of her history of thrombophlebitis
   E. not prescribe estrogen because of her hypertension

2. The increase in facial hair noted in postmenopausal women is a direct consequence of

   A. increased levels of testosterone
   B. increased levels of androstenedione
   C. increased sensitivity of the hair follicles
   D. increased luteinizing hormone (LH)
   E. a decrease in the estrogen/androgen ratio

3. A 53-year-old white woman with type 2 diabetes has been undergoing hormonal replacement for her hot flashes. These are unbearable unless she takes at least 1.25 mg per day of conjugated equine estrogen. Previously, the patient had not been taking a progestin. She would prefer not to have withdrawal bleeding. Of the following regimens listed, the one that will most likely meet her request and still provide protection to the endometrium is

Estrogen & amount	Number of estrogen days/month	Progestin & amount	Number of progestin days/month
A. Conjugated equine estrogen 0.625 mg	First 25	Medroxyprogesterone 2.5 mg	First 10
B. Estrone sulfate 0.625 mg	First 25	Medroxyprogesterone 5 mg	Last 10
C. Estrone sulfate 1.25 mg	First 21	Medroxyprogesterone 10 mg	Last 14
D. Micronized estradiol 2 mg	Continuous	Medroxyprogesterone 5 mg	First 12
E. Esterified estrogen 1.25 mg	Continuous	Methyltestosterone 2.5 mg	Continuous

4. A 67-year-old gravida 5, para 5, has urgency, urge incontinence, and stress incontinence. The stress incontinence is confirmed by urodynamic testing. Urinalysis results are normal, and the urine culture is negative. The patient has a pale atrophic vagina. She takes no medication or vitamin supplementation and otherwise feels well. At this point you should

   A. perform retropubic suspension
   B. perform vaginal hysterectomy and anterior colporrhaphy
   C. start a β-adrenergic agent
   D. start an anticholinergic agent
   E. start vaginal estrogen

5. The mean age of menopause for nonsmoking women in the United States is

   A. 45
   B. 47
   C. 49
   D. 51
   E. 53

6. In a patient whose major complaint is hot flashes that greatly interfere with her daily life, you would expect to find all the following except

   A. less than ideal body weight
   B. decreased estrone
   C. decreased estradiol
   D. increased sex hormone–binding globulin (SHBG)–bound estradiol
   E. increased follicle-stimulating hormone (FSH)

7. In those women at risk for osteoporosis who are not properly treated, the percentage of lost bone mass each year after menopause is

   A. 0.25%–0.5%
   B. 1%–2%
   C. 3%–4%
   D. 5%–6%
   E. 8%–10%

8. Estrogen replacement therapy causes

   A. adenocarcinoma of the endometrium
   B. hypertension
   C. thrombosis
   D. a thickened vaginal epithelium
   E. ductal carcinoma of the breast

9. Multiple prospective and retrospective studies have considered the likelihood of endometrial cancer in women who have been undergoing estrogen replacement. The main conclusion reached is that postmenopausal estrogen is associated with a(n)

   A. endometrial adenocarcinoma that is relatively undifferentiated
   B. relative risk of more than 5.0 of developing adenocarcinoma of the endometrium
   C. risk of adenocarcinoma of the endometrium that has no correlation with the length of therapy
   D. risk of adenocarcinoma of the endometrium that has no correlation with the dose of estrogen prescribed
   E. higher risk in those women who have taken oral contraceptives before menopause

10. A 42-year-old woman complains of hot flashes. Her periods are fairly regular, every 26 to 30 days. Flow lasts 3 to 7 days. In the past, her periods were exactly 28 to 29 days and flow lasted 3 to 4 days. A serum FSH level was elevated, and the serum progesterone was 10 ng/mL. Your advice would be that this patient should

    A. stop worrying about contraception
    B. use progestin supplementation
    C. consider herself menopausal
    D. undergo LH determination
    E. begin estrogen supplementation

11. Of the several women listed below, which one is unlikely to experience hot flashes?

    A. a 50-year-old 45,X who had been taking 1 mg of micronized estradiol daily until 3 months ago
    B. a 55-year-old Caucasian woman, 5 feet 2 inches tall, 100 pounds
    C. a 50-year-old Asian woman, 5 feet tall, 85 pounds
    D. a 38-year-old Caucasian woman, 5 feet 4 inches tall, 180 pounds, who has just undergone total abdominal hysterectomy and bilateral salpingo-oophorectomy
    E. an 18-year-old woman with pure gonadal dysgenesis who has just undergone total abdominal hysterectomy and bilateral salpingo-oophorectomy

12. Postmenopausal serum levels of

    A. calcium are decreased
    B. phosphorus are decreased
    C. calcitonin are decreased
    D. parathyroid hormone are increased
    E. 1,25-dihydroxyvitamin D are increased

13. The histologic appearance of the ovaries of a 49-year-old woman who had her last normal menstrual period 1 year ago would reveal

    A. lack of ovarian follicles
    B. proliferation of the theca
    C. proliferation of the granulosa
    D. degeneration of the stroma
    E. absence of surface epithelial cysts

14. A typical 55-year-old woman who has hot flashes describes them to you. She is likely to tell you that hot flashes

    A. have interfered with her activities for 6 to 7 years
    B. are occasionally followed by profuse perspiration
    C. come on gradually over a 15-minute period
    D. rarely occur more than once in 24 hours
    E. last 10 to 15 minutes

15. The diagnosis of osteoporosis in trabecular bone can be accurately established by all the following except

    A. computed tomography (CT)
    B. single-photon absorptiometry
    C. dual-photon absorptiometry
    D. x-ray examination
    E. dual-energy x-ray absorptiometry (DEXA)

16. The major mechanism responsible for the reduction in cardiovascular disease noted in women receiving estrogen replacement is

    A. decreased LDL cholesterol
    B. increased HDL cholesterol
    C. increased serum triglycerides
    D. decreased total cholesterol
    E. direct action on the arterial wall

17. The addition of 10 to 12 days of a synthetic progestin to a cyclic postmenopausal estrogen regimen

    A. renders it less effective in the prevention of hot flashes
    B. negates the beneficial effect that estrogen has on bone density
    C. enhances the beneficial effect that estrogen has on serum lipids
    D. may cause mild depression and irritability
    E. prevents vaginal atrophy

18. A factor that appears to affect the age of a woman's menopause is

    A. weight
    B. use of oral contraceptives
    C. number of term pregnancies
    D. smoking
    E. age at menarche

19. FSH is elevated in the postmenopausal woman because of decreased levels of

    A. estradiol
    B. estrone
    C. inhibin
    D. LH
    E. prolactin

20. A hot flash is followed by

    A. increases in digital perfusion
    B. increases in peripheral skin temperature
    C. decreases in LH
    D. decreases in heart rate
    E. decreases in cortisol

21. A number of complaints, such as anxiety and worry about oneself, have been attributed to menopause. Recent studies suggest that postmenopausal patients who receive exogenous estrogen improve because the estrogen

    A. increases prolactin
    B. decreases testosterone
    C. increases plasma β-endorphin
    D. increases estrogen receptors
    E. decreases LH

22. A 60-year-old gravida 4, para 4, woman whose last period was 10 years prior and who is postmenopausal presents for her annual examination. Her medical history and physical examination are unremarkable. Because of her intolerance of progesterone agents, she has been on only conjugated estrogen, 0.625 mg/day, for the past 8 years. She denies any vaginal bleeding. In addition to routine examination and Pap smear, one of the following should be done *except*

    A. endometrial sampling
    B. nothing
    C. progesterone challenge test
    D. sonohystogram
    E. transvaginal ultrasonography for endometrial stripe

23. A 50-year-old woman, gravida 2, para 2, whose last period was 3 months ago, complains of increasingly severe hot flashes that are markedly compromising daily activity. Her medical and surgical history findings are negative except for a diagnosis of a deep venous thrombophlebitis during her second pregnancy at age 32. This occurred after some trauma and was treated with anticoagulation for the remainder of the pregnancy and for a few months postpartum. She is now interested in estrogen replacement therapy. Management should be

A. estrogen replacement only
B. estrogen and progesterone replacement
C. no hormonal treatment of the flashes
D. oral contraceptives, low dose
E. referral for herbal alternatives

24. A 49-year-old gravida 0, para 0, presents for evaluation for hormone replacement therapy. Although the patient is currently healthy, she has a strong family history for multiple medical problems. She is knowledgeable about the issues of hormone replacement therapy and breast cancer, osteoporosis prevention, and lipid status. She wants to know more about other possible side effects of hormone replacement therapy. She should be told that there is an association with hormone replacement therapy use and an increase in

A. colon cancer
B. gallbladder disease
C. hypertension
D. non–insulin-dependent (type 2) diabetes
E. weight gain

DIRECTIONS:

for Questions 25–29: For each numbered item, select the one heading most closely associated with it. Each lettered heading may be used once, more than once, or not at all.

25–27. For the following, select the percent affected without hormonal replacement.

(A) 5%
(B) 10%
(C) 15%
(D) 20%
(E) 25%

25. Caucasian or Asian women who experience spinal compression fractures by age 60

26. 80-year-old women with a hip fracture who die from the hip fracture or its complications within 6 months

27. 80-year-old white women who will experience hip fractures

28–29. For the following, select the daily dose.

(A) 0.3 mg
(B) 0.625 mg
(C) 2.5 mg
(D) 700 mg
(E) 1500 mg

28. The minimum amount of conjugated equine estrogen that will prevent osteoporosis in patients who ingest at least 1500 mg of calcium in their diet or through calcium supplementation

29. The minimum recommended amount of daily supplemental vitamin D necessary to retard osteoporosis

DIRECTIONS:

for Questions 30–40: Select the one best answer or completion.

30. Factors known to increase the risk of osteoporosis include all the following except

A. a diet high in alcohol
B. early spontaneous menopause
C. cigarette smoking
D. obesity
E. sedentary lifestyle

31. In the postmenopausal woman, androstenedione

A. is secreted primarily by the ovary
B. is secreted primarily by the adrenal
C. is converted to β-estradiol in peripheral body fat
D. acts as an estrogen

32. **Compared with the bone loss that occurs with aging, which of the following patterns characterizes the bone loss associated with estrogen withdrawal?**

	Cortical bone	Trabecular bone
A.	Unchanged	Unchanged
B.	Slightly increased	Markedly increased
C.	Markedly increased	Slightly increased
D.	Markedly increased	Markedly increased
E.	Markedly decreased	Markedly decreased

33. **Of the following, which has the highest level of dietary calcium?**

    A. chocolate milk, 1 cup
    B. cottage cheese, low-fat, 1 cup
    C. ice cream, vanilla, 1 cup
    D. frozen yogurt, vanilla, 1 cup
    E. nonfat yogurt, plain, 8 ounces

34. **A 51-year-old woman, gravida 1, para 1, presents with perimenopausal complaints including hot flashes. She has multiple risk factors for osteoporosis but is very hesitant to take estrogen replacement because of fears of breast cancer. Her only family history of breast cancer is a maternal grandmother, in whom the diagnosis was made when she was 73 years old. Which of the following statements regarding breast cancer is most correct?**

    A. Addition of progesterone to estrogen replacement therapy clearly protects from breast cancer.
    B. Baseline risk of breast cancer is decreased in obese women.
    C. Her positive family history clearly adds additional risk.
    D. Risk of mortality from breast cancer found in current estrogen uses is increased.
    E. The small reported increased risk of breast cancer may be a detection bias.

35. **A 49-year-old patient who is 5 feet 9 inches tall and weighs 155 pounds (70 kg) is concerned about the possibility of weight gain if she begins estrogen therapy. You should advise her that estrogen replacement therapy is associated with**

    A. a decrease in body weight and body fat
    B. a decrease in body weight and an increase in body fat
    C. no change in body weight or body fat
    D. an increase in body weight and body fat
    E. an increase in body weight and a decrease in body fat

36. **A 52-year-old woman with a history of migraine headaches seeks your opinion regarding the impact of menopause. You should advise her that studies indicate that menopause is associated with**

    A. a significant increase in migraine headaches
    B. a mild increase in migraine headaches
    C. no change in the frequency of migraine headaches
    D. a mild decrease in migraine headaches
    E. a significant decrease in migraine headaches

37. **Oral estrogen-testosterone therapy is associated with**

    A. increased HDL cholesterol levels
    B. increased libido
    C. increased frequency of acne
    D. decreased LDL cholesterol levels
    E. decreased hair growth

38. **Menopause that occurs before the age of 45 is most closely associated with which of the following factors?**

    A. smoking
    B. low body weight
    C. early menarche
    D. chromosomal abnormality
    E. prolonged lactation

39. **A 53-year-old woman presents for consultation regarding continuing estrogen replacement therapy. Her history is remarkable for a total abdominal hysterectomy for dysfunctional uterine bleeding at age 42. When she was 49, she had a "mild heart attack" and was found to have elevated lipids. She was placed on statins, low-dose aspirin, exercise, and estrogen replacement therapy since she was also perimenopausal. She has done well on the regimen. She now hears in the news that estrogen replacement therapy in patients with known cardiac disease increases their risk of death. This patient should be**

    A. advised to switch to herbal estrogen preparations that have not been shown to have this effect
    B. instructed to immediately discontinue the use of estrogen replacement therapy
    C. reassured and encouraged to continue on her current dose
    D. told that the news reports are wrong and to ignore them

40. A 55-year-old woman, gravida 1, para 1, whose last period was 5 years ago is currently not on hormone replacement therapy because of the diagnosis of stage II breast cancer 3 years ago. The patient is doing well with only rare hot flashes. However, at a recent health fair, she has a screening DEXA scan and has brought the report for interpretation and management as indicated. Her T-score is –2.90 and her Z-score is –2.0. Given this report, management should consist of

A. bisphosphonate therapy
B. estrogen replacement therapy
C. increased exercise, calcium, and vitamin D
D. reassurance that this is a normal report for her age

ANSWERS

1. **A,** Pages 1240–1242, 1246–1250. This patient's hot flashes are an indication for estrogen replacement. There is no contraindication to its application in the history. Although the use of high-dose oral contraceptive agents has been associated with hypertension, postmenopausal estrogen therapy has not. This is due in part to the potency and formulation of the estrogens involved. Studies demonstrate that postmenopausal estrogen users have improved lipid profiles. There is evidence that the use of progestin lowers the chances of endometrial cancer in postmenopausal estrogen users; however, this is not a concern for this patient because of her hysterectomy. Depending on the formulation, progesterone may have an adverse effect on serum lipids. In vitro studies demonstrate increased mitotic activity in breast tissue with progestin exposure. This suggests a potential deleterious effect on the human breast. Until additional studies are available, it appears prudent not to add a progestin to the postmenopausal hormonal therapy of a patient who has undergone hysterectomy.

2. **E,** Pages 1220–1221. The postmenopausal levels of testosterone and androstenedione are not elevated, and in fact generally decline, though not to the degree that occurs for estrogen. Although LH is increased in the postmenopausal woman, it is not directly associated with hirsutism. The physiologic process of a decrease in the estrogen/androgen ratio is the cause of the increased facial hair growth that frequently occurs after menopause.

3. **D,** Pages 1246–1248. The patient has demonstrated that she currently requires 1.25 mg/day of conjugated equine estrogen to adequately control her hot flashes. Later, the amount can be reduced to 0.625 mg/day. The dosage of 0.625 mg/day is the amount necessary to retard development of osteoporosis. In the control of hot flashes, 2 mg/day of micronized estradiol is equivalent to 1.25 mg/day of conjugated equine estrogen or 1.25 mg/day of estrone sulfate. It has been demonstrated that for postmenopausal women receiving 0.625 mg of conjugated equine estrogen, 2.5 mg of medroxyprogesterone reduced nuclear and cytosol estrogen receptor levels to those found before estrogen administration. With a daily dose of 1.25 mg of conjugated equine estrogen, 5 mg of medroxyprogesterone was necessary to decrease the receptor synthesis to the same degree. Estrogen may be given every day of the month continually, and the progestin may be given daily for the first 10 to 13 days of the month with the combined regimen. The continuous estrogen regimen frequently results in breakthrough bleeding during the first 6 months, but with longer use nearly all women remain amenorrheic. Given this patient's request, continuous estrogen therapy would appear to be the appropriate approach at this time. Another approach, suggested by Weinstein and colleagues, would be to administer both continuous estrogen and progestin. The combination of 1.25 mg esterified estrogen and 2.5 mg of methyltestosterone is distributed under the trade name Estratest. The addition of testosterone has been advocated to increase libido. There is concern that the use of testosterone will have a deleterious effect on lipid metabolism and possibly cause hirsutism.

4. **E,** Pages 1223–1224. The trigone of the bladder and the urethra are embryologically derived from

estrogen-dependent tissue, and estrogen deficiency can lead to their atrophy, producing symptoms of urinary urge incontinence, dysuria, and urinary frequency. With a decrease of elastic tissue around the vagina caused by estrogen deficiency, a urethrocele may develop. Although operative correction ultimately may be needed, local estrogen should be tried first since it may relieve the symptoms. Estrogen should be given before operation to thicken the vaginal mucosa. This patient might also benefit from Kegel exercises. Because vaginal administration of estrogen results in irregular systemic absorption, for long-term prevention of vaginal atrophy and for osteoporosis and atherosclerosis, the patient is best treated with oral or transdermal estrogen after 2 to 3 weeks of vaginal estrogen. It should be noted that it may take up to 6 months of therapy for atrophic changes to completely resolve.

5. **D,** Page 1217. The mean age of menopause is 51.4 years. The 95% confidence limits are between ages 45 and 55 years. Menopause is defined as the cessation of menstruation for at least 6 months because of depletion of ovarian follicles.

6. **D,** Pages 1224–1227. Postmenopausal women with hot flashes have lower circulating estrone and estradiol levels, less total body weight, and a lower percentage of ideal body weight compared with persons without hot flashes. Postmenopausal women with hot flashes also have less SHBG-bound estradiol.

7. **B,** Page 1228. In short, frail, thin-skinned, sedentary women who do not receive hormonal therapy, about 1% to 2% of bone mass is lost each year after menopause.

8. **D,** Pages 1240–1244. An association between the use of estrogen and adenocarcinoma of the endometrium, hypertension, and thrombosis has been established. The association with breast cancer is controversial. An association is not the same as cause and effect. Furthermore, the development of these complications is highly dependent on the dosage, mode of administration, length of treatment, and type of estrogen. For example, 2.5 mg of conjugated equine estrogen causes less of an increase in the liver's production of binding globulin than does 30 mg of ethinyl estradiol, the estrogen used in many contraceptive pills. One such globulin is angiotensinogen, which when converted to angiotensin is associated with an increase in blood pressure. Patient predisposition is also likely to be a factor in these complications. The potency of an estrogen depends on the effect used to measure potency (ie, factors such as vaginal thickness and lipid concentration). Estrogen does thicken the vaginal epithelium.

9. **B,** Pages 1244–1246. Since 1975, many studies have addressed the question of the relative risk of estrogen users for endometrial adenocarcinoma. These have been both prospective and retrospective investigations. Several reviews have critiqued these studies. Given this information, it would appear that the relative risk for patients who have taken an estrogen without a progestin is 3 to 7. The endometrial cancer that develops in estrogen users is nearly always well-differentiated and is usually cured by simple hysterectomy. The risk increases with increasing duration of the use of estrogen and with increased dosage. It has been reported that prior oral contraceptive use of 1 year or longer negated some of the increased risk of endometrial cancer in postmenopausal women who were receiving only estrogen.

10. **E,** Pages 1219–1221. About 5 years before actual menopause, FSH is elevated because of lack of negative feedback. This effect occurs because although a serum estradiol may be in the normal range, the total estrogens from cycle to cycle are decreased. The low estrogen is responsible for this patient's hot flashes. Since her progesterone level is normal, this patient is still ovulating. Although the situation is unlikely, she can still become pregnant. Obtaining a serum LH would not be cost-effective. Given the FSH, the LH level is predictable. This woman would benefit from low-dose estrogen supplementation, 0.3 mg of conjugated equine estrogen, 0.3 mg of estrone sulfate, or 0.5 mg of micronized estradiol from the fifth day after menstruation begins until the onset of the next menses. Also, oral contraceptive pills are an option if the patient is a nonsmoker with no contraindications to oral contraceptive use and needs contraception.

11. **E,** Pages 1224–1227. A woman who has had low estrogen levels throughout her life, such as an 18-year-old with pure gonadal dysgenesis, will not experience hot flashes. This is true even if her gonads are removed. If a woman without any ovaries, such as the 50-year-old 45,X, were to receive estrogen, she would probably experience hot flashes when the estrogen is stopped. The change in estrogen levels leads to alterations in the hypothalamus that are probably mediated through the central nervous system. Hot flashes do not persist in most women for more than 2 to 3 years, and it is uncommon for hot flashes to last more than 5 years after menopause. Ninety-five percent of women are menopausal by the age of 55 years. When the change in estrogen levels is not gradual but sudden, such as occurs after castration, the person is more likely to experience symptomatic hot flashes. Postmenopausal women with hot flashes have lower circulating estrone and

estradiol levels, less total body weight, and a lower percentage of ideal body weight compared with those without hot flashes.

12. **C,** Pages 1229–1231. Although the mechanism whereby estrogen prevents a decrease in bone density is not precisely known, it has been determined that postmenopausal serum levels of calcium and phosphorus are slightly increased. Serum levels of parathyroid hormone and the active form of vitamin D (1,25-dihydroxyvitamin D) are decreased, as is calcium absorption. In addition, calcitonin levels are lowered. Serum calcium levels are maintained within a fairly narrow range, and they are regulated in part by parathyroid hormone production. Parathyroid hormone increases serum calcium levels by three mechanisms: bone resorption, tubal resorption of calcium in the kidney, and production of an enzyme (1-α-hydroxylase) that changes vitamin D from its inactive form to its active form and thereby increases calcium absorption from the gut. It has been postulated that estrogen, androgens, and progestins block the action of parathyroid hormone on bone resorption, reducing the amount of calcium reabsorbed from the bone. Estrogen increases calcitonin levels, and calcitonin prevents bone resorption. Human osteoblast cells have estrogen receptors, and it may be through a receptor phenomenon that estrogen therapy decreases bone loss. Bone formation in women with osteoporosis is normal.

13. **A,** Page 1219. The basic feature of menopause is depletion of ovarian follicles with degeneration of the granulosa and theca cells. As theca cells degenerate, they fail to react to endogenous gonadotrophins. As a result, less estrogen is produced, and there is a decrease in the negative feedback on the hypothalamic-pituitary axis. In contrast with the follicular cells, the stroma cells of the ovary continue to function and are the major source of androgens. Other structural features of the "aged" ovary are obliterative arteriolar sclerosis and surface epithelial cysts.

14. **B,** Pages 1224–1227. Hot flashes do not persist in most women for more than 2 to 3 years, and it is uncommon for a woman to have hot flashes that last more than 5 years after menopause. About half of women with flashes experience at least one a day, and about 20% experience more than one a day. These flashes frequently occur at night; they awaken the person and then produce insomnia. A hot flash is a sudden explosive systemic physiologic phenomenon that takes place over a period of 30 seconds to 5 minutes. The flash is preceded by an increase in digital perfusion, which is followed by increases in peripheral skin temperature, which sometimes includes profuse perspiration.

15. **B,** Page 1229. At least 25% of the bone needs to be lost before osteoporosis can be diagnosed by routine x-ray examination. Dual-photon absorptiometry and CT effectively measure bone density in trabecular bone. DEXA is the most reliable method of measuring bone density. It is precise and can be completed in a short time. Because an anteroposterior projection is used, dual-photon absorptiometry measures not only the mainly trabecular bone of the vertebral body but also the cortical bone of the posterior processes, which does not contribute to the development of osteoporotic fractures. DEXA is based on a lateral projection technique. The technique of single-photon absorptiometry can be used only to measure the density of structures composed primarily of cortical bone—that is, bones in the axial skeleton such as the radius, femur, or os calcis. Since postmenopausal osteoporosis affects trabecular bone more rapidly than it does cortical bone, use of single-photon absorptiometry on bones in the limbs can fail to detect the presence of loss of trabecular bone in the thoracic spine because the density of the bone being measured may remain within the normal range.

16. **E,** Pages 1238–1240. Although numerous studies have shown that the administration of oral conjugated equine estrogens and of other oral estrogens raises triglyceride and serum HDL cholesterol levels and lowers LDL cholesterol levels, with minimal changes in total cholesterol levels, recent data support a direct effect on the arterial wall as the major mechanism of action of estrogen therapy. Oral estrogen administered for 9 weeks resulted in an improvement in flow-mediated, endothelium-dependent dilatation, probably by increasing the synthesis and release of nitric oxide. Other studies have reported that estrogen replacement therapy increases vascular antioxidant activity, preventing plaque formation, as well as reverses the constricting effect of acetylcholine on the coronary arteries.

17. **D,** Pages 1246–1248. The addition of a progestin to estrogen therapy does not appear to cause an increase of any other systemic disease and acts synergistically with estrogen to cause a slight increase in bone density. The use of synthetic progestins may slightly reverse the beneficial effect of estrogen on serum lipids. This effect on lipids is most pronounced with 19-norprogestins. Progestin is active alone in the treatment of hot flashes. Estrogen and progestin together do not cancel each other; they constitute effective treatment for hot flashes. A progestin may have an adverse effect on the vaginal and urethral mucosa, may produce undesired central nervous system symptoms, and may adversely affect mood and the sense of

well-being. Some patients taking norethindrone have reported depression, anxiety, and irritability.

18. **D,** Pages 1218–1219. The age at which menopause occurs is genetically predetermined. It is related to the number of primordial follicles the woman has at the time of birth. A woman is constantly attempting to mature follicles even prior to puberty. Therefore, the age of menopause is not related to the number of prior ovulations; it is not affected by pregnancy, lactation, use of oral contraceptives, or failure to ovulate spontaneously. It is also not related to race, socioeconomic conditions, education, height, weight, age at menarche, or age at the last pregnancy. The age of menopause may be affected by smoking because it has been reported that cigarette smokers experience an earlier spontaneous menopause than do non-smokers.

19. **C,** Page 1219. After menopause, circulating estradiol levels are generally less than 15 pg, whereas FSH levels are greater than 40 mIU/mL and LH levels are also increased. Administration of large amounts of oral or parenteral estrogen will not cause FSH levels to return to premenopausal concentrations because release of FSH is controlled mainly by circulating inhibin levels. Since inhibin levels decline with absent ovarian follicular activity, FSH remains elevated even when estrogen replacement is given.

20. **B,** Pages 1224–1227. A hot flash is preceded by an increase in digital perfusion, which is followed by increases in peripheral skin temperature, circulating norepinephrine and LH levels, and heart rate. With each flash, there are increases in LH, adrenocorticotropic hormone, and cortisol but not in FSH or estradiol. The LH increase is an effect of the change in the hypothalamic-pituitary axis, not a cause of the hot flash, because patients without a pituitary gland also have hot flashes. Infusing a patient with LH will not cause a hot flash.

21. **C,** Pages 1227–1228. The following symptoms improve in women who receive postmenopausal estrogen: vaginal dryness, poor memory, anxiety, and worry about oneself. In addition, an increase in optimism and good spirits has been noted in psychological testing. Thus, estrogen improves psychological symptoms in addition to relieving the hot flash and allowing the patient to sleep better. Postmenopausal women have lower levels of plasma β-endorphin (β-EP) and β-lipotrophin (β-LPH) than do women of reproductive age. Administration of estrogen to postmenopausal women increases plasma β-EP and β-LPH to normal levels. The modulation of these peptide levels by estrogen may be one mechanism whereby estrogen replacement therapy improves mood and sense of well-being because lowered endorphin

levels have been associated with symptoms of depression.

22. **B,** Pages 1249, 1244–1246. Because unopposed estrogen increases a woman's risk of endometrial cancer by more than seven times, an assessment of the development of endometrial hyperplasia is warranted. This can be done in a number of ways. Ultrasound imaging of the endometrial stripe, with or without saline contrast, helps to determine potential risks. Also, an endometrial sampling via any number of sampling curettes can be done. An inexpensive method is a progesterone challenge test. If a patient has endometrial hyperplasia, she will experience a withdrawal bleed unless she has cervical stenosis. The lack of a bleed is reassuring that the endometrial lining is atrophic.

23. **B,** Pages 1241–1242. Estrogen or estrogen-progesterone use is associated with decreased levels of circulating fibrinogen and factor VII, as well as plasminogenic activator inhibitor, compared with levels obtained in postmenopausal women not taking estrogen. Other studies suggest that estrogen replacement therapy reduces platelet aggregation. These hematologic findings suggest that the postmenopausal use of estrogen should not increase the risk of deep venous thrombophlebitis. However, the results of several more recent case-control studies consistently found that postmenopausal estrogen users were two to four times more likely to experience an episode of deep venous thrombophlebitis predominantly in the first use. If the patient has an inherited thrombotic abnormality, this risk is likely greater. Since this patient had a trauma-related deep venous thrombophlebitis, it is unlikely that she has a coagulopathy, and thus estrogen replacement therapy or hormone replacement therapy is reasonable. Since she has a uterus, progesterone should be added. Oral contraceptives may place a patient at a slightly higher risk than hormone replacement therapy for deep venous thrombophlebitis. Since this patient is menopausal, she should not be given oral contraceptives as first-line therapy.

24. **B,** Pages 1241–1242. Although estrogen is often blamed for many problems, it also provides many advantages, particularly in the lower doses used in the peri- and postmenopausal phases. The occurrences of hypertension and non–insulin-dependent diabetes are lower in women on hormone replacement therapy. The rate of weight gain is lower in women on hormone replacement therapy than in women not on any replacement. Also, women not on replacement therapy seem to have a greater shift of the adipose to a more central distribution, which increases the risk of cardiovascular problems. There is a 33% decrease

in the rate of colon cancer in users of hormone replacement therapy. There is not a similar decrease in rectal cancer occurrence. There is a statistically increased risk of gallbladder disease in postmenopausal estrogen users, with a twofold higher rate of cholecystectomy.

25–27. 25, **E**; 26, **C**; 27, **D**; Page 1228. By age 60, 25% of Caucasian and Asian women experience spinal compression fractures. Loss of bone mass in cortical bone occurs at a much slower rate than in trabecular bone. Thus, osteoporotic fractures of the femur usually do not begin until about age 70 or 75. By age 80, 20% of all Caucasian women have experienced hip fractures; of these, about 15% die from the fracture itself or from complications within 6 months.

28–29. 28, **A**; 29, **D**; Pages 1230–1235. The minimum dose of estrogen needed to prevent osteoporosis in women with adequate calcium and vitamin D is probably 0.3 mg of conjugated equine estrogen or the equivalent. In addition to estrogen replacement, calcium supplementation and weight-bearing exercises are of ancillary benefit in preventing postmenopausal osteoporosis. The addition of vitamin D has not been shown to be useful in the prevention of osteoporosis. Vitamin D should be supplemented only in patients with insufficient vitamin D intake or those not exposed to sunlight, such as institutionalized women. Supplementation should be kept at a level of 600 to 800 mg per day.

30. **D**, Page 1228. Factors known to increase the risk of osteoporosis include
    a. Caucasian or Asian race
    b. Reduced weight for height
    c. Early spontaneous menopause
    d. Early surgical menopause
    e. Family history of osteoporosis
    f. Diet: low calcium intake, low vitamin D intake, high caffeine intake, high alcohol intake, and high protein intake
    g. Cigarette smoking
    h. Endocrine disorders such as diabetes mellitus, hyperthyroidism, and Cushing disease
    i. Sedentary lifestyle

    Obesity is associated with a number of health hazards, but it is not by itself a risk factor for osteoporosis. In fact, being slightly overweight may be somewhat protective if the patient otherwise is healthy and active.

31. **B**, Page 1221. Ninety-five percent of postmenopausal androstenedione is produced by the adrenal gland, whereas 5% comes from the ovary. Androstenedione is an androgen that is converted to estrone in the peripheral body fat. This rate of conversion increases as a person ages. Although both the estrogen levels and androgen levels decrease postmenopausally, the estrogen levels decrease dramatically. This means that the androgen levels, although lower, are more dominant in their effect, thus resulting in increasing hirsutism. However, because of the overall decrease in androgen, a postmenopausal patient may notice decreasing libido due to the lower androgen levels.

32. **B**, Page 1228. With estrogen deficiency, bone density decreases most rapidly in trabecular bone. Cortical bone loss is slower but still accelerated compared with that caused by aging alone.

33. **E**, Pages 1232–1233; Table 42–4. Of the items listed, the highest level of dietary calcium is provided by nonfat yogurt, which contains 452 mg. The next richest source is chocolate milk, which supplies 284 mg. This is followed by frozen yogurt (249 mg) and ice cream (176 mg). Although cottage cheese is a reasonable source of dietary calcium, 1 cup supplies only 154 mg.

34. **E**, Pages 1242–1244. The studies are still conflicting, but it appears that there may be a slightly increased risk with women on estrogen replacement. This risk is possibly increased with the addition of progesterone. The presence of a family history that is not in a first-degree relative does not appreciably affect a patient's risk. An often understressed risk for breast cancer is obesity. In fact in women with body mass indexes greater than 26, the risk gained from weight exceeds the risk from estrogen replacement therapy. It appears that diagnosis is conferred earlier in women on hormone replacement therapy, who thus receive earlier subsequent treatment of breast cancer with resultant decreased mortality. Some of the confusion regarding risks of hormone replacement therapy may be due to detection bias because of the more frequent use of mammograms in women receiving hormone replacement than with nonusers.

35. **C**, Pages 1221–1222. Although there is a normal small increase in body weight after menopause, the use of estrogen replacement therapy itself is not associated with alteration of body weight or fat composition. Estrogen replacement does prevent the shift of body fat from peripheral sites to the abdomen, which occurs after menopause in untreated women.

36. **E**, Page 1227. Migraine headaches usually improve or disappear after menopause, whereas tension-type headaches remain unchanged or worsen.

37. **C**, Pages 1227–1228. Although many patients and physicians think that testosterone therapy improves libido, studies indicate that this is most closely associated with parenteral therapy and that oral therapy does not have this effect. Oral testosterone therapy is associated with a decrease in HDLs and an increase in LDLs while increasing

the incidence of hair growth and acne. A recent clinical trial comparing the effects of transdermal testosterone administered by a patch in women with bilateral oophorectomy found an increase in libido and frequency of intercourse compared with placebo. The transdermal patch did not alter serum lipids or increase acne or hair growth.

38. **D,** Pages 1218–1219. Premature menopause is most closely associated with alterations in the X chromosome. It is not related to environmental factors or reproductive history. Although women who smoke do have a lower age of menopause, the change in age brought on by smoking is generally in the range of only 2 years.

39. **C,** Page 1237. This patient is probably referring to the recent large 5-year clinical trial, which looked at hormone replacement therapy compared with placebo in women with preexisting cardiovascular disease. The study found that there was an increase of cardiovascular events during the first year of the study of hormone users. However, this increase leveled in the second year and was decreasing compared with placebo by the fifth year. Thus, there is no reason to stop hormone replacement in women who have been using the hormones for more than 1 year.

40. **A,** Pages 1242–1244. Although some doctors might prescribe replacement for a patient with a history of stage I breast cancer or who is beyond 5 years from diagnosis, it is not the ideal approach at this point. However, the patient is demonstrating significant osteoporosis and not just osteopenia with these results. Although exercise, calcium, and, if indicated, vitamin D will slow loss, they are not likely to halt it or to regain bone. Bisphosphates suppress bone reabsorption and reduce the incidence of vertebral and nonvertebral fractures. Another possibility for this patient is tamoxifen or selective estrogen receptor modulators (SERMs). Such agents may have suppressive effects against the breast cancer while conferring some estrogenic effect on the bone.